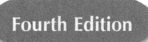

Fourth Edition

Understanding and Managing
VISION DEFICITS

The new fourth edition of *Understanding and Managing Vision Deficits: A Guide for Occupational Therapists* provides practitioners not only with a comprehensive understanding of vision and how vision problems can impact on the practice of occupational therapy, but also invaluable guidance on how to effectively manage clients with these issues.

The book presents a three-part model of vision to inform readers' understanding of the issues, and management across a range of eye conditions:

- Visual integrity: Includes visual acuity (clarity), the optics of the eye, and eye health.
- Visual efficiency skills: Includes focusing, eye teaming, and eye movements.
- Visual information processing skills: Includes the ability to analyze, interpret, and respond to visual information.

Covering key topics such as vision problems related to acquired brain injury and learning disorders among children with special educational needs, the new edition has been thoroughly updated to the latest findings in vision research, while there are also new chapters on using an interprofessional collaborative approach to client care, and how remediation can be integrated into occupational therapy principles to create occupation-based remedial vision rehabilitation.

A unique collaboration between the professions of occupational therapy and optometry together, and including a glossary of key terms and a sample vision screening report form, this is a key text for health care professionals to provide the ultimate in patient care.

Mitchell Scheiman, FCOVD, FAAO, is a nationally known optometric educator, lecturer, author, and private practitioner. He graduated from the New England College of Optometry, Boston, MA, in 1975 and completed a residency in vision therapy at the State University of New York College of Optometry in 1976. He has specialized in vision therapy for the past 50 years. Dr. Scheiman is currently Senior Associate Dean of Research at the Pennsylvania College of Optometry at Drexel University.

Fourth Edition

Understanding and Managing

VISION DEFICITS

A Guide for Occupational Therapists

Mitchell Scheiman

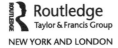

Routledge
Taylor & Francis Group

NEW YORK AND LONDON

Designed cover image: Tinhouse Design

Fourth edition published 2025
by Routledge
605 Third Avenue, New York, NY 10158

and by Routledge
4 Park Square, Milton Park, Abingdon, Oxon OX14 4RN

Routledge is an imprint of the Taylor & Francis Group, an informa business

First edition published by SLACK Incorporated 1996
Third edition published by SLACK Incorporated 2011

ISBN: 9781638220961 (hbk)
ISBN: 9781032882871 (pbk)
ISBN: 9781003526841 (ebk)

DOI: 10.4324/9781003526841

Typeset in Times New Roman
by codeMantra

Contents

About the Author

Mitchell Scheiman, FCOVD, FAAO, is a nationally known optometric educator, lecturer, author, and private practitioner. He graduated from the New England College of Optometry, Boston, MA, in 1975 and completed a residency in vision therapy at the State University of New York College of Optometry in 1976. He has specialized in vision therapy for the past 50 years. Dr. Scheiman is currently a Professor and Senior Associate Dean of Research at the Pennsylvania College of Optometry at Drexel University. He has written three books for optometrists, covering the topics of binocular vision and vision therapy, pediatric optometry, and learning-related vision problems, and he has published more than 240 articles in the professional literature. He is a Diplomate in Binocular Vision and Perception and a Fellow in the College of Optometrists in Vision Development.

Dr. Scheiman has a long and close relationship with occupational therapists. He is the founder of Vision Education Seminars, a company that develops and provides continuing education programs about vision to occupational therapists. In the past 35 years he has lectured to more than 9,000 occupational therapists. His wife, Maxine Scheiman, who recently retired, was an occupational therapist for more than 30 years.

Contributing Authors

Sarah D. Appel, *OD, FAAO (Chapters Eleven and Twelve)*
Retired Optometric Educator and Low Vision Specialist
Diplomate in Low Vision Rehabilitation (American Academy of Optometry)

Elise B. Ciner, *OD, FAAO (Chapters Eleven and Twelve)*
Professor of Optometry
Pennsylvania College of Optometry at Drexel University
Elkins Park, Pennsylvania

Amber Fessler, *OTD, MS OTR/L (Chapters Thirteen and Fourteen)*
Private Practice
Rapid City, South Dakota

Beth I. Fishman, *OTR, COVT (Chapter Ten)*
Private Practice
Centennial, Colorado

Lynn Fishman Hellerstein, *OD, FCOVD, FAAO (Chapters Nine and Ten)*
Adjunct Professor
Pacific University College of Optometry
Illinois College of Optometry
Southern College of Optometry
Private Practice
Centennial, Colorado

Marcy Graboyes, *ACSW, LSW (Chapter Twelve)*
Retired after more than 40 years as a social worker and educator in the William Feinbloom
Vision Rehabilitation Center

Alicia Reiser, *OTD, MS OTR/L, ADHD-RSP (Chapter Thirteen and Fourteen)*
Private Practice
Bethlehem, Pennsylvania

Preface to the Fourth Edition

Thirteen years have passed since the publication of the third edition of this book, and as can be expected, there have been many new developments in vision care and occupational therapy. The primary goal of this new fourth edition is to ensure that this book continues to be an up-to-date resource for occupational therapists about vision, enabling them to develop a comprehensive understanding of vision, to appreciate the various effects vision problems can have on the practice of occupational therapy, and to more effectively manage patients with vision disorders.

The most important changes are the inclusion of two new chapters written by occupational therapists who have taken advanced courses in remedial vision rehabilitation at Salus University. Afterwards, they returned to their practices and incorporated their new education into clinical practice. In Chapter Thirteen Drs. Fessler and Reiser write about using an interprofessional collaborative approach for the successful care of the person. In Chapter Fourteen they talk about how to take the information provided in earlier chapters about vision therapy for eye movement and vision information processing disorders and combine that with occupational therapy treatment principles and create occupation-based remedial vision rehabilitation.

Some of the general changes in each chapter include updated figures, incorporation of new research, and updated references. Several areas required more extensive updates. For example, there have been very important developments in vision therapy research over the past 13 years, with a number of randomized clinical trials published since 2011.

The final change is elimination of the chapters related to low vision rehabilitation. Remedial vision rehabilitation is a separate field from low vision rehabilitation, and we felt that the field of low vision rehabilitation requires more than just the few chapters we had added in the previous edition. There are full textbooks available that discuss low vision therapy for occupational therapists.

Preface to the Third Edition

The primary goal of this new edition is to ensure that this book continues to be an up-to-date resource for occupational therapists about vision, enabling them to develop a comprehensive understanding of vision, to appreciate the various effects vision problems can have on the practice of occupational therapy, and to more effectively manage patients with vision disorders. Eight years have passed since the publication of the Second Edition and, as can be expected, there have been many new developments in vision care.

Some of the general changes in each chapter include updated figures, incorporation of new research, and updated references. Several areas required more extensive updates. For example, there have been very important developments in vision therapy research over the past 8 years with a number of randomized clinical trials published since 2005. Another area of significant change is in traumatic brain injury. As a result of the wars in Iraq and Afghanistan, more than 30,000 soldiers have returned to the United States with injuries requiring rehabilitation. Over 50% of those returning with injuries due to traumatic brain injury have significant vision problems. Studies have shown that binocular vision, accommodation, eye movements, and visual field disorders are prevalent in this population. If left undetected and uncorrected these problems can interfere with the patient's ability to regain independence in activities of daily living. We have incorporated updated information about research and treatment of the vision conditions that are prevalent after traumatic brain injury.

Finally, occupational therapy continues to emerge as one of the important professions involved in the care of patients with visual impairment. Legislative changes in the past decade have created an atmosphere in which occupational therapists can be more easily reimbursed for low vision rehabilitation. These factors combined with the aging of the population and an increase in the prevalence of visual impairment have created a very strong interest from occupational therapists in topics such as the low vision evaluation, low vision aids, and low vision rehabilitation. As a result, we have updated the three chapters related to low vision in this Third Edition.

My hope is this book will continue to bring the professions of occupational therapy and optometry closer together, which will ultimately lead to the best possible care for patients being treated by both professions.

Preface to the Second Edition

The first edition of this book was written to meet a perceived demand for information about vision by occupational therapists. The response to this book during the past 4 years has been outstanding and demonstrates that there is indeed very strong interest from occupational therapy about vision problems and intervention strategies for these problems.

The need for a second edition became apparent shortly after completion of the first edition. In the past few years, occupational therapy has emerged as one of the professions involved in the care of patients with visual impairment. This emergence has been a gradual process and has evolved for at least two reasons. First, occupational therapists are uniquely trained to care for patients with low vision. Low vision problems significantly affect an individual's ability to perform activities of daily living. Helping individuals regain independence in activities of daily living is the distinctive skill of occupational therapists. In addition, legislative changes in the past few years have created an atmosphere in which occupational therapists can be more easily reimbursed for low vision rehabilitation. These factors combined with the aging of the population and an increase in the prevalence of visual impairment have created a very strong interest from occupational therapists in topics such as low vision evaluation, low vision aids, and low vision rehabilitation.

To meet this need, I have added three new chapters that specifically address the area of low vision. These chapters are written by experienced clinicians from optometry, occupational therapy, and the three other important low vision professions: rehabilitation teachers, orientation and mobility instructors, and teachers of the visually impaired.

Chapter Fourteen is an introductory chapter and provides an overview of the low vision evaluation, low vision aids, and low vision rehabilitation from an optometric viewpoint. Chapter Fifteen describes the various professional disciplines involved in low vision rehabilitation and how occupational therapy fits into the team of rehabilitation professionals. This chapter also provides detailed information about environmental assessment and modification for individuals with low vision. The final chapter on low vision is written by an occupational therapist who has developed a low vision rehabilitation program in her rehabilitation facility. It is a practical presentation of how an occupational therapist can develop a low vision specialty. It includes information about necessary competencies for treating low vision patients, educational opportunities for occupational therapists to gain these competencies, becoming certified in low vision, generating patient referrals, marketing low vision rehabilitation services, documentation, reimbursement issues, and billing.

The original 15 chapters have all been revised and updated based on recommendations from reviewers and changes that have occurred in theory, diagnosis, and treatment over the past 4 years.

Preface to the First Edition

My primary goal for writing this book is to create a resource for occupational therapists about vision, enabling them to develop a comprehensive understanding of vision, to appreciate the various effects vision problems can have on the practice of occupational therapy, and to manage patients with vision disorders more effectively. There can be little argument that occupational therapists evaluate and treat patients with a high prevalence of vision disorders. For example, adults with traumatic brain injury and cerebrovascular accident and children with pervasive developmental disabilities, cerebral palsy, mental retardation, learning disorders, and traumatic brain injury are all commonly seen by occupational therapists. One of the major health concerns present in all of these patients is vision problems.

In some instances, these vision problems may be primary and may prevent any meaningful progress. In other cases, the vision problem is not the key factor but, if left untreated, may interfere with the occupational therapy care process, leading to less than optimal treatment outcomes.

A second motive for writing this book is to develop a text that will help the professions of optometry and occupational therapy relate to and understand each other more effectively. In recent years, a number of authors have described several striking similarities between optometry and occupational therapy. These include a strong emphasis on investigating the relationship between physical and cognitive deficiencies and performance on activities of daily living, the importance of therapeutic intervention, and the importance of eliminating underlying skills problems. At the same time, the differences between the professions are also obvious, each having its own unique perspectives and strengths. These similarities and differences have led many individual professionals from optometry and occupational therapy to realize that, in some instances, optimal care for patients requires a joint effort between the two professions.

Although optometry and occupational therapy have traditionally not worked in the same clinical settings, this is occurring more often. Optometrists are becoming part of the health care team in rehabilitation settings, providing both direct care and, in some cases, consultative services. In the private sector, more and more optometrists and occupational therapists are working together in practices to meet the needs of their patients. Continuing education courses for occupational therapists about vision, visual perception, and vision therapy are becoming commonplace.

From my own personal experience being married to a pediatric occupational therapist and having interacted with many therapists in early intervention programs, rehabilitation hospitals, and school-based programs, I know that in many cases occupational therapists are anxious to acquire as much knowledge as possible about vision and that they recognize its importance in the care of their patients. I have often been asked to lecture about vision problems, screening procedures to help determine if such problems exist, and even information on intervention when these problems are present.

The objectives of this book are to meet these needs. The first five chapters of the book are designed to provide background information about vision. After the introductory chapters, Chapters Three through Five develop an understanding of the complexity of vision and present a three-component model, including acuity, refraction, eye health, visual efficiency disorders, and visual processing problems. Chapter Six describes a screening battery that can be used in a variety of settings by occupational therapists to screen for visual acuity, refractive, visual efficiency, and visual information processing problems. The screening procedures described can generally be done in a short period of time and without an investment in expensive instrumentation.

Chapter Seven reviews the management of refractive, visual efficiency, and visual information processing problems. This chapter is not designed to teach occupational therapists to perform optometric vision therapy. The optometric viewpoint is that vision therapy should be performed by optometrists or under the supervision of optometrists. However, there are several ways in which the occupational therapist can help in the management of patients with vision disorders. This chapter is designed to accomplish several objectives regarding intervention. The first goal is to provide information about how optometrists treat various vision disorders using lenses, prism, and vision therapy. The second objective is to provide detailed suggestions about how the occupational therapist can work along with the optometrist when treating children who are also being treated for a vision disorder. The final goal is to provide several treatment sequences that can be used by occupational therapists to supplement the vision therapy being performed by an optometrist in the areas of eye movements and visual information processing skills.

Chapters Eight through Twelve provide detailed information about common vision problems in three very important populations: those with developmental disabilities, children and adults who have experienced traumatic brain injury, and children with learning disabilities. Chapter Thirteen provides details about visual field deficits and neglect, two of the more common and enigmatic vision disorders occurring after cerebrovascular accident and traumatic brain injury. Chapter Fourteen presents a four-step inter-relationship model for optometrists and occupational therapists.

The final chapter, written by two experienced pediatric occupational therapists, provides a frame of reference for occupational therapists interested in managing patients with vision problems. The entire text has been reviewed by occupational therapist Maxine Scheiman to ensure accuracy and relevance for occupational therapists. In addition, it has been peer reviewed by occupational therapists.

My hope is that, by developing a better understanding of vision, this book will serve to bring the two professions closer together, which will ultimately lead to the best possible care for patients being treated by both professions.

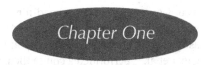

Chapter One

Background Information

Mitchell Scheiman

The Importance of Vision for Occupational Therapists

Occupational therapy is concerned with a person's ability to participate in desired life tasks, including caring for one's self, working, going to school, playing, and living independently. If a person's ability to perform these tasks is affected by an illness, disease, or disability, occupational therapy can be important in improving the individual's quality of life.[1] The premise of this book is that, given the high prevalence of vision disorders in the patients they serve, occupational therapists must understand the complexity and importance of vision and how visual deficits can interfere with occupational therapy, to be maximally effective in achieving these goals.

Reading, writing, and driving, for example, are three important functional skills that are very dependent on normal visual function.[2,3] There is a strong overflow to most other daily tasks. Vision problems may interfere with mobility, filling out forms, dressing, eating, locating objects, shopping, cooking, grooming, and managing finances. Hemiplegic patients with visual field deficits and/or visual neglect have also been shown to be accident prone.[4] This type of behavior may prolong treatment programs and may affect how the therapist grades the patient's level of competence in various activities of daily living. Visual scanning disorders may be one of the key factors causing the accident prone behavior.[5] In children, vision problems may interfere with learning to read, write, and play. Studies have also looked at the importance of vision for normal social interaction and found that a significant amount of social interaction involves nonverbal communication, which is often based on recognition of facial cues during conversation. Vision problems can, therefore, interfere with conversation and can cause social interaction problems for both adults and children. Recognizing faces and facial expressions is a common problem after traumatic brain injury or cerebrovascular accident.[6] It is not unusual for brain injury patients to miss important social cues, become more passive during conversation, and retreat from normal social interaction. Clearly, a change in visual processing can affect all aspects of a person's functioning.

Pediatric occupational therapists care for children with a wide variety of problems, including cerebral palsy, Down syndrome, other types of intellectual disabilities, spina bifida, low birth weight syndrome, pervasive developmental delay, sensory integrative dysfunction, and child abuse and neglect. Studies have shown that most of these patients have a high prevalence of vision

DOI: 10.4324/9781003526841-1

disorders, which creates a need for a comprehensive understanding of vision.[7–22] The most common conditions found in these children include optical problems such as hyperopia, myopia, and astigmatism; strabismus; amblyopia; nystagmus; optic atrophy; and visual processing problems.[12] Ciner et al.[21] performed a comprehensive visual examination on 135 preschool children at an early intervention program in Philadelphia. These children had various mentally and physically handicapping conditions, including Down syndrome, cerebral palsy, history of parental substance abuse, failure to thrive, and unlabeled developmental delays. They found that 60% of this population had significant vision problems. Strabismus was the most common condition, followed by refractive conditions such as hyperopia, myopia, and astigmatism.

For occupational therapists working with adults, the most common patients seen are those who have experienced cerebrovascular accidents, traumatic brain injury (TBI), and spinal cord injuries. Gianutsos reported that nearly half of the people admitted to a long-term rehabilitation facility after brain injury had visual system deficits, primarily in the area of binocular vision and accommodation.[19,20] Suchoff et al.[21] evaluated 62 consecutive patients entering a rehabilitation hospital with acquired brain injury (mean age: 49, range: 19 to 70). They found a high prevalence of vision disorders including problems with eye teaming (42%), eye movement (40%), focusing (10%), external eye disease (23%), glaucoma (19%), and visual field defects (32%). Ciuffreda et al.[22] reported on a retrospective study of 220 patients with traumatic brain injury or stroke and found that 90% of the individuals with traumatic brain injury and 86.7% with stroke had ocular motor dysfunction. Accommodative and binocular vision problems were most common in the traumatic brain injury group while cranial nerve palsy and strabismus were most common in the stroke population. Most recently several authors[23–25] reported on the frequency of vision problems in combat-injured inpatient and outpatient military personnel. Convergence, accommodative, and eye movement dysfunction were common in both populations. In these studies the most common vision problem found in both populations was a binocular vision problem called convergence insufficiency. Other commonly reported vision problems include reduced visual acuity, decreased contrast sensitivity, visual field deficits and neglect, strabismus, ocular motor dysfunction, accommodative dysfunction, and reduced stereopsis.[26–40]

Whether working with children or adults, occupational therapists often manage patients who have vision disorders. Unfortunately, visual deficits are not always recognized in the evaluation process or taken into consideration in therapy. Warren,[41] Bouska et al.,[42,43] and Gianutsos[44] have all expressed concern that there appears to be little systematic consideration of a patient's visual profile in occupational therapy. Gianutsos[44] suggests that there "is a real delivery system vacuum." After brain injury, patients generally fail to articulate complaints due to impaired subjective experience or reduced cognition.[44] Bouska et al.[42] also suggest that vision problems are not routinely detected in rehabilitation settings. They describe the patient who is labeled confused, clumsy, anxious, uncooperative, or unmotivated by professionals who are unaware that vision deficits may be the cause of the patient's behavior. When vision is addressed, it is usually from a strictly medical perspective, with attention given only to visual acuity and eye health. Chapters Three through Five will fully develop the concept that vision is more than good visual acuity and eye health.

Because visual function is dynamically interwoven within functional task performance,[44] ignoring visual deficits is likely to result in invalid assessment, faulty clinical reasoning, and, ultimately, ineffective treatment. The following are examples of how a visual deficit can interfere with occupational therapy and why a comprehensive vision examination is important before beginning occupational therapy:

- A 3-year-old child was referred for occupational therapy because she could not maintain eye contact, had poor fine motor skills, could not follow directions, could not sit still, and feared movement-based activities. The occupational therapy evaluation revealed low tone, tactile hyposensitivity, postural insecurity, and poor fine motor skills. A treatment plan was designed to deal with each of these problems. Although some progress was noticed, the therapist felt that the child still had great difficulty maintaining eye contact and concentrating on tasks, particularly if the task involved small objects. Finally, a vision evaluation was performed, and a very high degree of hyperopia (farsightedness) was found. The presence of high hyperopia would be expected to cause blurred vision and an inability to remain focused on a near activity for even short periods of time. Eyeglasses were prescribed, and occupational therapy proceeded much more effectively.

- A learning disabled, 7-year-old second grader was referred for a school occupational therapy consultation because the child frequently lost his place when reading, reread the same line, and showed a lack of interest in reading. The occupational therapist performed an evaluation and found normal sensory motor integration skills and visual processing. Tests to probe the area of scanning and tracking revealed mild problems, and treatment was designed to improve these skills. Little progress was achieved after six months of intervention. A visual evaluation revealed a significant binocular vision disorder called convergence insufficiency. What was overlooked in this case was that the child's behavior was characteristic of a child with a binocular vision (eye teaming) disorder. Inefficient use of the two eyes together as a team can mimic the symptoms and signs of a tracking or scanning problem. This child required a program of optometric vision therapy to improve binocular vision.

- An occupational therapist was treating a 74-year-old woman after a cerebrovascular accident. The therapist was struggling to help this patient regain independence in daily activities. She appeared fearful of walking in new environments and also had great difficulty localizing objects and reaching for things. An optometric evaluation revealed the presence of an inferior visual field deficit along with intermittent double vision. This patient required prism in her glasses to treat the double vision and occupational therapy to teach her how to compensate for the visual field deficit.

In each of these three cases, the vision problem may have been the primary factor interfering with progress for the patient. An attempt to continue occupational therapy without an evaluation and appropriate treatment of the vision problem would lead to frustration for both the therapist and the patient and less-than-optimal progress. In other cases, the vision problem may not be the key factor, but if left untreated, may interfere with the occupational therapy care process and lead to less-than-optimal treatment outcomes.

Vision is our most far-reaching sense, and it is clear that vision is critical for most activities of daily living. It is evident that for an occupational therapist to be maximally effective, a comprehensive understanding of vision is important.

Optometry and Occupational Therapy

The Eye Care Professions

There are two primary providers in the eye care profession. The differences between the two professions are significant and are related to the respective educational and clinical training programs for each profession. An *ophthalmologist* is a medical doctor who specializes in diseases of the eye and eye surgery. The initial training for an ophthalmologist is similar to any other medical doctor and has a heavy emphasis on disease. Following completion of medical school and an internship, the physician enters a residency and fellowship training program to specialize in ophthalmology. This period of training can last another 3 to 8 years, with a continuing focus on disease. The treatment approaches that are emphasized are medication and surgery. Rehabilitation of the visual system using vision therapy, lenses, low vision devices, or prism is not an important part of training. In fact, in many instances, negative opinions about visual rehabilitation are developed during this period of specialization.[45]

An *optometrist* is a primary health care provider who specializes in the examination, diagnosis, treatment, and management of diseases and disorders of the visual system, the eye, and associated structures, as well as the diagnosis of related systemic conditions.[46] To become an optometrist, an individual must graduate from a 4-year college program and then enter a 4-year program in a college of optometry. The emphasis in both didactic and clinical education is different from the ophthalmological residency programs. Although optometrists are also educated to diagnose and treat eye disease, a significant portion of the educational program deals with the concept of vision and its relationship to performance in play, school, work, and sports.

The optometrist is taught to evaluate the visual system in a manner that allows diagnosis of visual conditions that can interfere with performance and affect the quality of life. An integral concept in the optometric curriculum that is absent in ophthalmological training is that the status of the visual system is directly related to the environment and to how the individual uses their eyes. With increased close work such as reading and computer work, the visual system becomes more susceptible to disorders of accommodation, binocular vision, and refractive error. In fact, optometric theory suggests that many of the common vision problems that are prevalent in society are actually caused by the excessive close work that all of us experience in modern society.[47] Finally, optometrists are taught that rehabilitation using lenses, prism, low vision devices, and vision therapy is indeed an effective alternative to help patients become more comfortable and productive in school and work.[48] Many hours in the typical optometric curriculum are devoted to the study of the use of vision therapy to rehabilitate a wide variety of vision disorders.

Although all optometrists receive this training, only a percentage choose to offer this service in practice. Optometrists who offer vision therapy and vision rehabilitation in practice often have completed additional residency training or have passed comprehensive examinations designed to assess their level of expertise in these areas. The two organizations that administer such examinations are the American Academy of Optometry (Binocular Vision, Perception, and Pediatric Optometry Section) and the College of Optometrists in Vision Development (COVD). Optometrists successfully completing the examination process for the American Academy of Optometry are called Diplomates in Binocular Vision, Perception, and Pediatric Optometry. Approximately 50 optometrists in the United States have achieved this status. Optometrists successfully completing the examination process for COVD are called Fellows of COVD (FCOVD). Approximately 500 optometrists in the United States are FCOVDs, and about another 700 optometrists are associate members of COVD. Another organization that has established a certification process is the Neuro-Optometric Rehabilitation Association International (NORA). This organization is focused on advancing the art and science of the rehabilitation of the neurologically challenged individual and has a membership list of optometrists with an interest in vision therapy and vision rehabilitation after acquired brain injury.

There are also other optometrists who have expertise in the area of vision therapy but have not passed the examinations administered by these three organizations. My advice is to first look for an optometrist with at least one of the credentials described above to help you manage your patients. All three organizations maintain lists of these optometrists, including their addresses and phone numbers. The organizations' details are included at the end of this chapter. You can also access these membership directories from the Web sites of these organizations. If you are unable to find a local optometrist who has been certified by one of these three organizations, there is an additional organization—the Optometric Extension Program—that has a membership list of optometrists with an interest in vision therapy and vision rehabilitation. While members of this organization have a strong interest in these areas, they may not have passed any additional testing to certify their competence.

These differences in educational experience and clinical training explain the experiences of many therapists relative to the eye care professions. I have often heard occupational therapists comment about the frustration they experience when attempting to help a patient who they suspect may have a vision problem. For example, a therapist may refer a child for an eye examination because of concern about tracking or focusing skills. Depending on the doctor to whom the child is referred, it would not be unusual for the child to be sent back with completely contradictory reports. One doctor might suggest that there is no vision problem, that visual acuity is 20/20, that glasses are unnecessary, and that the eyes are healthy. The other doctor agrees that acuity is normal, glasses are not required, and the eyes are healthy, but reports the presence of a significant binocular vision problem that can explain the therapist's observations.

This lack of uniformity in vision care is confusing to therapists and to the public and may lead to lack of identification and treatment of vision disorders that can interfere with occupational therapy. The differences in approach between optometry and ophthalmology are important, and even within the optometric profession, philosophical differences may be significant. It is critical, therefore, that therapists seeking meaningful information about a patient's or client's visual status make the referral to an eye care professional who has training and expertise in the areas of binocular vision, vision and learning, and vision therapy. This will most likely require a referral to an optometrist who is either a FCOVD or a Diplomate in Binocular Vision, Perception, and Pediatric Optometry. Another acceptable credential is completion of a residency in pediatric optometry or vision therapy.

Optometry and Occupational Therapy Similarities and Differences

In recent years, a number of authors have described several striking similarities between optometry and occupational therapy.[49-51] These include a strong emphasis on the relationship between physical and cognitive deficiencies and performance in activities of daily living; the importance of therapeutic intervention, including both remedial and adaptive approaches; and the importance of eliminating underlying skills problems.

Optometrists routinely try to find relationships between vision disorders and problems with learning, work, and play. This is remarkably similar to occupational therapy's consistent concern about the effects of dysfunction on activities of daily living. Occupational therapy is the art and science of directing man's participation in selected tasks to restore, reinforce, and enhance performance.[52] The goals of optometric intervention are similar and revolve around restoring normal visual function to enhance performance in everyday tasks. When it is clear that there is a relationship between a diagnosed condition and performance, both occupational therapists and optometrists use all available treatment options to try to eliminate the interference or to teach the patient how to compensate for the problem. In some cases, this involves an adaptive approach to capitalize on the patient's remaining strengths and, in other cases, a remedial approach to restore normal function. The goal of treatment for both professions is ultimately to improve the patient's quality of life. As an optometrist, I was elated when I discovered another profession with such a strong commitment to the restoration and enhancement of function and performance.

At the same time, differences between the professions are also apparent, with each having its own unique perspectives and strengths. Occupational therapists generally use activities of daily living to improve function, while optometrists work directly with the affected function. Optometrists test and treat disorders of the peripheral visual system, such as eye movements, accommodation, and binocular vision. Occupational therapists may screen for these disorders but do not generally treat them, with the exception of some work with eye movements. Optometric testing tends to concentrate primarily on higher-level functioning at the level of the cerebral cortex, while occupational therapists may focus more on lower-level brainstem functions of the vestibular and proprioceptive system and how they are organized and processed.[51] Optometrists stress the predominance of the visual system in treatment, while occupational therapists stress the importance of the vestibular system and sensory motor integration. These similarities and differences have led many individual professionals from optometry and occupational therapy to realize that, in some instances, optimal care for patients requires a joint effort between the two professions.[49–51]

Optometry and occupational therapy have traditionally not worked in the same clinical settings. However, this is occurring more often. Optometrists are becoming part of the health care team in rehabilitation settings, providing both direct care and, in some cases, consultative services.[53–56]

In the private sector, more and more optometrists and occupational therapists are working together in practices to meet the needs of their patients. Continuing education courses for occupational therapists about vision, visual perception, and vision therapy are becoming commonplace.

Understanding Vision

Optometric Model of Vision

When people are asked to define good vision, they generally respond with one of the following three answers:

1. Good vision is the ability to see 20/20 or to see clearly.

2. Good vision means having healthy eyes and not needing glasses.

3. Good vision means that I am able to pass the school vision screening or the eye test at my doctor's office.

While an individual with "good vision" would certainly see clearly, have 20/20 vision, have healthy eyes, and pass a vision screening, there is much more that must be considered when answering this question. In addition to clear vision, an individual must have the ability to use their eyes for extended periods of time without discomfort, be able to analyze and interpret the incoming information, and be able to respond to what is being seen.

Optometric authors have developed models of vision that tend to emphasize that vision is a learned process dependent upon how the child interacts with their environment and that, in particular, it is related to a child's motor development. Hendrickson stressed that instead of asking what vision is, we should be asking what vision is for.[57] Suchoff[58] proposed an answer to this question, stating that "A primary mission of vision in the human organism is the organization and manipulation of space." This concept that vision is used to interact with and not just receive information is central to the optometric concept of vision. Getman[59] described vision as "The learned ability to see for information and performance. Vision is the ability to understand the things we cannot touch, taste, smell, or hear. Vision is the process whereby we perceive space as a whole." Another emphasis in optometric models of vision has been the important role of movement. Movement has been called the key to learning, thinking, and vision.[57] Skeffington said, "Thinking is a movement pattern. Vision is a movement pattern."[60] This emphasis on movement and motor skills is one of several key similarities in the philosophy that links optometry and occupational therapy.

One of my key objectives in writing this book is to demonstrate to the reader the complexity of vision and how vision disorders can impact on the occupational therapy process. To accomplish this, I will present the Three Component Model of Vision, which goes beyond 20/20 visual acuity, good optics, and normal eye health. The individual must also have normal binocular vision, accommodation, ocular motility, and visual information processing skills and be able to respond to the environment. The Three Component Model of Vision presented in Chapters Three through Five, therefore, consists of three distinct but interrelated components, which are visual integrity (acuity, refraction, and eye health); visual efficiency (accommodation, binocular vision, and eye movements); and visual information processing (visual spatial, visual analysis, and visual motor integration skills).

Although I will present these three components separately, they are closely related and interdependent. Disorders and delayed development in one component invariably will affect function in the other areas. Once the reader understands the complexity of vision, it should be apparent why occupational therapy and optometry should work closely together.

Directory of Optometrists With Expertise in Vision Therapy and Vision Rehabilitation

American Academy of Optometry, Diplomates in Binocular Vision, Perception, and Pediatric Optometry
http://aaopt.org/section/bv/diplomates/index.asp

College of Optometrists in Vision Development
www.covd.org

Neuro-Optometric Rehabilitation Association, International
http://nora.cc/

References

1. American Occupational Therapy Association. *Occupational Therapy Services for Children With Visual Dysfunction.* Bethesda, MD: Author; 1994.
2. Lorenze EJ, Cancro R. Dysfunction in visual perception with hemiplegia: its relation to activities of daily living. *Arch Phys Med Rehabil.* 1962;43:514–517.
3. Weinberg J, Diller L. On reading newspapers by hemiplegics—denial of visual disability. *Proc 76th Ann Con Am Psychol Assoc.* 1968;3:655–656.
4. Diller L, Weinberg J. Evidence for accident prone behavior in hemiplegic patients. *Arch Phys Med Rehabil.* 1970;51:358–363.
5. Diller L, Weinberg J. Attention in brain damaged people. *J Educ.* 1968;150:20–27.
6. Hier DB, Mondlock J, Caplan LR. Behavioral abnormalities after right hemisphere stroke. *Neurol.* 1983;33:337–344.
7. Scheiman M. Assessment and management of the exceptional child. In: Rosenbloom AA, Morgan MW, eds. *Pediatric Optometry.* Philadelphia, PA: JB Lippincott; 1990:388–419.
8. Kirschen M. A study of visual performance of mentally retarded children. *American Journal of Optometry and Archives of the American Academy of Optometry.* 1954;31:282–286.
9. LoCascio GP. A study of vision in cerebral palsy. *Am J Optom Physiol Opt.* 1977;54:332–335.
10. LoCascio GP. A longitudinal study of vision in cerebral palsy. *Am J Optom Physiol Opt.* 1984;61:689–692.
11. Scheiman M. Optometric findings in children with cerebral palsy. *Am J Optom Physiol Opt.* 1984;61:321–327.
12. Lyle WM, Woodruff ME, Zuccaro VS. A review of the literature on Down syndrome and an optometrical survey of 44 patients with the syndrome. *Am J Optom Physiol Opt.* 1972;49:715–721.
13. Pesch RS, Nagy DK, Caden B. A survey of the visual and developmental abilities of the Down syndrome child. *J Am Optom Assoc.* 1978;49:1031–1036.
14. Shapiro MB, France TD. The ocular features of Down syndrome. *Am J Ophthalmol.* 1985;99:659–665.
15. Clements DB, Kausal K. A study of the ocular complications of hydrocephalus and meningomyelocele. *Trans Ophthalmol Soc UK.* 1970;40:383–394.
16. Gottlieb DD, Allen WA. Incidence of visual disorders in a selected population of hearing impaired students. *J Am Optom Assoc.* 1985;56:292–297.
17. Ciner EB, Macks B, Schanel-Klitsch E. A cooperative demonstration project for early intervention vision services. *Occup Ther Pract.* 1991;3:42–56.
18. Akinci A, Oner O, Bozkurt OH, et al. Refractive errors and ocular findings in children with intellectual disability: a controlled study. *Journal of AAPOS.* 2008;12:477–481.
19. Gianutsos R, Ramsey G. Enabling survivors of brain injury to receive rehabilitative optometric services. *J Vis Rehab.* 1988;2:37–58.
20. Gianutsos R, Ramsey G, Perlin R. Rehabilitative optometric services for survivors of brain injury. *Arch Phys Med Rehabil.* 1988;69:573–578.
21. Suchoff IB, Kapoor N, Waxman R, Ference W. The occurrence of ocular and visual dysfunctions in an acquired brain-injured patient sample. *J Am Optom Assoc.* 1999;70:301–308.
22. Ciuffreda KJ, Kapoor N, Rutner D, et al. Occurrence of oculomotor dysfunctions in acquired brain injury: a retrospective analysis. *Optometry.* 2007;78:155–161.

23. Goodrich L, Kirby J, Cockerham G, Ingalla SP, Lew HL. Visual function in patients of a polytrauma rehabilitation center: a descriptive study. *J Rehabil Res Dev.* 2007;44:929–936.
24. Brahm KD, Wilgenburg HM, Kirby J, Ingalla S, Chang CY, Goodrich GK. Visual impairment and dysfunction in servicemembers with TBI. *Opt Vis Sci.* 2009;86:817–825.
25. Stelmack JA, Frith T, Van Koevering D, Stelmack TR. Visual function in patients followed at a Veterans Affairs polytrauma network site: an electronic medical record review. *Optometry.* 2009;80:419–424.
26. Kwatny E, Bouska MJ. *Visual System Disorders and Functional Correlates: Final Report.* Philadelphia, PA: Temple University Rehabilitation Research and Training Center #8; 1980.
27. Mitchell R, MacFarlane A, Cornell E. Ocular motility disorders following head injury. *Aust Orthop J.* 1983;20:31–36.
28. Cohen M, Groswasser Z, Barchadski R, Appel A. Convergence insufficiency in brain-injured patients. *Brain Inj.* 1989;3:187–191.
29. Schlageter Gray B, Hall K, Shaw R, Sammet R. Incidence and treatment of visual dysfunction in traumatic brain injury. *Brain Inj.* 1993;7:439–448.
30. Elisevich KV, Ford RM, Anderson DP, et al. Visual abnormalities with multiple trauma. *Surg Neurol.* 1984;22:565–575.
31. Tierney DW. Visual dysfunction in closed head injury. *J Am Opt Assoc.* 1988;59:614–622.
32. Padula WV. Head injury causing post trauma vision syndrome. *N Engl J Optom.* 1988;Dec:16–21.
33. Krohel GB, Kristan RW, Simon JW, et al. Post-traumatic convergence insufficiency. *Ann Ophthalmol.* 1986;18:101–104.
34. Roca PD. Ocular manifestations of whiplash injuries. *Ann Ophthalmol.* 1972;4:63–73.
35. Uzzell BP, Dolinskas CA, Langfitt TW. Visual field defects in relation to head injury severity. *Arch Neurol.* 1988;45:420–424.
36. Rutner D, Kapoor N, Ciuffreda KJ, et al. Occurrence of ocular disease in traumatic brain injury in a selected sample: a retrospective analysis *Brain Inj.* 2006;20(10):1079–1086.
37. Jones, SA, Shinton, RS. Improving outcome in stroke patients with visual problems. *Age Ageing.* 2006;35:560–565.
38. McKenna K, Cooke, DM, Fleming J, et al. The incidence of visual perceptual impairment in patients with severe traumatic brain injury. *Brain Inj.* 2006;20(5):507–518.
39. Suchoff, IB, Kapoor, N, Ciuffreda KJ, et al. The frequency of occurrence, types, and characteristics of visual field defects in acquired brain injury: a retrospective analysis. *Optometry.* 2008;79:259–265.
40. Rowe F. Visual perceptual consequences of stroke. *Strabismus.* 2009;17:24–28.
41. Warren M. Identification of visual scanning deficits in adults after cerebrovascular accident. *Am J Occup Ther.* 1990;44:391–399.
42. Bouska MJ, Kauffman NA, Marcus SE. Disorders of the visual perceptual system. In: Umphred DA, Jewell MJ, eds. *Neurological Rehabilitation.* St. Louis, MO: CV Mosby; 1985:552–585.
43. Bouska MJ, Gallaway M. Primary visual field deficits in adults with brain damage: management in occupational therapy. *Occup Ther Pract.* 1991;3:1–11.
44. Gianutsos R. Working relationships between psychology and optometry. *J Beh Optom.* 1991;2:30–36.
45. American Academy of Ophthalmology. *Policy Statement: Learning Disabilities, Dyslexia, and Vision.* San Francisco, CA: American Academy of Ophthalmology; Revised 2009.
46. American Optometric Association. *Position Statement on Vision Therapy.* St. Louis, MO; 1999.
47. Skeffington AM. *Introduction to Clinical Optometry. Santa Ana, CA: Optometric Extension Program Foundation, Optometric Extension Program Postgraduate Courses.* Vol 37, Oct 1964–Sept 1965.
48. Scheiman M, Wick B. *Clinical Management of Binocular Vision.* 3rd ed. Philadelphia, PA: JB Lippincott; 2008.
49. Cool SJ. Occupational therapy and functional optometry: an interaction whose time has come? *Sensory Integration Special Interest Newsletter.* 1987;10:1–6.
50. Appelbaum SA. Sensory integration: optometric and occupational therapy perspectives. *Optom Ext Program Curriculum II.* 1988;61(1–12).
51. Hellerstein LF, Fishman B. Vision therapy and occupational therapy: an integrated approach. *Sensory Integration Special Interest Newsletter.* 1987;10:4–5.
52. Hopkins HL, Smith HD. *Occupational Therapy.* 6th ed. Philadelphia, PA: JB Lippincott; 1983:27.
53. Mastrangelo R. Visionary effort: OT and optometry join hands. *OT Week.* 1990;6(28):1–2.
54. Breske S. Opening eyes to vision deficits in rehab. *Advance for Occupational Therapists*; 1995.
55. Schlageter K, Shaw R. Vision therapy. *OT Week.* 1991;5(31):12–13.
56. Scheiman M. The eyes have it. *Advance for Physical Therapists and Rehab Medicine.* 2000;October 1:61–62.
57. Hendrickson H. *Vision Development in Man—A Review. Vision and Learning.* St. Louis, MO: American Optometric Association; 1976:21–45.
58. Suchoff I. *Visuo-Spatial Development in the Child: An Optometric Theoretical and Clinical Approach.* New York, NY: State University of New York; 1981.
59. Getman GN, Hendrickson H. The needs of teachers for specialized information on the development of visuomotor skills in relation to academic performance. In: Cruickshank WM, ed. *The Teacher of Brain Injured Children.* New York, NY: Syracuse University Press; 1966:156–157.
60. Skeffington AM. *The Low Acuity Emmetrope Who Constricted Her Visual System.* Duncan, OK: Clinical Optometry, Optometric Extension Program; 1972:45(1,3).

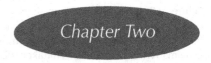
Review of Basic Anatomy, Physiology, and Development of the Visual System

Mitchell Scheiman

Basic Anatomy and Physiology of the Visual System

This chapter is designed to provide a review of the basic anatomy and physiology of the visual system. Space limitations prevent a comprehensive discussion of this topic. Readers requiring more in-depth information about these topics should review the text provided in the Reference of this chapter.

Orbit, Eyelids, Eyeball

A traditional method of describing the anatomy of the eye is to begin with the outermost structures and move inward. The orbit of the eye, which is a bony recess in the skull, contains a number of major structures, including the eyeball, the optic nerve, the muscles of the eye, and their nerves and blood vessels. The eyeball, which is about 2.5 cm long, is suspended in the orbital cavity in such a way that the six ocular muscles can move it in all directions.

The eyelids protect the eyes from injury and excessive light and keep the cornea moist. As illustrated in Figure 2.1, the upper eyelid partially covers the iris, whereas the entire inferior half of the eye is normally uncovered. The eyelids are covered internally by the highly vascular palpebral conjunctiva. The palpebral conjunctiva continues onto the eyeball and is called the bulbar conjunctiva. Inflammation of either the bulbar or palpebral conjunctiva is referred to as conjunctivitis, commonly called pink eye. Conjunctivitis can be secondary to bacterial, viral, or allergic etiology. Infection of the conjunctiva is generally self-limiting, but occasionally conjunctivitis can lead to inflammation of the cornea as well.

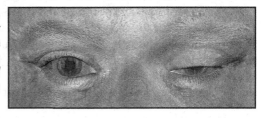

Figure 2.1. The upper eyelid partially covers the iris, whereas the entire inferior half of the eye is normally uncovered. (Reprinted with permission from Scheiman M, Scheiman M, Whittaker SG. *Low Vision Rehabilitation: A Practical Guide for Occupational Therapists.* Thorofare, NJ: SLACK Incorporated; 2007.)

DOI: 10.4324/9781003526841-2

Figure 2.2. The anterior one-sixth of the outer coat of the eye is the transparent structure called the cornea. (Reprinted with permission from Scheiman M, Scheiman M, Whittaker SG. *Low Vision Rehabilitation: A Practical Guide for Occupational Therapists.* Thorofare, NJ: SLACK Incorporated; 2007.)

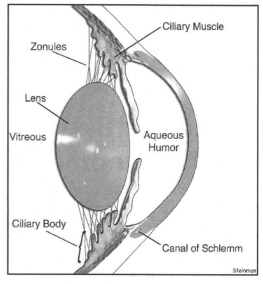

The bulbar conjunctiva covers the white portion of the eye called the sclera. The sclera is the external coat of the eye and is a white tissue covering the posterior five-sixths of the eye. The anterior one-sixth of the outer coat of the eye is the transparent structure called the cornea (Figure 2.2). The cornea is an extremely important structure of the eye because it is the key optical component responsible for refraction of light that enters the eye. It is an unusual tissue because it is clear and has no blood vessels. The cornea is susceptible to infection from bacterial, viral, fungal or allergic causes, and inflammation of the cornea is referred to as keratitis. Severe inflammation, a corneal burn due to exposure to toxic substances, or trauma to the cornea can all lead to scarring and loss of transparency of the cornea. This can then lead to a loss of vision if the scarring is located in the central portion of the cornea. Reduced visual acuity secondary to central corneal scarring is a disease condition that may be encountered by occupational therapists in clients who have experienced head trauma. Other common age-related problems of the anterior part of the eye that affect vision and cause discomfort include blepharitis (chronic inflammation of the lids) and dry eye. These can be managed medically but with varying success.

Directly behind the cornea is a clear, watery fluid called the aqueous humor, which is produced in the posterior chamber and fills the anterior chamber of the eye (see Figure 2.2). The aqueous is continuously produced by the ciliary body and provides nutrients for the avascular cornea and lens. After passing through the pupil from the posterior chamber into the anterior chamber, the aqueous is drained off through the canal of Schlemm (see Figure 2.2).

Lens

The lens is a transparent, flexible structure that is held in position by zonular fibers (see Figure 2.2). It is located posterior to the iris and anterior to the vitreous humor. Like the cornea, the lens is both transparent and avascular and is another key part of the refractive system of the eye. To accommodate or focus on objects, the lens must change shape. The ciliary muscle contracts, and this allows the lens to thicken, enabling the individual to focus. As an object moves away, the ciliary muscle relaxes, the lens becomes thinner, and the focusing system relaxes. The lens of the eye is the structure that gradually loses its transparency as a person ages. This loss of transparency and development of opacities is referred to as cataracts.

Figure 2.3. Cross-section of the eye. (Reprinted with permission from Scheiman M, Scheiman M, Whittaker SG. *Low Vision Rehabilitation: A Practical Guide for Occupational Therapists*. Thorofare, NJ: SLACK Incorporated; 2007.)

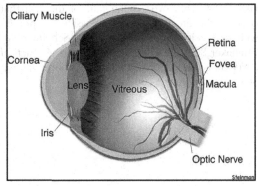

Vitreous

The vitreous body is located behind the lens (Figure 2.3). It consists of a jelly-like substance called vitreous humor, in which there is a meshwork of collagen fibrils. Vitreous humor is a colorless, transparent gel. It consists of 99% water and forms four-fifths of the eyeball. In addition to transmitting light, it holds the retina in place and provides support for the lens. In contrast to the aqueous humor, it is not continuously replaced.

Choroid

The eyeball has three concentric coats. The first or outermost coat, the sclera, was described above. The middle coat is a heavily pigmented, vascular layer consisting of the iris, ciliary body, and the choroid. The iris, which is the colored portion of the eye, is located between the cornea and the lens. The eye color depends on the amount and distribution of pigment in the iris. The iris is a contractile diaphragm that has a central, circular aperture for transmitting light, which is called the pupil. The size of the iris continually varies to regulate the amount of light entering the eye through the pupil. The ciliary body lies between the iris and the choroid. This structure secretes aqueous humor. The ciliary body also contains the ciliary muscle, which can contract or relax to permit accommodation or focusing of the eye. The choroid is a dark brown membrane and is also part of this middle coat of the eye. It continues from the ciliary body and covers the entire posterior portion of the eye. The choroid attaches firmly to the retina and contains the venous plexus and layers of capillaries that are responsible for nutrition of the retina.

Retina

The most internal coat of the eye is the retina, which is a thin, delicate membrane. The retina is the posterior portion of the eye and there is a circular depressed area called the optic nerve (see Figure 2.3). This is where the optic nerve enters the eye and its fibers spread out in the neural layer of the retina. Because it contains nerve fibers and no photoreceptor cells, the optic disc is insensitive to light. For this reason it is sometimes referred to as the blind spot. Another very important structure just lateral to the optic disc is the fovea (Figure 2.4). The fovea is the part of the eye that contains the area of most acute vision. Whenever we look at an object we must aim the eye so that the image of the object is focused on the fovea. Smooth eye movements, called pursuits, and jump eye movements, called saccades, are both designed to allow the individual to use the fovea.

The retina is composed of ten layers including the pigment epithelium, which is closest to the choroid and the photoreceptors (cones and rod photoreceptors). Beneath the pigment epithelium of

Figure 2.4. The fovea is the part of the eye that contains the area of most acute vision. (Reprinted with permission from Scheiman M, Scheiman M, Whittaker SG. *Low Vision Rehabilitation: A Practical Guide for Occupational Therapists.* Thorofare, NJ: SLACK Incorporated; 2007.)

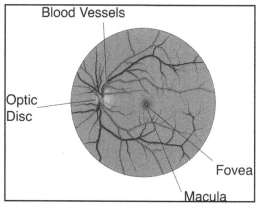

Figure 2.5. Beneath the pigmented epithelium of the retina are the ten layers of the retina. (Reprinted with permission from Scheiman M, Scheiman M, Whittaker SG. *Low Vision Rehabilitation: A Practical Guide for Occupational Therapists.* Thorofare, NJ: SLACK Incorporated; 2007.)

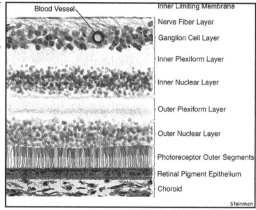

the retina are the ten layers of the retina (Figure 2.5) from the outside (furthest from the retina) to the inside (closest to the retina):

- Sclera (white part of the eye)
- Large choroidal blood vessels
- Choriocapilaris
- Bruch's membrane (separates the pigment epithelium of the retina from the choroid)

Note that light must pass through all layers of the retina to reach the photoreceptors where the visual process begins. Diseases such as macular degeneration or diabetic retinopathy that affect the clarity of retina or swelling that affects the shape of the retina will have a profound effect on vision.

Photoreceptors (Cones and Rods)

Light causes a chemical reaction in cones and in rods, beginning the visual process. Activated photoreceptors stimulate bipolar cells, which in turn stimulate ganglion cells. The impulses continue into the axons of the ganglion cells, through the optic nerve, and to the visual cortex at the occipital lobe of the brain.

There are about 6.5 to 7 million cones in each eye, and they are sensitive to bright light and to color. The highest concentration of cones is in the macula. The center of the macula contains only cones and no rods. The highest concentration of rods is in the peripheral retina, decreasing in density up to the macula. Rods do not detect color, which is the main reason it is difficult to tell the color of an object at night or in the dark. Defective or damaged cones results in color deficiency, whereas defective or damaged rods result in problems seeing in the dark and at night.

Muscles of the Orbit and Their Innervation

Six extraocular muscles attach to each eye and allow movement in all directions of gaze. There are four rectus muscles—the superior, inferior, lateral, and medial recti muscles—and two oblique muscles—the inferior and superior oblique muscles.

Each of the six muscles has one position of gaze in which it exerts the main influence on eye position. Figure 2.6 illustrates the various positions of gaze that are evaluated clinically. The diagram also displays the muscle that is primarily responsible for movement into each position of gaze. This diagram is the basis for the clinical evaluation of eye muscle problems. For example, if a client has difficulty moving their eyes down and to the right, the two possible muscles involved would be the right inferior rectus and the left superior oblique. The left superior oblique moves the left eye down and to the right and the right inferior rectus moves the right eye down and to the right. To determine which of the two remaining muscles is at fault requires additional clinical testing.

Three cranial nerves supply innervation to the six extraocular muscles. The third cranial nerve innervates the superior, inferior, medial recti, and the inferior oblique muscle. The fourth cranial nerve supplies innervation to the superior oblique, and the sixth cranial nerve innervates the lateral rectus.

Diplopia, or double vision, is a very common symptom of clients treated by occupational therapists, particularly after cerebrovascular accident or head trauma. Diplopia occurs when the object at which the individual is looking stimulates the fovea of one eye and a non-foveal part of the retina of the other eye. Thus, diplopia suggests misalignment of the eyes. There are a number of disorders that can lead to diplopia. Brain injury from stroke or trauma that affects the midbrain or cerebellum area often affects both balance and eye movements. Among the more common problems are cranial nerve palsies. The most common nerve palsies seen by occupational therapists are sixth and fourth nerve palsies.

The most common causes of fourth nerve palsy are head trauma and vascular problems. Fourth cranial nerve palsy can be unilateral or bilateral and can affect the superior oblique muscle. Bilateral fourth nerve palsy is often seen following vertex blows to the head, such as those that occur in motorcycle accidents. The presence of a fourth nerve palsy causes the eye with the affected muscle to drift upward. The client has difficulty looking down and to the right if it is a left superior oblique problem, and down and to the left if it is a right superior oblique problem.

Sixth cranial nerve palsies are the most frequently reported ocular motor nerve palsies. The nerve has the longest intracranial course of any nerve and is often subject to embarrassment with raised intracranial pressure. The causes include vascular disease, trauma, elevated intracranial

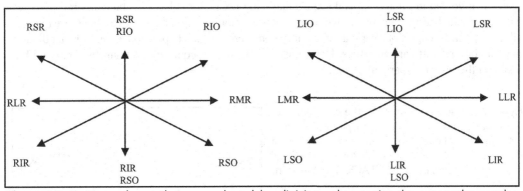

Figure 2.6. Positions of gaze that are evaluated by clinicians when testing the extraocular muscles. (RSR=right superior rectus, RLR=right lateral rectus, RIR=right inferior rectus, RSO=right superior oblique, RMR=right medial rectus, RIO=right inferior oblique, LSR=left superior rectus, LLR=left lateral rectus, LIR=left inferior rectus, LSO=left superior oblique, LMR=left medial rectus, LIO=left inferior oblique.)

pressure and neoplasm. The sixth nerve innervates the lateral rectus. A sixth nerve palsy will interfere with the client's ability to abduct the eye (move the eye away from the nose).

Visual Pathways

One of the most common vision problems occupational therapists encounter after acquired brain injury is visual field deficits. One of the most common is a right or left field loss referred to as a homonymous hemianopsia. To understand why a client would lose vision to just one side, it is necessary to understand how visual information travels from the retina to the visual cortex. Vision begins with the capture of images focused by the optical media on photoreceptors of the retina. The fibers from the upper half of each retina enter the optic nerve above the horizontal meridian, and those from the lower half enter below the horizontal meridian. Fibers from the periphery of the retina lie peripherally in the optic nerve, and fibers from the fovea lie centrally. This arrangement persists throughout the entire course of the visual pathways from the optic nerve through the chiasm, the optic tracts, and optic radiations.

Visual information from the right field strikes the nasal half of the retina of the right eye and the temporal half of the retina of the left eye. Similarly, visual information from the left field strikes the nasal half of the retina of the left eye and the temporal half of the retina of the right eye (Figure 2.7). When the fibers from each optic nerve reach the optic chiasm, a decussation takes place. The fibers from the temporal part of the retina remain on the temporal or outside aspect of the chiasm and are called uncrossed fibers (see Figure 2.7). The nasal fibers of the retina cross over in the chiasm and are called crossed fibers. After leaving the chiasm, the fibers form the optic tract. Thus, all visual information originating from the right field travels in the left optic tract, and all of the visual information originating from the left field travels in the right optic tract. The fibers in the upper half of the tract originate from the upper half of the two retinas, and the fibers from the lower half of the tract come from the lower half of the two retinas. The fibers from the optic tract synapse in the lateral geniculate body. The cells of the lateral geniculate body give rise to new fibers which form the optic radiation. These fibers then proceed to the cells of the visual cortex (see Figure 2.7). Any lesion that affects the visual pathway on only the right or left side after this decussation takes place will affect either the left visual field or right visual field.

Vision Areas of the Brain

The brain is divided into several different lobes. Starting anteriorly are the frontal lobes, which are responsible for decision making, planning ahead, emotional tone, abstract thinking, and carrying out intentions. Immediately behind them and in front of the motor area is the prefrontal cortex, which is involved in organizing and sequencing complex motor behavior. The temporal lobes are associated with hearing and also provide some contribution to vision. The parietal lobes are responsible for tactile recognition. Parietal lobe injury commonly results in perceptual deficits that disrupt ambulation and self-care activities. Hemisensory neglect is a common problem in clients with a lesion in the posterior parietal cortex.

Figure 2.7. Visual pathway from the optic nerve to the visual cortex. (Reprinted with permission from Scheiman M, Scheiman M, Whittaker SG. *Low Vision Rehabilitation: A Practical Guide for Occupational Therapists*. Thorofare, NJ: SLACK Incorporated; 2007.)

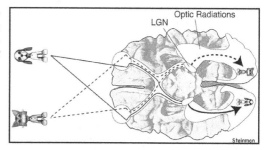

The occipital lobe contains the visual cortex, with nerve pathways leading to higher centers in the parietal and temporal lobes, where visual sensations acquire meaning. Lesions in the visual cortex and in associated areas can produce visual and perceptual problems. The cerebellum integrates the smooth coordination of muscular activity. If it is damaged, general motor clumsiness occurs. This may interfere with manual dexterity and other forms of fine muscular performance, as well as eye movement control. Dysfunction within the cerebellum yields problems with equilibrium, motor control, body image, laterality, and sometimes with reading and speech.

All of the visual fibers end in the striate area of the cortex which is called area 17. Area 17 is considered to be the primary visuosensory area in humans. Outside of area 17 and closely following its contours are two other areas that are concerned with visual reactions as well. These are called areas 18 and 19. Most physiologists agree that vision is a function of higher parts of the brain than just the visual cortex. The message relayed to area 17 enables a person to see. It does not enable a person to recognize what they see or to recall things that have been seen. These functions are dependent on other parts of the brain. In order for a person to be able to interpret the sensory information reaching area 17, the message must be sent on to the two secondary visual areas and areas 18 and 19. Area 18 is concerned exclusively with the recognition of objects, animate or inanimate, but is not concerned with the recognition of written or printed symbols of language. Area 19 is concerned with the recall of visual memory relating to objects but not to language symbols.

Two parallel routes carry visual information from the occipital lobe to the prefrontal lobe and the frontal eye fields. Fibers from these two routes distribute fibers to many other areas along each route before terminating in the prefrontal cortex and in the frontal eye fields. The first route is the superior route via the parietal and frontal lobes. The other route is the inferior route via the temporal and frontal lobes.

Summary

Since low vision is a condition in which visual acuity is reduced because of eye disease, it is important to have a basic understanding of the anatomy and physiology of the eye and visual system. We urge readers who feel a need for more detail to refer to the Bibliography provided at the end of this chapter.

Reference

Lens AI, Coyne Nemeth S, Ledford JK. *Ocular Anatomy and Physiology*. 2nd ed. Thorofare, NJ: SLACK Incorporated; 2008.

Three Component Model of Vision, Part One
Visual Integrity

Mitchell Scheiman

The Three Component Model of Vision that will be described in Chapters Three through Five consists of three components:

1. Visual integrity (visual acuity, optics of the eye, and eye health)
2. Visual efficiency (accommodation, binocular vision, and eye movements)
3. Visual information processing (visual spatial, visual analysis, and visual motor integration skills)

Visual integrity, discussed in this chapter, involves the ability to see clearly at all distances and deals with the optical system and eye health.

Visual Acuity

Definition

Visual acuity is a measure of the resolving power of the eye. Because visual acuity testing is so popular, most people are familiar with the concept of 20/20 visual acuity. An individual with 20/20 acuity is considered to have normal ability to see small detail at the distance tested. The numerator refers to the testing distance at which the subject recognizes the stimulus, and the denominator refers to the distance at which the letter being viewed could be identified by a patient with normal visual acuity. For example, 20/100 suggests that a patient with normal visual acuity could identify the letter presented at a distance of 100 feet. The actual individual being tested could only see this letter at 20 feet, indicating that the visual acuity is reduced relative to the normal finding. In traditional vision screenings, visual acuity below the level of 20/30 to 20/40 is considered cause for referral. However, clinically, any deviation from 20/20 is considered a problem, and, in the course of the vision evaluation, the clinician must determine the basis for the loss of visual acuity.

DOI: 10.4324/9781003526841-3

Classification of Visual Acuity Disorders

There is no classification of visual acuity disorders because these problems are actually always secondary to other conditions. Reduced visual acuity can occur secondary to a wide variety of conditions, including myopia, hyperopia, astigmatism, accommodative disorders, binocular vision disorders, amblyopia, eye disease, and psychogenic causes.

Clinical Assessment

Visual acuity testing is performed by every type of eye care professional and is repeated at every eye examination. In addition, visual acuity testing is often performed by family physicians, pediatricians, and school nurses. There are three methods of assessing visual acuity. The variable for these methods is the type of target used. The three methods are recognition acuity, resolution acuity, and detection acuity.

The recognition acuity format is a visual acuity task in which the patient is asked to "recognize" and identify a series of targets. Most people have experienced this type of visual acuity testing. The standard Snellen Acuity Chart (Figure 3.1) is an example of this format. In almost all clinical examinations, this is the general format used to assess visual acuity.

A second possible testing format would be to use resolution acuity. This is a task in which the patient is required to locate and "resolve" a difference between two targets. The most common

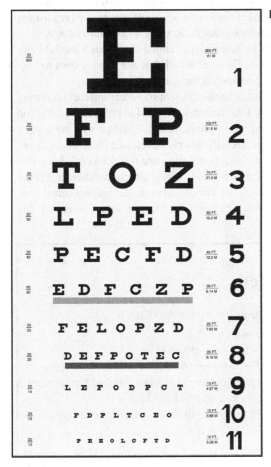

Figure 3.1. The standard Snellen Acuity Chart.

example of this is called preferential looking. In this approach, the child is asked to resolve or differentiate a black-and-white striped stimulus from a homogeneous gray target.

The final general format is called a detection acuity task. In this approach, the patient is asked to "detect" and find a target. For example, the patient may have to find a small black dot on a white background. The smallest black dot that can be seen is considered the highest level of visual acuity for the patient. The detection acuity format is rarely used. It has potential value when assessment with a recognition acuity format is not possible.

There are many clinical tests available for visual acuity assessment. Most use the recognition format described previously. Visual acuity testing is generally a subjective evaluation in which the patient must identify visual stimuli presented at distance or at near. The test that is most widely used is the Snellen Acuity Chart (see Figure 3.1). This procedure is used for adults and children who can recognize and recall all the letters of the alphabet. Most children from first grade and above can be evaluated with the Snellen Acuity Chart. Children who have trouble with letter recognition or children who are nonverbal must be evaluated using other tests. Adults after cerebrovascular accident or traumatic brain injury are often difficult to evaluate with a standard Snellen Acuity Chart because of cognitive, perceptual, memory, and visual problems.

Three alternative approaches have been developed to enable clinicians to evaluate visual acuity in patients unable to respond to the Snellen Acuity Chart. These include the use of numbers, pictures, and charts that limit the number of letters; tests that minimize or eliminate verbal interaction; and tests that rely on the behavioral observation of the examiner. As Table 3.1 illustrates, clinical tests are now available that allow optometrists to assess the visual acuity of any patient regardless of age or cognitive ability. For example, infants can be evaluated as early as 1 month of age.

Figure 3.2 shows a test that uses pictures. The picture chart is called the Allen Visual Acuity Chart and is rather easy to administer. It has a serious flaw because it has not been shown to correlate well with the Snellen Acuity Chart, which is considered the standard measure.

Figures 3.3a through 3.3c illustrate other tests that limit the amount of verbal interaction during visual acuity testing. The Tumbling E Test (see Figure 3.3a) requires the child to point in the direction in which the "E" is pointing. The child simply points up, down, right, or left. Children who are 5 years old and younger often have difficulty with this test because of a poorly developed sense of direction.

The two tests that are most effective in the preschool population are the Broken Wheel Test and the Lea Symbols Test. These tests can be used when brain injury affects number and letter recognition. With the Broken Wheel Test (see Figure 3.3b), the examiner holds up two cards. One has a car with broken wheels while the other card has a picture of a car with intact wheels. If the

Table 3.1

Acuity Tests

Test Type	Name of Test	Appropriate for Age Group
Traditional	Snellen Acuity Chart	6 years to adult
Limits verbal interaction	Tumbling E Test	5- to 6-year-old children
Limits verbal interaction	Broken Wheel Test	2½- to 6-year-old children, TBI and CVA patients
Limits verbal interaction	Lea Symbols Test	2½- to 6-year-old children, TBI and CVA patients
Limits verbal interaction	Allen Visual Acuity Chart	2½- to 6-year-old children
Limits verbal interaction	Teller Acuity Cards	18 to 36 months with operant conditioning
Eliminates need for verbal interaction	Teller Acuity Cards	1 to 18 months

Notes: CVA=cerebrovascular accident, TBI=traumatic brain injury.

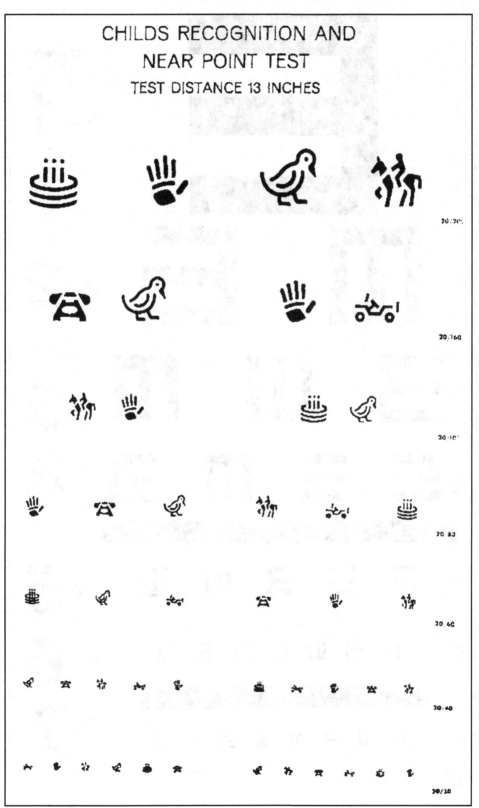

Figure 3.2. The Allen Visual Acuity Chart.

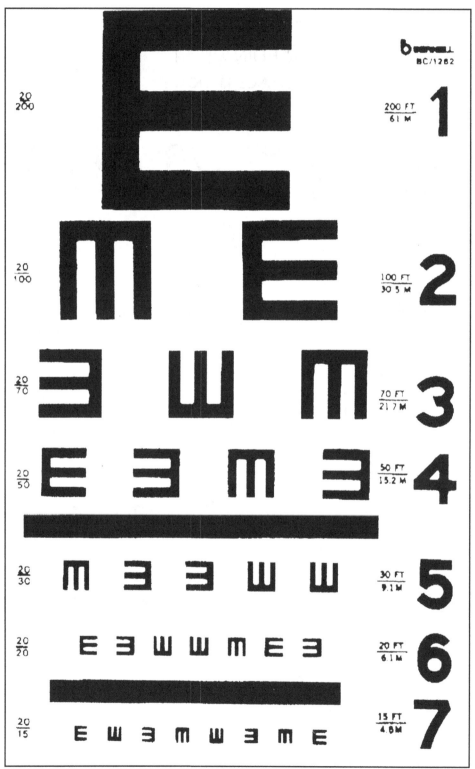

Figure 3.3a. The Tumbling E Test.

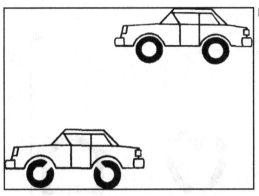

Figure 3.3b. The Broken Wheel Test.

child can see the small gap in the wheel, they are able to identify which card has the car with broken wheels. The child is taught to point to the car with broken wheels. The cars become smaller as does the gap in the wheel.

The Lea Symbols Test (see Figure 3.3c) is also extremely effective with children 2½ to 6 years of age. The examiner places the wooden puzzle with four pieces (apple, circle, square, and house) on the child's lap. The child is taught to point or hold up the block that matches the shape to which the examiner points. As soon as it is clear that the child understands the task, the examiner selects smaller and smaller targets until the child can no longer accurately match the shape. The Lea Symbols Test comes in several versions, allowing clinicians to select the version that is most appropriate for the patient's developmental level.

Figure 3.4 illustrates visual acuity testing in very young infants. The procedure is called forced-choice preferential looking, and the specific test displayed is the Teller Acuity Cards. This is an example of a resolution acuity task discussed above. The entire procedure is based on the fact that, when presented with two stimuli, infants will "prefer" to look at the stimulus with a pattern rather than a stimulus without a pattern. In order to evaluate acuity, the conditions must be ideal. The child must be comfortable, dry, well rested, and fed. The testing should be performed in a room without distractions, and it is preferable to use the setup illustrated in Figure 3.5. With the infant on the parent's lap and facing the examiner, the examiner holds up a card that has two stimuli. One has vertical lines, and the other matches the first stimulus in luminance but has no lines. If the infant can "see" the lines, they will be able to see a difference between the two stimuli and will, therefore, prefer to view the stimulus with lines. The examiner must observe the infant's behavior and will notice that the child tends to look at or prefer one stimulus over the other. The examiner continues to change the cards, choosing cards with narrower vertical lines until the child no longer appears to show a preference for one stimulus and spends an equal amount of time looking from one to the other. This test has been widely studied and is considered a reliable and valid assessment of visual acuity in the hands of an experienced clinician with the following exception[1]—researchers have reported that this test may overestimate the visual acuity in cases of strabismic amblyopia and macular disease.[2] In these cases, the results must be interpreted with caution.

Preferential looking acuity works well with young infants. However, around the age of 18 to 24 months, children no longer seem attracted enough to these stimuli to maintain attention during this task. Researchers and clinicians[3] have developed a modification called operant preferential looking to permit older infants and toddlers to be tested. This is illustrated in Figure 3.6. The key modification is the use of operant conditioning theory. The child is taught that if they point to the stimulus with the stripes, they will receive a reward. Most clinicians use bits of cereal as a reward. Each time the child correctly identifies the stimulus with stripes, they receive the reinforcement.

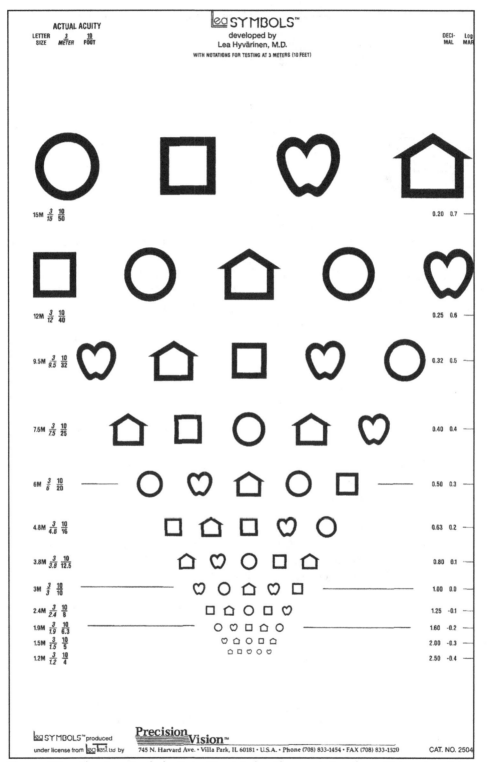

Figure 3.3c. The Lea Symbols Test. (Reprinted with permission from Vision Associates, www.visionkits.com.)

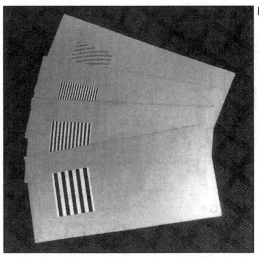

Figure 3.4. The Teller Acuity Cards.

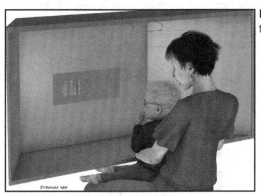

Figure 3.5. Preferential looking acuity procedure with the infant on the parent's lap and facing the examiner.

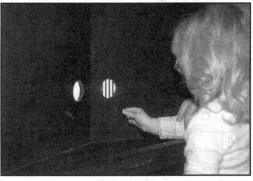

Figure 3.6. Operant preferential looking procedure. The child is taught that if they point to the stimulus with the stripes, they will receive a reward.

Studies have also demonstrated the effectiveness of this procedure. Forced-choice and operant preferential learning have also been used effectively with special populations such as mentally disabled adults.

The important message is that optometrists now have the ability to evaluate visual acuity in virtually any patient regardless of age or cognitive ability.

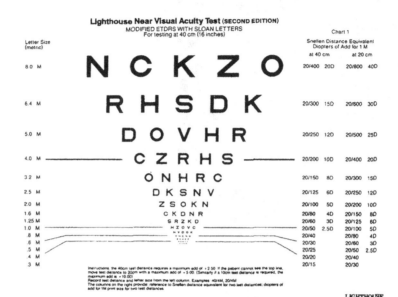

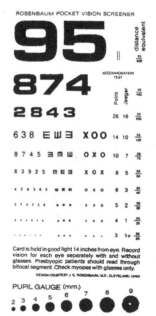

Figure 3.7. Variety of near point visual acuity cards.

Visual acuity can also be tested at near. Figure 3.7 illustrates a variety of near point visual acuity cards that are available. Essentially, they are simply reduced versions of the distance visual acuity charts.

Development of Visual Acuity

Researchers have used two different methods to study the development of visual acuity in infants and young children. One method is an electrophysiological approach using visually evoked potentials, and the other is the behavioral method called forced-choice preferential learning described previously. The electrophysiological approach simply requires the child to look at a video display of a flickering checkerboard pattern. The cortical response to this changing stimulus is recorded using electrodes placed on the scalp over the occipital pole.

There are significant differences between the results obtained from the two methods. Both approaches indicate that infants are born with very poor visual acuity and suggest that visual acuity is approximately 20/400 to 20/800 in newborns. The electrophysiological approach, however, suggests that the visual acuity reaches adult levels (20/20) by 6 months of age.[4,5] Studies using forced-choice preferential learning indicate that visual acuity is about 20/50 to 20/60 at 6 months, about 20/100 by 12 months, and slowly improves to 20/20 by 5 years of age.[6–8] Despite the differences in results, both research methods demonstrate that there is a very rapid period of development in visual acuity between birth and 6 months of age. The first 6 months of life are, therefore, very important in the development of visual acuity and many other aspects of the visual system.

When discussing the development of the visual system, it is important to mention the concept of plasticity and sensitivity. As described above, the infant is born with poor acuity. With normal stimulation during the first five years of life, however, acuity develops to adult levels. This time period has been referred to as the sensitive period of visual development, and it is the time frame during which the visual system is plastic and capable of developing normally. However, it is also the time period during which any disorder or interference will severely impact the normal developmental process. The first 6 months of life is the period of most rapid development in acuity, accommodation, and binocular vision and is sometimes referred to as the critical period. This is the period of maximum sensitivity to interference.

The presence of uncorrected or undetected vision problems during the first 5 to 6 years of life will interfere with the development of visual acuity and binocular vision, and with other aspects of the visual system. This is the basis for the recent recommendation of the American Optometric Association (AOA). The AOA now recommends the first full eye examination by an optometrist at the age of 6 months, the second examination at age 3, and the next at 6 years of age.

Significance of Visual Acuity Disorders for Occupational Therapy

Reduced visual acuity does not occur as an isolated problem. Acuity that is less than expected for a given age level is always related to other vision problems or eye disease. Reduced visual acuity, therefore, can be thought of as a sign that another vision anomaly is present. The presence of undetected poor visual acuity in both eyes in young children can have a devastating effect on development and on the child's ability to interact with their environment. It is important to understand that reduced visual acuity has this effect only if it is present in both eyes. If there is a loss of vision in only one eye, the child will use the eye with normal acuity, and generally there will be no interference with functional performance. From a clinical standpoint, of course, loss of acuity in one eye, called amblyopia, is very significant and requires aggressive treatment. It does not affect the child's ability to interact with their environment, however, and would be unlikely to interfere with occupational therapy. It is also important to remember that the quality of the patient's vision is also critical for performance. It is possible for a patient to have reasonably good vision but still have significant and legitimate complaints about the quality of vision.

> ### Table 3.2
> # Reduced Visual Acuity: Symptoms and Effect on Function
>
> •
>
> *Blurred vision at far or near*
> - Need to move closer to objects of interest
> - Lack of interest in the environment
> - Lack of interest in reading
> - Difficulty with writing tasks
> - Difficulty locating objects for grooming, self-care, cooking
> - Trouble with driving
> - Difficulty with mobility
> - Fear of new environments
> - Squinting
> - Inability to recognize faces
> - Difficulty with social interaction
> - Avoidance of visual tasks

Reduced visual acuity will have a significant effect on rehabilitation of either a child or an adult. Reading, writing, and driving, for instance, are three tasks that are almost totally dependent on vision. Whether the occupational therapist is working with a developmentally delayed child or with a patient recovering from cerebrovascular accident or head trauma, reduced visual acuity will generally interfere with progress. It is critical for the therapist to be sensitive to this possibility and to make an appropriate referral for an evaluation and treatment of the reduced acuity.

Signs, Symptoms, and Significance of Visual Acuity Disorders for Occupational Therapy

The signs and symptoms of visual acuity are summarized in Table 3.2. The primary problems that therapists will observe are a need for the patient to move closer to objects of interest, lack of interest in the environment, difficulty with mobility, fear of new environments, squinting, and avoidance of visual tasks.

Contrast Sensitivity

Definition

An important topic that is related to visual acuity is contrast sensitivity. While visual acuity tests enable the therapist to estimate how well someone can see small high-contrast objects, contrast sensitivity testing enables the therapist to estimate how well someone can see larger low-contrast objects. Contrast sensitivity is related to visual acuity but provides information that is not as well captured by visual acuity measurement.[9] Contrast sensitivity is strongly associated with reading performance,[10] mobility,[11,12] driving,[13,14] face recognition,[14,15] and activities of daily living.[15,16] Contrast sensitivity testing tells us about the quality of the available vision when viewing larger objects. For instance, it is possible for a client to have reasonably good visual acuity but still complain of problems such as dim, foggy, or unclear vision or sensitivity to bright light. Visual acuity only allows us to evaluate one limited aspect of the person's ability to see. Contrast sensitivity is a measure of how faded or washed out an image can be before it becomes indistinguishable from a uniform field. A person with impaired contrast sensitivity might describe the problem by saying, "it is like looking through a dirty windshield when I drive." People with reduced contrast sensitivity often are very particular about lighting. They usually are glare sensitive or can see best over only a very narrow range of light intensity.

Contrast sensitivity determines the lowest contrast level that can be detected by a client for a given size target. Contrast can vary from no contrast (0%) to highest contrast (100%). For example, high-quality print has 85% to 95% contrast, while paper currency has only 55% to 60% contrast.

Examples of Low Contrast in Activities of Daily Living

- Communication: We need to use information from the faint shadows on people's faces to recognize facial expressions.

- Orientation and mobility: We need to see low-contrast forms such as the curb, faint shadows, and the last step of carpeted stairs when walking. When driving, we need to function in low-contrast conditions such as seeing in dusk, rain, fog, snowfall, and at night.

- Reading: When reading we may encounter poor-quality copies, newsprint, and older books with poor contrast.

- Kitchen tasks: When cutting certain foods such as chicken, onion, or other light-colored objects on a white or light-colored cutting board, we may encounter low-contrast situations.

Classification of Contrast Sensitivity Disorders

There is no classification of contrast sensitivity disorders because these problems are always secondary to other conditions. Reduced contrast sensitivity can occur secondary to a wide variety of conditions, including amblyopia, and a wide variety of eye diseases.

Clinical Assessment

Contrast sensitivity testing can be performed at both distance and near using the instrumentation shown in Figures 3.8a through 3.8e. One test used for older children and adults is illustrated in Figure 3.8a. To use this device, the examiner asks the patient to observe the sample gratings at the bottom of the chart. The four possible responses (left, right, up, and blank) should be reviewed. With one eye occluded, the patient is instructed to begin with the top row and identify the orientation of as many of the circular patches as possible. This is repeated for all five rows of the chart. As Figure 3.8a illustrates, the contrast decreases as the patient views from left to right.

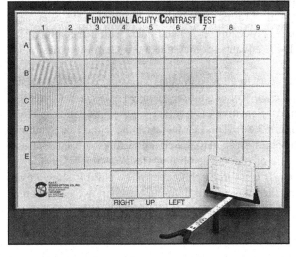

Figure 3.8a. Contrast sensitivity testing. The patient is instructed to begin with the top row and identify the orientation of as many of the circular patches as possible.

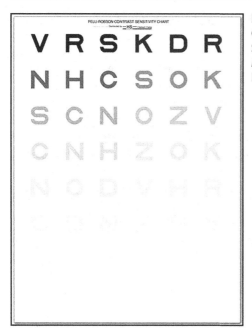

Figure 3.8b. The Pelli-Robson Contrast Sensitivity Chart. (Reprinted with permission from Scheiman M, Scheiman M, Whittaker SG. *Low Vision Rehabilitation: A Practical Guide for Occupational Therapists*. Thorofare, NJ: SLACK Incorporated; 2007.)

In recent years, however, letter contrast sensitivity testing has become the preferred method in clinical settings because it is easy to administer and clients are familiar with the use of letters to test vision.[17] The Pelli-Robson Contrast Sensitivity Chart has been a popular method of testing letter contrast sensitivity (see Figure 3.8b).[18] It is a large wall-mounted chart, arranged in eight rows of two triplets each. The three letters within each triplet have constant contrast, whereas the contrast across triplets, reading from left to right, and continuing on successive lines, decreases in contrast. The client reads the letters across and down the chart, as in standard letter acuity measurement. Instead of the letters decreasing in size, however, they decrease in contrast.

Although widely used by researchers, it has not been widely used by clinicians for a variety of reasons.[17] First, it is inconvenient for testing in small clinical spaces, as it requires a large amount of wall space devoted to it. Second, it is difficult to arrange lighting that will illuminate such a large area uniformly. Third, a wall-mounted chart is difficult to keep clean and free of defects.[17]

Recently, Arditi[17] reported on a new letter contrast sensitivity test called the Mars Letter Contrast Sensitivity Test (see Figure 3.8c). It is similar to the Pelli-Robson but has greater accuracy due to its finer contrast decrements and scoring procedure, it is hand-held, with a recommended viewing distance of 50 cm, and is portable. These advantages may make this chart more desirable in a clinical setting.

Tests have also been developed in recent years to allow clinicians to evaluate contrast sensitivity in infants, young children, and developmentally or cognitively delayed patients.[19] Currently available tests include the Lea Symbols Contrast Sensitivity Chart (see Figure 3.8d) and the Hiding Heidi Contrast Sensitivity Chart (see Figure 3.8e). The Lea test uses the same Lea symbols described earlier for visual acuity testing. The child is asked to match the pictures at each contrast level. This test is effective for children 3 years or older. The Hiding Heidi Contrast Sensitivity Chart can be used with even younger children. It is a forced-choice test. The child is shown two pictures, one with a homogeneous pattern and the other with a light-contrast happy face. When a repeatable response is elicited to the light-contrast figure, testing continues with reduced-contrast figures.[19]

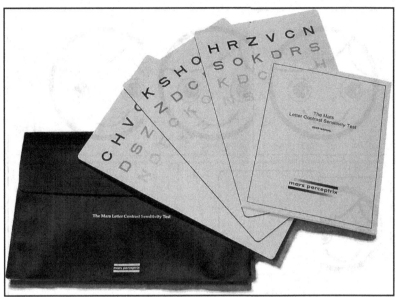

Figure 3.8c. The Mars Letter Contrast Sensitivity Test. (Reprinted with permission from Scheiman M, Scheiman M, Whittaker SG. *Low Vision Rehabilitation: A Practical Guide for Occupational Therapists*. Thorofare, NJ: SLACK Incorporated; 2007.)

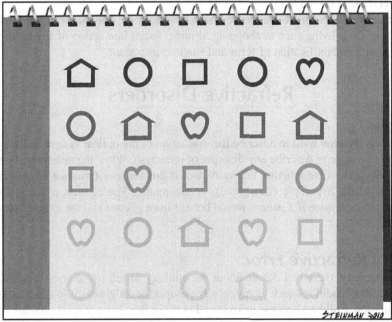

Figure 3.8d. The Lea Symbols Contrast Sensitivity Chart used to evaluate contrast sensitivity in infants, preverbal children, and developmentally and cognitively delayed patients.

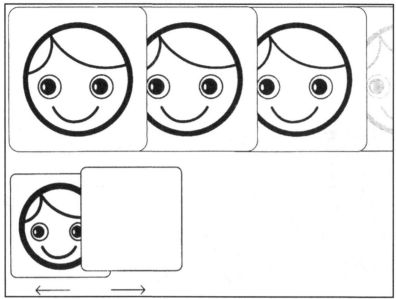

Figure 3.8e. The Hiding Heidi Contrast Sensitivity Chart used to evaluate contrast sensitivity in infants, preverbal children, and developmentally and cognitively delayed patients.

Significance of Contrast Sensitivity Disorders for Occupational Therapy

Contrast sensitivity problems can cause vision to seem hazy, dim, or cloudy and will interfere with activities of daily living such as shopping, driving, social interaction of any kind, and almost any activity in which identification of form and shape is important.

Refractive Disorders

Definition

Refraction is the term used to describe the evaluation of the optical system of the eye. We use the term *refractive error* to describe any disorder of refraction. When the optometrist performs the "refraction," they determine whether the individual is emmetropic (absence of refractive error), myopic (nearsighted), hyperopic (farsighted), or astigmatic. The refraction is the examination procedure used to determine if a patient would benefit from glasses and the exact prescription that is appropriate.

Etiology of Refractive Error

Within optometry, there is a debate about the etiology of refractive error. Traditional theory attributes refractive conditions such as myopia, hyperopia, or astigmatism to genetics and random biological variation. Children become nearsighted because they have parents who are nearsighted. Because refractive conditions are genetically determined, treatment involves correction of the refractive condition with appropriate lenses. Advocates of this theory dismiss any attempts to reduce or modify the problem using special lenses, prism, or vision therapy procedures.

Other models attribute the development of refractive problems and many other vision disorders to the extensive near work demands imposed by our society. The most popular model is

Skeffington's near point stress model.[20] He suggests that refractive, binocular, and accommodative disorders develop because near work creates demands that are incompatible with our physiology. Proponents of this model have developed therapeutic regimens that stress prevention and remediation using special lens prescriptions, prism, and vision therapy.[21]

In spite of many years of research, this debate continues without a definitive answer. My philosophy at this time is that both theories are probably partially correct. I believe that there are certainly cases of refractive error that have a genetic basis. Usually, very high degrees of myopia, hyperopia, or astigmatism that have an early onset would fit into this category. Such cases are best treated in the traditional mode using corrective lenses without any attempt to eliminate or alter the refractive error. On the other hand, it is clear that there are also many cases in which the refractive condition may be secondary to environmental factors. Older children who develop myopia as they become heavily involved with reading or young adults who develop myopia in college or after entering the work force are examples of individuals who may have refractive disorders secondary to environmental demands. Studies have reported that there is a constellation of clinical findings that suggest when clinicians should attempt to prevent, control, or eliminate myopia using lenses, prism, or vision therapy.[22-25] This topic will be covered in more depth in Chapter Seven.

Classification of Refractive Conditions

EMMETROPIA

The word emmetropia is used to describe the condition in which there is an absence of refractive error. In emmetropia, the light rays entering the eyes focus right on the retina. Figure 3.9 illustrates how the light rays entering the eye are perfectly focused on the retina in emmetropia. In such a case, the patient is neither nearsighted nor farsighted and does not have astigmatism. Emmetropia is not necessarily considered normal, expected, or desirable. In fact, the average person is slightly hyperopic. A finding of emmetropia can be an indication that the patient's visual system is changing and is becoming myopic.

MYOPIA (NEARSIGHTEDNESS)

Myopia is a condition in which the light rays entering the eye focus in front of the retina. In myopia, the vision is blurred at distance but clear at near. Figure 3.10 illustrates the reason why a patient with myopia experiences blurred vision. The light rays entering the eye are focused in front of the retina because the optics of the eye are too strong relative to the length of the eye. The myopic eye has a longer axial length than the emmetropic or hyperopic eye. The human eye can make no internal adjustment to overcome the optical problem associated with myopia. An individual with myopia can squint, which actually does allow improved vision, but this is generally considered an unacceptable way to regain clarity because it can cause discomfort and is cosmetically unacceptable. Squinting helps compensate for the blur associated with myopia because it creates a pinhole effect. Any attempted focusing adjustment will simply make the blurred vision worse. Thus, a patient with myopia will have to move closer to the object they are trying to view. Table 3.3 lists the signs and symptoms associated with myopia.

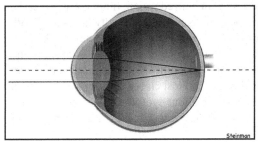

Figure 3.9. Light rays entering the eye are perfectly focused on the retina in emmetropia. (Reprinted with permission from Scheiman M, Scheiman M, Whittaker SG. *Low Vision Rehabilitation: A Practical Guide for Occupational Therapists.* Thorofare, NJ: SLACK Incorporated; 2007.)

Figure 3.10. The light rays entering the eye are focused in front of the retina in myopia causing blurred vision. (Reprinted with permission from Scheiman M, Scheiman M, Whittaker SG. *Low Vision Rehabilitation: A Practical Guide for Occupational Therapists.* Thorofare, NJ: SLACK Incorporated; 2007.)

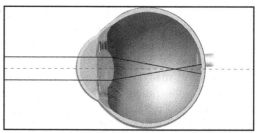

Table 3.3

Myopia: Symptoms and Effect on Function

- Blurred vision at far
- Need to move closer to objects of interest
- Lack of interest in the environment
- Squinting

Figure 3.11a. The light rays entering the eye are focused behind the retina in hyperopia causing blurred vision. (Reprinted with permission from Scheiman M, Scheiman M, Whittaker SG. *Low Vision Rehabilitation: A Practical Guide for Occupational Therapists.* Thorofare, NJ: SLACK Incorporated; 2007.)

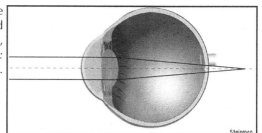

HYPEROPIA (FARSIGHTEDNESS)

Hyperopia is a condition in which light rays entering the eye focus behind the retina and the individual must accommodate to see clearly (Figure 3.11a). This need to accommodate requires the use of muscular effort. The amount of effort necessary is greater when the individual looks at near. Figure 3.11b illustrates that to see clearly, a person with hyperopia must contract the ciliary muscle to change the shape of the lens in the eye and regain clarity. Contraction of the ciliary muscle leads to a change in focus and is referred to as accommodation. The effort that is necessary to accommodate is directly related to the degree of hyperopia. A very high degree of hyperopia requires so much muscular effort that it cannot be overcome and results in blurred vision. If not corrected early, very high degrees of hyperopia can lead to amblyopia (loss of vision) and difficulty interacting with the environment. Moderate degrees of hyperopia can be overcome using accommodation. The constant need for accommodation, however, requires the use of muscular effort and leads to signs and symptoms, such as blurred vision, eyestrain, tearing, burning, inability to concentrate and attend, avoidance of visual tasks, and the need to move the object of interest closer or farther away. Small degrees of hyperopia are generally successfully overcome without symptoms. Remember that a low degree of hyperopia is considered normal, expected, and desirable. Table 3.4 lists the signs and symptoms associated with hyperopia.

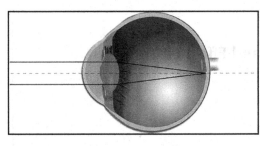

Figure 3.11b. To see clearly, a person with hyperopia must contract the ciliary muscle to change the shape of the lens in the eye and regain clarity. (Reprinted with permission from Scheiman M, Scheiman M, Whittaker SG. *Low Vision Rehabilitation: A Practical Guide for Occupational Therapists*. Thorofare, NJ: SLACK Incorporated; 2007.)

Table 3.4

Hyperopia: Symptoms and Effect on Function

- Blurred vision at near
- Blurred vision at far if the degree of hyperopia is great
- Discomfort when reading
- Tearing
- Headaches associated with reading
- Avoidance of close work
- Moves objects away from eyes to read

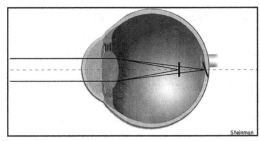

Figure 3.12. The effect of astigmatism on the light rays focusing on the retina. (Reprinted with permission from Scheiman M, Scheiman M, Whittaker SG. *Low Vision Rehabilitation: A Practical Guide for Occupational Therapists*. Thorofare, NJ: SLACK Incorporated; 2007.)

ASTIGMATISM

Astigmatism is a condition in which vision is blurred and distorted at both distance and near. An astigmatic eye is not spherical. Rather, it has an oval shape, and this causes the light rays entering the eye to focus at two different points. Figure 3.12 illustrates the effect that astigmatism has on the light rays focusing on the retina. In order to see clearly, a person with astigmatism will attempt to accommodate. While accommodation may improve clarity, it is never completely successful for a person with astigmatism, and the effort that is necessary to accommodate may lead to discomfort. As discussed above for hyperopia, the degree of accommodation necessary is related to the degree and type of astigmatism. In some cases of astigmatism, accommodation has no beneficial effect on clarity. A very high degree of astigmatism generally cannot be overcome and results in blurred vision. If not corrected early, such problems can lead to amblyopia (loss of vision) and difficulty interacting with the environment. Moderate degrees of astigmatism can sometimes be overcome using accommodation. The constant need for accommodation, however, requires the use of muscular effort and leads to signs and symptoms, such as blurred vision, eyestrain, tearing, burning, inability to concentrate and attend, avoidance of visual tasks, and the need to move the object of interest closer or farther away. Small degrees of astigmatism are common and are generally successfully overcome without symptoms. Table 3.5 lists the signs and symptoms associated with astigmatism.

Table 3.5

Astigmatism: Symptoms and Effect on Function

- Blurred vision at distance and near
- Discomfort when reading
- Tearing
- Headaches associated with reading
- Avoidance of close work
- Moves objects away from eyes to read

ANISOMETROPIA

Anisometropia is not another type of refractive error. Rather, the term refers to a condition in which there is a significant difference in the magnitude of the refractive error between the two eyes. Anisometropia can be present along with myopia, hyperopia, or astigmatism. The following are four common examples of anisometropia:

1. A patient has a mild degree of hyperopia in the right eye and a moderate or high degree of hyperopia in the left eye.
2. A patient has a mild degree of myopia in the right eye and a moderate or high degree of myopia in the left eye.
3. A patient has a mild degree of astigmatism in the right eye and a moderate or high degree of astigmatism in the left eye.
4. A patient has a mild to moderate degree of hyperopia in one eye and a mild to moderate degree of myopia in the other.

The significance of anisometropia is that the difference in refractive error between the two eyes interferes with binocular vision. The visual cortex receives images from each eye that differ in clarity and size, and this makes it difficult for the brain to fuse or merge the information from the two eyes. In such cases, the visual cortex generally will learn to suppress or ignore the information coming from the eye with the greater degree of refractive error. If the condition occurs during the sensitive period of visual development described earlier in the chapter, suppression will lead to loss of vision in the eye with the greater degree of refractive error. This loss of vision is referred to as amblyopia, which will be described in detail in Chapter Four.

Clinical Assessment

Like visual acuity, refraction is also a test that is performed by all eye care professionals. There are two general methods of evaluating the refractive status of the eye. These include objective and subjective methods. Subjective tests can only be successfully performed with cooperative, attentive patients with reasonable cognitive ability. These tests can generally be performed with any person with a developmental age of 7 years or older. Objective testing, however, can be successfully performed at any age and for virtually any patient.

Subjective Refraction Techniques

Most adults have had an eye examination at least once in their lives, and, if they have, they are likely to remember the subjective refraction portion of the examination. The instrumentation used is illustrated in Figure 3.13. This instrument, called the phoropter, contains numerous lenses and allows the optometrist to find the combination of lenses that will provide the

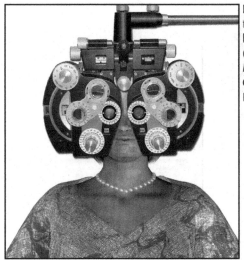

Figure 3.13. The phoropter is an instrument used to find the combination of lenses that will provide the best possible vision for any patient being examined. (Reprinted with permission from Scheiman M, Scheiman M, Whittaker SG. *Low Vision Rehabilitation: A Practical Guide for Occupational Therapists.* Thorofare, NJ: SLACK Incorporated; 2007.)

best possible vision for any patient being examined. The procedure is very subjective, and the optometrist will ask questions such as, "Which is better, choice one or choice two?" or "Does this lens make the letters look clearer or just blacker and smaller?" This subjective approach works well for most of the population but is generally not used with children below the age of 6 or 7 or with patients who have attention problems, perceptual and cognitive disorders, or other special needs. It is clear, therefore, that many patients who are treated by occupational therapists will be unable to be evaluated using subjective refraction procedures. Fortunately, excellent objective techniques are available and produce accurate results in the hands of an experienced clinician.

Objective Refraction Techniques

The instrument illustrated in Figure 3.14 is called a retinoscope. This instrument permits the optometrist to accurately and objectively assess refractive status in virtually any patient. The optometrist directs the light from the retinoscope into the patient's eye and views the light that is reflected out of the eye. As the optometrist moves the retinoscope from side to side, they interpret the movement of the reflected light. Lenses are used to alter the movement of light and help the clinician determine the refraction and necessary eyeglass prescription. The procedure generally requires less than 1 minute per eye. It can be performed with or without eye drops. With a cooperative, intelligent patient with good attention, I always begin the refraction using retinoscopy. The subjective refraction is then performed to refine these results.

If a subjective refraction is not possible, clinical decisions can be made with confidence from the objective refraction alone. Thus, it is possible to determine if an individual has a refractive error such as myopia, hyperopia, or astigmatism even if they are unable to respond subjectively. A newborn child can be examined using this procedure, and an experienced clinician can confidently assess the refractive status of the eye.

Another objective refraction procedure can be performed using a computerized device called an automated refractor. The instrument is relatively expensive and provides the same type of information as the very inexpensive retinoscope. It also may require the patient to be attentive, to place their chin and forehead against the instrument, and to accurately fixate for a relatively long period of time. As a result, it has little value in the evaluation of patients unable to respond to subjective testing, even though this is an objective of the procedure. The typical patient seen by occupational therapists could not be tested with an automated refractor.

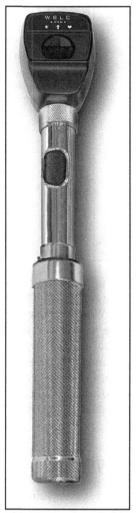

Figure 3.14. The retinoscope can be used to accurately and objectively assess refractive status in virtually any patient. (Reprinted with permission from Scheiman M, Scheiman M, Whittaker SG. *Low Vision Rehabilitation: A Practical Guide for Occupational Therapists*. Thorofare, NJ: SLACK Incorporated; 2007.)

Refractive Error: Developmental Changes

The development of refractive error has been studied extensively. Before 1970, most of the research was performed with children starting from age 5 or so. In the past 20 years, however, new techniques have been developed that allow researchers and clinicians to evaluate vision in infants and preverbal children. This has led to a more complete understanding of the developmental changes that occur in the refractive status of the eye.

These studies have demonstrated that the most active period for changes in refractive error is the first 4 years of life. In particular, large fluctuations are common in astigmatism and anisometropia.[26] Studies have shown that large amounts of astigmatism are common in children below the age of 3 years.[6,26–29] In fact, Gwiazda et al.[27] found that about 50% of infants between 9 and 32 weeks old have a significant degree of astigmatism. The magnitude of the astigmatism declines over the first few years of life so that the incidence of astigmatism is about 10% by 5 to 6 years of age.

All investigations show a bell-shaped curve distribution of refractive error with wide variability during infancy. This variability diminishes between the first and second years of life, with only small changes occurring thereafter.[30,31] Newborn infants tend to have a low to moderate degree of hyperopia with an incidence of about 35%. Most authors agree that hyperopia may increase during the first year of life; then there is a general reduction in the magnitude of hyperopia sometime after the age of 1 year.[19] Myopia is unusual in infants and preschool children, and at the age of 6 the incidence of myopia is only about 3.7%.[29] Children with very mild degrees of hyperopia or emmetropia at 5 or 6 years old develop mild to moderate myopia between ages 7 and 13. Others may develop mild myopia, or myopia may increase between ages 18 and 21.[32] Extreme ametropias are most often congenital and relatively stable.

Signs and Symptoms of Refractive Disorders and Significance of Refractive Disorders for Occupational Therapy

The significance of refractive disorders on progress in occupational therapy varies with the type of problem, the magnitude of the refractive error, and the age of the patient. In the adult population, most patients will have had several eye examinations, and as a general rule, any significant refractive error will already have been detected. In spite of this, it is important that the occupational therapist not assume that the glasses that were used before a stroke or head trauma are still appropriate. Studies have shown that changes in eyeglasses are sometimes necessary after cerebrovascular accident and traumatic brain injury, particularly for hyperopia and presbyopia, because of disorders of accommodation.[33,34] This issue is discussed in more detail in Chapters Nine and Ten.

For the pediatric population, the issue of refractive error and its effect on therapy is very significant. Studies have shown that children with these problems have a high incidence of refractive disorders. For example, the incidence of refractive disorders in children with mental retardation has been reported to be 50% to 80%; in children with cerebral palsy, 50% to 70%; and in children with Down syndrome, 43% to 65%.[35] In addition, a high percentage of children being seen by occupational therapists may never have had a comprehensive vision evaluation. Studies show that only about 31% of children between ages 6 and 16 are likely to have had an eye examination within the past year, while below the age of 6, only about 14% are likely to have had an eye examination.[36] Many parents still believe that between the pediatrician and school vision screenings, all of the vision care needs of their children are being met. This is an unfortunate misconception that may lead to late detection of significant vision disorders and negative effects on overall development. And certainly with children who have mentally and multi-handicapping conditions, the visual system should be functioning at the best possible level.

Researchers have studied the effect of correction of refractive error in mentally and multi-impaired people. These studies are very significant and demonstrate important changes in ability to identify objects and people; improved eye-to-eye contact; improved performance in activities such as catching, kicking, and throwing a ball; improved posture while eating; and in fine motor control, such as reaching and grasping for objects, stacking blocks, stringing beads, and cutting paper.[37] Any occupational therapist would be thrilled to see such changes in their patient, and occupational therapy would certainly proceed more effectively.

HIGH DEGREES OF REFRACTIVE ERROR IN BOTH EYES

If a child has a high degree of refractive error in both eyes and it is not corrected with eyeglasses, amblyopia can develop, leading to difficulty seeing and problems with mobility. Any therapy task requiring good visual skills will be compromised. Amblyopia affects both far and near tasks.

MODERATE DEGREES OF REFRACTIVE ERROR IN BOTH EYES

Moderate degrees of refractive error present in both eyes and left uncorrected generally do not lead to a loss of vision. Rather, any task that requires good vision will be much more difficult for the patient because of the need to use excessive effort to overcome the refractive error. Symptoms related to this type of problem are generally directly related to the amount of detail in the task and the amount of sustained attention and concentration required of the patient to complete the task. The effects of moderate degrees of uncorrected refractive error may be more severe for adults than children because children have a greater ability to accommodate than adults.

SIGNIFICANT DEGREES OF REFRACTIVE ERROR IN ONLY ONE EYE

This condition is referred to as anisometropia and if undetected or untreated can lead to ambly-opia in the eye. We call this condition anisometropic amblyopia. Although amblyopia is a serious vision problem with significant implications for the visual function in the affected eye, there are generally no effects on performance because the patient still has adequate vision in the dominant or good eye. Thus, with both eyes open, the patient is able to see clearly and has normal ocular motility function and accommodation. The only potential problems that might exist are a mild decrease in stereopsis (3-D vision) and other binocular vision skills. Although binocular vision is compromised in cases of anisometropic amblyopia, most people with this problem learn to ignore or suppress the information entering the amblyopic eye, and this prevents symptoms of double vision or eyestrain.

MYOPIA (NEARSIGHTEDNESS)

In the pediatric population, low (up to 1 diopter [D]) and moderate degrees (1 to 3 D) of myo-pia generally are insignificant in regard to their effect on therapy progress. Children with low to moderate myopia can often manage well by squinting and simply moving closer to the object of interest. Because these children tend to squint, they are generally easily identified as requiring help. High degrees (greater than 3 D) of myopia in young children, however, may interfere with motor development and lead to difficulty interacting with the environment. Children with undetected high myopia may be clumsy, fearful of activities involving movement through space, and slow to progress in therapy, and they may avoid all tasks that involve viewing distant objects. It is important to understand that even a child with a high degree of myopia may be able to see objects clearly if they are held very close to the eyes. Thus, holding objects very close to the face is a characteristic sign of uncorrected myopia. Because the negative effects of high myopia or other refractive error are so significant and easily treated, such problems certainly should be ruled out in all children with developmental, motor, or cognitive disorders.

In adults being treated after cerebrovascular accident or traumatic brain injury, the presence of refractive error must always be taken into consideration in treatment. In almost all cases, any significant myopia would have been previously detected and treated. Changes in refractive error occur after cerebrovascular accident or traumatic brain injury, and this has important implications for therapy. If an occupational therapist is working on activities of daily living such as cooking, shopping, writing checks, or driving, it is absolutely critical that the visual input be maximized. Visual information processing will certainly be compromised if the sensory input is affected. The occupational therapist should make sure that the patient is wearing their glasses correctly, and an eye examination should be performed to make sure that the prescription is up to date. Table 3.3 summarizes the signs and symptoms associated with myopia.

HYPEROPIA (FARSIGHTEDNESS)

In contrast to myopia, in which high degrees are of greater significance than low or moderate degrees of the disorder, with hyperopia, low (up to 1 D) and moderate degrees (1 to 3 D) of the condition can have a very deleterious effect on occupational therapy. Remember that an individual with hyperopia can accommodate to regain clear vision. Because the patient can regain clear vision with effort, they will be able to pass a typical vision screening that simply assesses visual acuity. Thus, an individual with low to moderate degrees of hyperopia will see clearly, but the effort that is necessary to accommodate can result in eyestrain, inability to attend and concentrate, headaches, and intermittent blurred vision. In some cases, the effort required to accommodate reflexively causes the eyes to turn inward (esophoria or esotropia), leading to intermittent or even constant double vision. The individual with low to moderate degrees of hyperopia, therefore, sees clearly but may feel uncomfortable and have difficulty sustaining attention. Because visual acuity is normal in such cases, the discomfort may not be attributed to a vision problem, and the individual may suffer for quite some time with an undiagnosed problem.

Occupational therapists often work with children with attention problems such as attention deficit hyperactivity disorder (ADHD). Because of their inability to concentrate and attend for reasonable periods of time, these children can be very difficult to successfully manage. In such cases, low to moderate degrees of hyperopia should certainly be ruled out as a possible contributing factor to the poor attention. Optometrists occasionally encounter patients who have been labeled as ADHD who have been functioning with moderate degrees of undetected hyperopia. When appropriate eyeglasses are prescribed, the attention problems dissipate.

Researchers have reported a significant relationship between hyperopia and visual perceptual skills.[38] These reports demonstrate a higher prevalence of visual perceptual disorders in children with moderate degrees of hyperopia than in children with myopia or emmetropia. Other studies have reported a higher prevalence of significant degrees of hyperopia in children with reading disorders.[39,40]

High degrees (greater than 3 D) of hyperopia cannot be overcome for extended periods of time and result in blurred vision. If not corrected early, such problems can lead to amblyopia (loss of vision) and difficulty interacting with the environment. Table 3.4 summarizes the signs and symptoms associated with hyperopia.

ASTIGMATISM

As with hyperopia, low (up to 1 D) and moderate degrees (1 to 3 D) of astigmatism can have a negative effect on occupational therapy. Patients with astigmatism may try to accommodate to regain clear vision. Unlike hyperopia, astigmatism can never completely be overcome by accommodating. The effort used to accommodate, however, can result in eyestrain, inability to attend and concentrate, headaches, and intermittent blurred vision. The individual with low to moderate degrees of astigmatism, therefore, will struggle with blurred vision and discomfort and may have difficulty sustaining attention. Because visual acuity is often borderline and may be just enough to pass a screening, the discomfort may not be attributed to a vision problem, and the individual may suffer for quite some time with an undiagnosed problem.

Low to moderate degrees of astigmatism should be ruled out as a possible contributing factor for any child with attention problems. High degrees (greater than 3 D) of astigmatism cannot be overcome and result in blurred vision. If not corrected early, such problems can lead to amblyopia (loss of vision) and difficulty interacting with the environment. Table 3.5 summarizes the signs and symptoms associated with astigmatism.

Eye Health Disorders

Classification

Eye health disorders are generally classified by the location of the disorder. The four main types of eye health problems are anterior segment, lenticular, posterior segment, and visual pathway disorders. Figure 3.15 is a cross-section of the human eye and illustrates the anterior and posterior portions of the eye. The anterior section includes all the structures from the front of the eye to the lens. The posterior segment includes all structures behind the lens to the optic nerve. Figure 3.16 is an illustration of the visual pathways from the optic nerve to the occipital cortex. Tables 3.6 through 3.9 summarize the most common eye disease conditions.

Figure 3.15. Cross-section of the human eye, illustrating the anterior and posterior portions of the eye. (Reprinted with permission from Scheiman M, Scheiman M, Whittaker SG. *Low Vision Rehabilitation: A Practical Guide for Occupational Therapists.* Thorofare, NJ: SLACK Incorporated; 2007.)

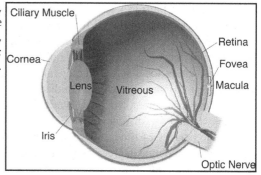

Figure 3.16. Illustration of the visual pathways from the optic nerve to the occipital cortex. (Reprinted with permission from Scheiman M, Scheiman M, Whittaker SG. *Low Vision Rehabilitation: A Practical Guide for Occupational Therapists.* Thorofare, NJ: SLACK Incorporated; 2007.)

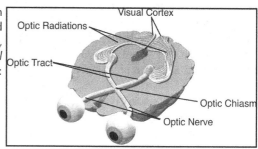

Table 3.6

Anterior Segment Disease

Condition	Description	Anatomical Structure
Ptosis	Drooping eyelid	Upper lid
Ectropion	Inferior eyelid does not make contact with the eyeball	Lower lid
Entropion	Inferior eyelid turns inward and lashes rub against eye	Lower lid
Basal cell carcinoma	Most common malignant tumor of the eyelid	Eyelid
Chalazion or hordeolum	Common lid lump in which there is an infection of a gland in the eyelid; the external type is sometimes referred to as a sty	Eyelid
Papilloma	Benign tumor of the eyelid	Eyelid
Blepharitis	Inflammation of the eyelid; common forms are bacterial, viral, or allergic blepharitis	Eyelid
Conjunctivitis	Inflammation of the conjunctiva; common forms are bacterial, viral, or allergic conjunctivitis	Conjunctiva
Scleritis	Inflammation of the sclera	Sclera
Keratitis	Inflammation of the cornea; common forms are bacterial, viral, or allergic keratitis	Cornea
Corneal abrasion	Injury to cornea; usually caused by a foreign body or contact lenses overwear	Cornea
Anterior uveitis	Inflammation of all or parts of the uvea including the iris and ciliary body	Iris and ciliary body
Hyphema	Accumulation of blood in the anterior chamber	Anterior chamber
Aniridia	Absence of the iris	Iris

Table 3.7

Disease of the Lens

Condition	Description	Anatomical Structure
Cataract	An opacity occurring in the normally transparent lens, causing reduced visual acuity; it is generally related to the aging process but can also occur as a result of trauma	Lens
Subluxation or dislocation of the lens	This can occur as a result of trauma or can be associated with a hereditary syndrome such as Marfan syndrome; the dislocation of the lens causes reduced visual acuity	Lens

Table 3.8

Posterior Segment Disease

Condition	Description	Anatomical Structure
Optic nerve atrophy	Loss of nerve fibers in the optic nerve; this can be acquired due to a variety of diseases or congenital	Optic nerve
Optic neuritis	Inflammation of the optic nerve head	Optic nerve
Papilledema	Swelling or edema of the optic disc secondary to elevated intracranial pressure	Optic nerve
Central retinal vein occlusion	A destructive retinal condition strongly associated with systemic disease or pressure on the optic nerve	Retina
Central retinal artery occlusion	Sudden, painless loss of vision due to occlusion of central retinal artery; it can be secondary to emboli from atheromatous plaques from the internal carotid artery, cardiac lesions	Retina
Diabetic retinopathy	Microaneurysms, retinal hemorrhages, and exudates due to disease of retinal vasculature secondary to diabetes	Retina
Retinopathy of prematurity	Retinal disease due to oxygen used to treat prematurity; it includes neovascularization, retinal dragging, scarring, retinal detachment	Retina
Age-related macular degeneration	Number one cause of blindness in the United States in people over 60; the patient experiences loss of vision, usually bilateral	Macula
Retinal detachment	The retina detaches from the choroid and leads to loss of vision if not repaired	Retina

Table 3.9

Disease Affecting the Visual Pathways

Condition	Description	Anatomical Structure
Glaucoma	Visual field defects caused by damage to retinal nerve fiber bundles at the optic nerve head; the deficits are generally paracentral, arcuate scotomas, or nasal steps.	Optic nerve
Opacities of ocular media	Generalized depression of sensitivity due to corneal opacities, cataracts, or vitreous opacities	Cornea, lens, vitreous
Optic nerve disease	Caused by monocular visual field defects; common problems include papilledema, optic neuritis, compressive optic neuropathy, drusen	Optic nerve
Optic chiasm disease	Characteristic bitemporal hemianopic defect commonly caused by a pituitary gland tumor	Optic chiasm
Retrochiasmal visual pathway disease	Hemianopic field defects	Optic tract, lateral geniculate body, optic radiations (temporal lobe, parietal lobe), visual cortex

Clinical Assessment of Eye Health Disorders

To evaluate the integrity of the health of the eyes, clinicians use diagnostic drugs, along with a variety of instrumentation that provides variable illumination and magnification. Instrumentation can range from inexpensive hand-held instruments such as the ophthalmoscope to very expensive, computerized equipment such as the laser ophthalmoscope. Equipment is available to permit assessment of all external and internal structures of the eye. To evaluate the internal structures of the eyes, clinicians must use a series of drugs designed to dilate the pupil. Dilation of the pupil allows the clinician to view the retina and other internal structures through a wider opening.

Clinicians can also evaluate the visual system beyond the retina, even though it cannot be directly viewed. Disorders in the visual pathways lead to visual field deficits that can be detected using visual field testing equipment. Disease in the visual pathways can also affect fixation ability, eye movements, convergence, binocular vision, pupillary response, eyelid function, and visual information processing skills. All of the areas are assessed in a comprehensive vision/eye health evaluation, and this information can be used to determine the integrity of the visual pathways.

Development of Anatomical and Physiological Characteristics of the Eye

After birth, the size of the eye continues to grow, and the most rapid growth is during the first two years of life. Between 2 and 5 years, the growth rate is reduced, and a slow progression occurs up to about 13 years of age.[41] Most of the important characteristics of the adult visual system are established before birth and the first few years thereafter. During this time, the neurons of the retina and visual pathways differentiate and make their permanent synaptic connections.

The retina is not fully developed at birth. The entire retina, and in particular the fovea, continues to develop until age 4 or 5 years. This initial immaturity probably accounts for the reduced visual acuity at birth and early infancy.[42] The central 5 degrees of the retina is immature at birth, though peripheral regions appear well developed and mature. Over the first few years of life, especially the first 6 months, the central retina develops very rapidly. During this early stage in life, the visual system is very susceptible to interference.

The optic nerve and optic tract are also not fully developed at birth. Some nerve fibers are myelinated at birth, but myelination proceeds rapidly up to 2 years of age and less rapidly thereafter.[43] The evidence that is available from anatomical and physiological studies suggests that there is a plastic or sensitive period in human visual development of the visual cortex that lasts from birth to 7 to 10 years of age at least. Very little is known about the developmental details of the many extrastriate visual areas in the cerebral cortex or the complex neural circuitry responsible for eye movements and eye-body coordination.[44]

Common Eye Diseases

This section reviews the four most common eye diseases the occupational therapist is likely to encounter.

Age-Related Macular Degeneration

DESCRIPTION

Age-related macular degeneration (AMD) is a degenerative, acquired disorder of the central retina, the macula, which usually occurs in patients over age 55, and results in progressive, sometimes significant, irreversible loss of central visual function from either fibrous scarring or atrophy of the macula. It is the leading cause of vision loss in the adult population.

The macula is located roughly in the center of the retina and is a small and highly sensitive part of the retina responsible for detailed central vision. The fovea is the very center of the macula. The normal macula has a characteristic appearance and is more heavily pigmented than the surrounding retina (Figure 3.17). The macula allows us to appreciate detail and perform tasks that require central vision such as reading, writing, recognizing faces, and driving. AMD is classified as either dry (nonexudative) or wet (exudative).

Dry (Nonexudative or Atrophic) Age-Related Macular Degeneration

Dry (nonexudative or atrophic) AMD accounts for 90% of all patients with AMD in the United States.[45] Most patients with dry AMD experience gradual, progressive loss of central visual function. This loss of vision is more noticeable during near tasks, especially in the early stages of the disease. In an estimated 12% to 21% of patients, dry AMD progresses to cause vision levels of 20/200 or worse.[46,47] Neovascularization is not present in dry AMD.

Wet (Exudative) Age-Related Macular Degeneration

Although wet AMD accounts for only 10% of patients with AMD, 90% of the AMD patients with significant vision loss have this form of the disease.[46,48] Wet AMD is characterized by the

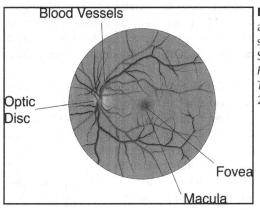

Figure 3.17. The normal macula has a characteristic appearance and is more heavily pigmented than the surrounding retina. (Reprinted with permission from Scheiman M, Scheiman M, Whittaker SG. *Low Vision Rehabilitation: A Practical Guide for Occupational Therapists.* Thorofare, NJ: SLACK Incorporated; 2007.)

Figure 3.18. Wet macular degeneration with bleeding in the macular area. (Reprinted with permission from Scheiman M, Scheiman M, Whittaker SG. *Low Vision Rehabilitation: A Practical Guide for Occupational Therapists.* Thorofare, NJ: SLACK Incorporated; 2007.)

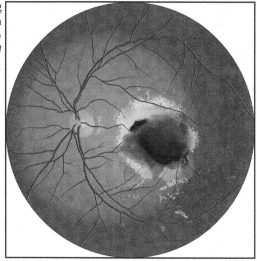

development of neovascularization in the choroid, leading to leakage of blood and subsequent elevation of the retinal pigment epithelium (Figure 3.18). Patients with wet AMD tend to notice a more profound and rapid decrease in central visual function. The leakage of blood from the new choroidal vessels causes distortion vision, central scotoma, and blurred vision.[49]

RISK FACTORS

Age is the most significant risk factor and clearly increases the risk of both developing AMD as well as of progressing to the late stages of the disorder.[50] Although age is a strong risk factor, AMD and vision loss do not inevitably occur with advancing age. People with an AMD-affected first-degree relative have a 50% lifetime risk of experiencing advanced AMD and vision loss, and tend to develop it earlier than those without a family history.[51] Smoking is associated with a four-fold increase in the risk of AMD and visual loss and, again, tends to promote earlier occurrence.[52] Studies have consistently implicated female gender as a risk factor. A relationship seems to exist between increased cumulative exposure to sunlight and ultraviolet radiation and wet AMD.[53] Weaker associations have been found with obesity, hypertension, macrovascular disease, raised cholesterol, and cataract surgery.

Dietary associations have also been found both with the signs of AMD and with progression to vision loss.[54–56] In a well-conducted, prospective study, dietary fat intake was systematically analyzed after correcting for other risk factors.[57] Vegetable fat intake had the strongest relationship with AMD progression, with a relative risk of 3.82 for the highest fat-intake quartile compared with the lowest quartile. Higher intakes of total fat and of saturated, monounsaturated, polyunsaturated, and trans-unsaturated fats all raised the relative risk of AMD progression about two-fold. Weekly fish intake and eating nuts two to three times a week were mildly protective. The implication is that a large shift away from vegetable oils, margarine, and fat-containing processed foods might reduce this epidemic of blindness in the elderly.

There is also evidence from a randomized controlled trial that high-dose dietary supplements of the antioxidants vitamin C, vitamin E, beta-carotene, and zinc can reduce the risk of progression from large or soft drusen to advanced AMD and visual loss by about 20% compared with controls over six years.[57] However, high-dose zinc can cause gastric irritation or anemia, and beta-carotene may possibly be associated with an increased risk of lung cancer among smokers. Uncontrolled studies suggest the antioxidants selenium, lutein, and zeaxanthin, which localize in the normal macula, may also help. There are as yet no studies to show whether dietary supplements are protective in patients in the early stages of dry AMD or in the 20% of patients who are at genetic risk.

It is not yet known whether major dietary adjustment and/or introduction of dietary supplements for large numbers of elderly people will be justified in terms of preventing blindness.

EFFECT ON VISION

Visual acuity varies with the extent of the degeneration and includes distortion, blurred vision (especially at near), and central scotoma. With dry AMD visual acuity can range from 20/20 to 20/400. Visual acuity with wet AMD is generally worse than 20/400. All patients with AMD have central visual field defects with normal peripheral vision. Patients with AMD almost never go totally blind. However, if AMD occurs in both eyes, the visual acuity loss along with the central scotoma significantly impair a person's ability to engage in activities of daily living and quality of life. High-resolution tasks such as reading, writing, sewing, telling time, taking care of financial issues, driving, and distinguishing colors and facial expressions become problematic. The consequences of AMD lead to loss of independence, lowered self-esteem, decreased mobility, increased risk of injury due to falls, and depression. Figures 3.19 and 3.20 illustrate what a patient might see with AMD and a macular scotoma.

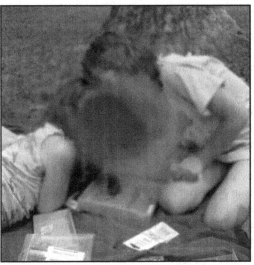

Figure 3.19. Visual problems associated with age-related macular degeneration and a macular scotoma. (Reprinted with permission from Scheiman M, Scheiman M, Whittaker SG. *Low Vision Rehabilitation: A Practical Guide for Occupational Therapists*. Thorofare, NJ: SLACK Incorporated; 2007.)

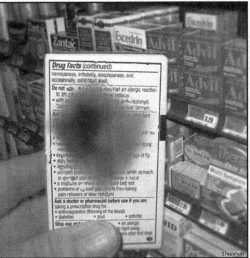

Figure 3.20. Visual problems associated with age-related macular degeneration and a macular scotoma. (Reprinted with permission from Scheiman M, Scheiman M, Whittaker SG. *Low Vision Rehabilitation: A Practical Guide for Occupational Therapists*. Thorofare, NJ: SLACK Incorporated; 2007.)

Some patients with AMD have a phenomenon called Charles Bonnet syndrome or visual hallucinations. This is an occasional complaint of patients with bilateral AMD and may occur spontaneously with no known external cause.

TREATMENT
Treatment of AMD includes various medical procedures to slow the progression of the disease and low vision rehabilitation including optical and non-optical devices, environmental changes, education, support groups, and training in eccentric viewing, scanning, and reading.

Dry Age-Related Macular Degeneration
There is no medical treatment for dry AMD that can restore vision loss. Patients who have early retinal changes such as small drusen or mild pigmentation changes may experience no symptoms or may notice slowly progressive changes in visual function. These patients are generally seen by an eye doctor every 6 months. Patients are instructed to return for further examination within 24 hours of the onset of new symptoms because 10% of patients with dry AMD progress to wet AMD. Studies have shown that early treatment of wet AMD may limit the extent of damage and vision loss.

Wet Age-Related Macular Degeneration
The principal aim of treatment of wet AMD is to preserve visual acuity and reduce the risk of additional severe vision loss for as long as possible. Recently, a new treatment for wet AMD, injection of drugs called angiogenesis inhibitors, has been shown to be effective in randomized clinical trials. It is not a cure for wet AMD but can prevent further loss of vision and may even improve vision to a small degree.

INJECTIONS WITH VASCULAR ENDOTHELIAL GROWTH FACTOR INHIBITOR
In December 2004, the Food and Drug Administration approved the latest treatment available for wet AMD using drugs known as vascular endothelial growth factor (VEGF) inhibitor. When these drugs (Lucentis [ranibizumab injection], Avastin [bevacizumab]) are injected into the vitreous humor of the eye, they have the capability of neutralizing a specific growth factor that promotes the growth of abnormal new blood vessels in eyes with AMD. The result is attack of both decrease of the vascular growth and leakage that are together responsible for the visual loss in wet AMD. These drugs have broad implications for treatment because it is effective in management of all types of new onset wet AMD. In fact, studies show that the use of these drugs can prevent severe visual loss (defined as loss of three lines of visual acuity on the Snellen eye chart) in as many as 70% of the treated patients during the period of follow-up.[58]

ANTIOXIDANTS
In a clinical trial researchers found that high levels of antioxidants and zinc significantly reduce the risk of advanced AMD and its associated vision loss.[57] In this study, patients at high risk of developing advanced stages of AMD lowered their risk by about 25% when treated with a high-dose combination of vitamin C, vitamin E, beta-carotene, and zinc. In the same high-risk group the nutrients reduced the risk of vision loss caused by advanced AMD by about 19%. For those study participants who had either no AMD or early AMD, the nutrients did not provide an apparent benefit.[57] It is important to understand that these nutrients are not a cure for AMD, nor will they restore vision already lost from the disease. However, it may delay the onset of advanced AMD. It is also important to understand that there is no evidence that this Age-Related Eye Disease Studies (AREDS) formulation is effective for those diagnosed with early-stage AMD. The study did not find that the formulation provided a benefit to those with early-stage AMD.

LOW VISION REHABILITATION
Although vision loss cannot be restored with medical treatment, low vision rehabilitation is an effective treatment that enables patients with dry AMD to function more effectively in activities

of daily living and regain independence in spite of the visual deficit. The occupational therapist's role in low vision rehabilitation includes instruction in the use of optical and non-optical assistive devices; modification of lighting, contrast, and other environmental factors; treatment to learn adaptive eye movement patterns, scanning, and reading skills; education; and involvement in support groups.[59]

Diabetic Retinopathy

DESCRIPTION

Diabetic retinopathy is the most serious vision-threatening complication of chronic diabetes mellitus. Although there has been extensive research over several decades, knowledge about the etiology of diabetic retinopathy is still incomplete. The vascular complications of diabetes involve all organ systems including the eye. In the eye, these vascular changes lead to bleeding of small blood vessels and exudative material (inflammatory substance) flowing into the eye (Figure 3.21).

RISK FACTORS

Having diabetes puts an individual at risk of retinopathy. The risk of diabetic retinopathy increases the longer the person has the disease. The duration of the diabetes is also the major determinant of the severity of retinopathy and progression. Other risk factors for diabetic retinopathy include poorly controlled blood sugar levels, high blood pressure, high blood cholesterol, pregnancy, obesity, and kidney disease.

EFFECT ON VISION

Patients with diabetic retinopathy experience decreased, fluctuating, or distorted vision; focusing problems; loss of color vision; and floaters. They frequently have impaired contrast sensitivity as well because of cataracts, cloudy vitreous, and retinal edema and are very glare sensitive and particular about lighting. They may also have a central scotoma due to effects of the diabetes on the macular area (maculopathy), loss of peripheral vision, and difficulty in dim light. Treatments (described below) often leave a client with a small island of good vision. They may see individual numbers or letters but not words. The treatments also produce scotomas in the periphery, "Swiss cheese" vision. Figure 3.22 illustrates the visual problems of a patient with diabetic retinopathy.

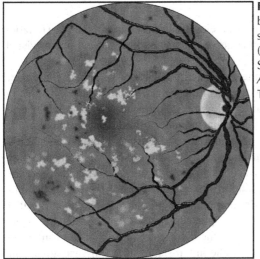

Figure 3.21. Vascular changes lead to bleeding of small blood vessels and exudative material (inflammatory substance) flowing into the eye in diabetic retinopathy. (Reprinted with permission from Scheiman M, Scheiman M, Whittaker SG. *Low Vision Rehabilitation: A Practical Guide for Occupational Therapists.* Thorofare, NJ: SLACK Incorporated; 2007.)

Figure 3.22. Visual problems associated with diabetic retinopathy. (Reprinted with permission from Scheiman M, Scheiman M, Whittaker SG. *Low Vision Rehabilitation: A Practical Guide for Occupational Therapists.* Thorofare, NJ: SLACK Incorporated; 2007.)

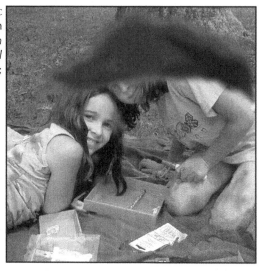

TREATMENT

During the early stages of diabetic retinopathy, no treatment is needed, unless macular edema is present. The current approach in the early stage emphasizes the early recognition of retinopathy, vigorous control of blood glucose, and direct therapy with laser photocoagulation and vitreous surgery.

As the disease progresses the retinopathy is treated with laser surgery. This procedure is called laser photocoagulation treatment. Laser photocoagulation treatment helps to shrink the abnormal blood vessels.

LOW VISION REHABILITATION

A hallmark of diabetic vision changes is impaired contrast sensitivity. Because of their fluctuating vision, these individuals usually respond well to electronic magnification, where contrast can be enhanced and magnification varied. Non-optical devices such as a glucose monitor and insulin-syringe aids are helpful to the patient.[59]

Glaucoma

DESCRIPTION

Glaucoma is a group of ocular diseases that cause an elevation of pressure in the eye (intraocular pressure) ultimately leading to progressive optic nerve damage and loss of peripheral visual function.

Figure 3.23 is an illustration of the front of the eye called the anterior chamber. The ciliary body is the structure that produces the fluid called aqueous fluid. This fluid is produced on a daily basis and flows to the front of the eye as illustrated in Figure 3.24. Because the eye is a closed structure, if new fluid is produced on a daily basis, an equal amount of fluid must drain out of the eye to maintain the proper intraocular pressure. Under normal conditions, the amount of aqueous fluid that is produced is equivalent to the amount that drains out on a daily basis, maintaining equilibrium and normal intraocular pressure. In glaucoma this equilibrium is disrupted. There are several reasons why a person may develop glaucoma; however, regardless of the cause, the ultimate problem is loss of this equilibrium causing a rise in intraocular pressure. When the intraocular pressure rises the nerve fibers exiting the eye through the optic nerve are compressed and damaged. The fibers that are generally affected in the beginning of the disease are those that carry information about our side vision (peripheral vision). Thus, in the initial stages of the disease, glaucoma

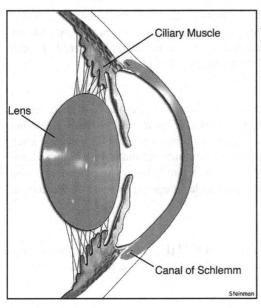

Figure 3.23. Anterior chamber of the eye. (Reprinted with permission from Scheiman M, Scheiman M, Whittaker SG. *Low Vision Rehabilitation: A Practical Guide for Occupational Therapists.* Thorofare, NJ: SLACK Incorporated; 2007.)

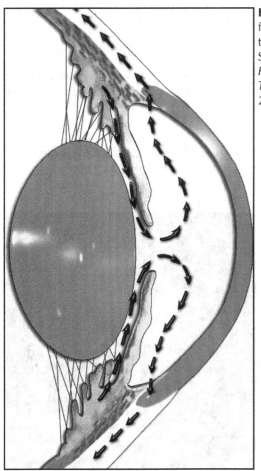

Figure 3.24. The ciliary body produces aqueous fluid that is produced on a daily basis and flows to the front of the eye. (Reprinted with permission from Scheiman M, Scheiman M, Whittaker SG. *Low Vision Rehabilitation: A Practical Guide for Occupational Therapists.* Thorofare, NJ: SLACK Incorporated; 2007.)

leads to a gradual loss of peripheral vision. In most cases of glaucoma, the disease is painless because the rise in pressure is very gradual. As a result, a person with glaucoma may be unaware of the problem until the loss of vision is advanced. Thus, routine eye examinations are important to rule out this disease and the best way to avoid the consequences of glaucoma.

RISK FACTORS

Age is a major risk factor for the development of glaucoma. The prevalence of glaucoma is four to ten times higher in the older age groups than in persons in their 40s.[60,61] Race is another major risk factor for primary open angle glaucoma. African Americans develop the disease earlier, do not respond as well to treatment, are more likely to require surgery, and have a higher prevalence of blindness from glaucoma than Caucasians.[61] Finally, a family history of glaucoma is also a significant risk factor. Ocular factors include high intraocular pressure, thinness of the cornea, and abnormal optic nerve anatomy.

EFFECT ON VISION

Left uncorrected, glaucoma causes a reduction in visual field (Figure 3.25), which may progress to total blindness. Central vision is generally unaffected until the end stage of the disease.

TREATMENT

Treatment of glaucoma usually begins with medications (pills, ointments, or eyedrops) that help the eye either drain fluid more effectively or produce less fluid. Several forms of laser surgery can also help fluid drain from the eye.

Cataract

DESCRIPTION

A cataract is an opacification or clouding of the lens in the eye that affects vision. Cataracts are very common in older people and can occur in either or both eyes. Figure 3.26 is an illustration of a cataract.

RISK FACTORS

The main risk for developing cataracts is aging. By age 65 about half of all Americans have developed some degree of lens clouding, although it may not impair vision. Other significant

Figure 3.25. Peripheral visual field loss associated with glaucoma. (Reprinted with permission from Scheiman M, Scheiman M, Whittaker SG. *Low Vision Rehabilitation: A Practical Guide for Occupational Therapists*. Thorofare, NJ: SLACK Incorporated; 2007.)

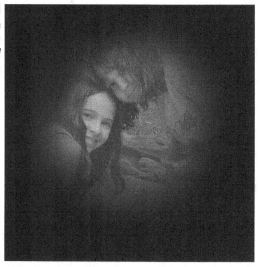

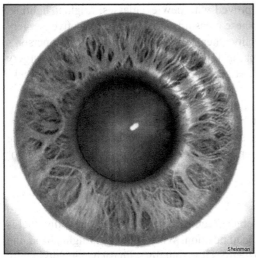

Figure 3.26. Opacification of the lens in cataract. (Reprinted with permission from Scheiman M, Scheiman M, Whittaker SG. *Low Vision Rehabilitation: A Practical Guide for Occupational Therapists.* Thorofare, NJ: SLACK Incorporated; 2007.)

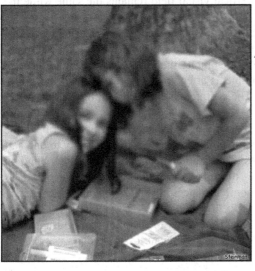

Figure 3.27. Visual problems associated with cataract. (Reprinted with permission from Scheiman M, Scheiman M, Whittaker SG. *Low Vision Rehabilitation: A Practical Guide for Occupational Therapists.* Thorofare, NJ: SLACK Incorporated; 2007.)

factors are diabetes, a family history of cataracts, previous eye injury or inflammation, previous eye surgery, prolonged use of corticosteroids, excessive exposure to sunlight, and smoking.

Effect on Vision

A cataract usually develops slowly and causes no pain. As a result, most people are unaware of its development until it begins to interfere with everyday activities. Symptoms of a cataract include blurry vision, increasing difficulty with vision at night, sensitivity to light and glare, poor contrast sensitivity, halos around lights, the need for brighter light for reading and other activities, frequent changes in eyeglass or contact lens prescription, fading or yellowing of colors, and double vision in a single eye. Figure 3.27 illustrates the effect of cataract on vision.

Treatment

The only effective treatment for a cataract is surgery to remove the clouded lens and replace it with a clear lens implant. The lens implant can correct refractive error as well. In some cases, one eye is corrected to focus at near and the other to focus at distance. Cataracts cannot be cured with medications, dietary supplements, exercise, or optical devices. However, in the early stages of cataract development the symptoms may be improved with new eyeglasses, brighter lighting, anti-glare sunglasses, or magnifying lenses. When these measures are no longer effective, surgery is necessary. Ophthalmologists treat cataract surgically when vision loss interferes with a person's activities such as working, driving, reading, or watching TV. Typically, if a person requires surgery on both eyes the surgery is performed on each eye at separate times, usually about 4 to 8 weeks apart.

Cataract removal is one of the most common, safest, and most effective types of surgery. Although cataract surgery is one of the most effective surgical procedures, there are potential risks including inflammation, infection, bleeding, swelling, retinal detachment, and glaucoma. Occasionally cataract surgery fails to improve vision because of conditions such as glaucoma or macular degeneration.

Visual Field Loss

The visual field is that portion of space where objects can be perceived while the individual is visually fixating on a single object in the straight-ahead position. When looking straight ahead, the normal visual field is 70 degrees vertically and 150 degrees horizontally with each eye individually (Figures 3.28 and 3.29). With both eyes open the vertical visual field remains the same while the horizontal visual field is now 180 degrees.

Visual field loss can occur after acquired brain injury that affects the visual pathway. This could be due to trauma, vascular causes, neoplasm, or it can occur secondary to surgical intervention for some other condition. Visual field disorders are among the most perplexing and difficult vision problems that therapists encounter. These problems affect mobility, reading, writing, activities of daily living, face recognition, and driving. The symptoms of visual field loss and its effect on performance are listed in Table 3.10.

As explained in Chapter Two, because of the anatomy of the visual pathway posterior to the optic chiasm (Figure 3.30), a common result is a complete or partial loss of sensitivity to one half of the visual field in each eye. This is referred to as a hemianopia meaning the patient is blind on one side of the visual field in both eyes. If the degree of loss of visual field is the same in both eyes it is referred to as a homonymous hemianopia. In some instances, a single quadrant is affected in which case it would be called a quadrantanopia.

Visual field loss is permanent and treatment is not designed to restore normal visual field; rather, it is designed to help the patient compensate for this permanent loss of vision.

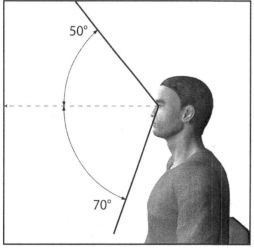

Figure 3.28. Vertical visual field is about 120 degrees in each eye. (Reprinted with permission from Scheiman M, Scheiman M, Whittaker SG. *Low Vision Rehabilitation: A Practical Guide for Occupational Therapists*. Thorofare, NJ: SLACK Incorporated; 2007.)

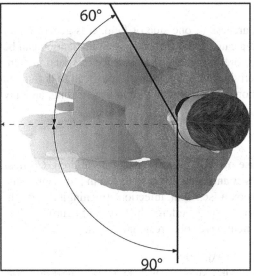

Figure 3.29. Horizontal visual field is about 150 degrees in each eye. (Reprinted with permission from Scheiman M, Scheiman M, Whittaker SG. *Low Vision Rehabilitation: A Practical Guide for Occupational Therapists.* Thorofare, NJ: SLACK Incorporated; 2007.)

Table 3.10

Visual Field Deficits: Symptoms and Effect on Function

Walking: Inferior field loss causes difficulty with mobility, trouble seeing steps or curbs, shortened and uncertain stride when walking, poor balance, a tendency to trail behind others when walking, a tendency to walk next to wall and hold onto wall with hands, a tendency to be anchored to ground, and discomfort in the middle of a room. Patient does not turn head as much, frequently bumps into things, and is disoriented when moving whether in car or walking

- Trouble identifying visual landmarks
- Superior field deficit causes difficulty seeing signs, worse if in wheelchair
- Leaves food on half of plate
- Misidentification of details, misreading of long words
- Difficulty with reading, misreads words, reads inaccurately, reads slowly, has difficulty with page navigation, cannot stay on line
- Difficulty with writing, cannot stay on line, inaccurate
- Self-grooming: Cannot find necessary items
- Dressing: Cannot find necessary items
- Telephone: Cannot take accurate messages
- Driving: Cannot drive usually
- Shopping: Cannot drive; cannot find items
- Emotional problems: Anxiety, reduced self-confidence, increased passivity, social isolation

---

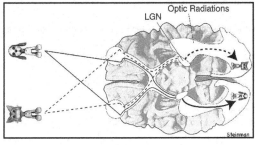

Figure 3.30. Anatomy of the visual pathway posterior to the optic chiasm. (Reprinted with permission from Scheiman M, Scheiman M, Whittaker SG. *Low Vision Rehabilitation: A Practical Guide for Occupational Therapists.* Thorofare, NJ: SLACK Incorporated; 2007.)

Visual Inattention/Neglect

Visual inattention is a passive, diminished awareness of one side of field. It is generally not due to a localized lesion as in hemianopia. Often the cause unknown and visual inattention can be present along with a visual field defect, or it can be present alone. The presence of visual inattention has a significant effect on rehabilitation and activities of daily living. It may lead to deficits in localization of objects, scanning, fixation, orientation, eating, dressing, mobility, reading, and any other visually based activities of daily living.

Cortical Visual Impairment

Cortical visual impairment is the leading cause of bilateral low vision in children. *Cortical visual impairment* replaces the term *cortical blindness* and is caused by a lesion in posterior visual pathways. This damage may be due to perinatal hypoxia-ischemia, infections (meningitis, encephalitis), or hydrocephalus. The diagnosis is based on physical findings, history, and neuroimaging. The majority of people with cortical visual impairment have some residual vision.

CHARACTERISTICS OF CORTICAL VISUAL IMPAIRMENT

Patients with cortical visual impairment may exhibit signs such as markedly short attention span, variable visual skills, frequent head turning when reaching for objects, close working distance, compulsive light gazing, photophobia (sensitivity to light), and eye pressing/poking.

PROGNOSIS IN CORTICAL VISUAL IMPAIRMENT

With early intervention some patients with cortical visual impairment may show improvement in visual skills.

Summary

Disorders of visual acuity, refraction, and eye disease are commonly diagnosed and treated by all eye doctors. Unfortunately, in many cases, an eye examination only includes an evaluation designed to detect these conditions. As the following two chapters will demonstrate, there are many more significant vision problems that must be considered.

References

1. Dobson V, MacDonald MA, Kohl P, et al. Visual acuity screening of infants and young children with the acuity card procedure. *J Am Optom Assoc.* 1986;57:284–289.
2. Mayer DL, Fulton AB, Rodier D. Grating and recognition acuities of pediatric patients. *Ophthalmology.* 1984;91:947–953.
3. Birch EE, Naegele J, Bauer JA, et al. Visual acuity of toddlers tested by operant preferential looking techniques. *Invest Ophthalmol Vis Sci.* 1980;20:210.
4. Marg E, Freeman DN, Peltzman P, Goldstein PJ. Visual Acuity development in human infants: evoked potential measurements. *Inv Ophthalmol.* 1976;15:150–153.
5. Sokol S. Measurement of infant visual acuity from pattern reversal evoked potentials. *Vision Res.* 1978;18:33–39.
6. Gwiazda J, Brill S, Mohindra I, Held R. Infant visual acuity and its meridional variation. *Vision Res.* 1978;18:1557–1564.
7. Dobson V, Teller DY. Visual acuity in human infants: a review and comparison of behavioral and electrophysiological studies. *Vision Res.* 1978;18:1469–1483.
8. Birch EE, Gwiazda J, Bauer JA, Jr., et al. Visual acuity and its meridional variations in children aged 7–60 months. *Vision Res.* 1983;23:1019–1024.
9. Haegerstrom-Portnoy G, Schneck ME, Lott LA, Brabyn JA. The relation between visual acuity and other spatial vision measures. *Optom Vis Sci.* 2000;77:653–662.
10. Whittaker SG, Lovie-Kitchin J. Visual requirements for reading. *Optom Vis Sci.* 1993;70:54–65.
11. Marron JA, Bailey IL. Visual factors and orientation-mobility performance. *Am J Optom Physiol Opt.* 1982;59:413–426.

12. Kuyk T, Elliott JL, Fuhr PS. Visual correlates of mobility in real world settings in older adults with low vision. *Optom Vis Sci.* 1998;75:538–547.

13. Wood JM, Troutbeck R. Elderly drivers and simulated visual impairment. *Optom Vis Sci.* 1995;72:115–124.

14. Owsley C, Sloane ME. Contrast sensitivity, acuity, and the perception of "real-world" targets. *Br J Ophthalmol.* 1987;71:791–796.

15. West SK, Rubin GS, Broman AT, et al. How does visual impairment affect performance on tasks of everyday life? The SEE Project. Salisbury Eye Evaluation. *Arch Ophthalmol.* 2002;120:774–780.

16. Rubin GS, Roche KB, Prasada-Rao P, Fried LP. Visual impairment and disability in older adults. *Optom Vis Sci.* 1994;71:750–760.

17. Arditi A. Improving the design of the letter contrast sensitivity test. *Invest Ophthalmol Vis Sci.* 2005; 46:2225–2229.

18. Pelli DG, Robson JG, Wilkins AJ. The design of a new letter contrast chart for measuring contrast sensitivity. *Clin Vis Sci.* 1988;2:187–199.

19. Ciner EB, Appel S, Graboyes M, Zambone AM. Low vision special populations I: the multiply impaired patient. In: Appel S, Brilliant R, eds. *Essentials of Low Vision Practice.* Boston, MA: Butterworth-Heinemann; 1999.

20. Skeffington AM. *Introduction to Clinical Optometry Optometric Extension Program Postgraduate Courses.* Santa Ana, CA: Optometric Extension Program Foundation; Oct 1964–Sept 1965.

21. Birnbaum MH. *Optometric Management of Nearpoint Vision Disorders.* Boston, MA: Butterworth-Heinemann; 1993.

22. Goss DA. Effect of spectacle correction on the progression of myopia in children: a literature review. *J Am Optom Assoc.* 1994;65:117–128.

23. Gwiazda J, Hyman L, Hussein M, et al. A randomized clinical trial of progressive addition lenses versus single vision lenses on the progression of myopia in children. *Invest Ophthalmol Vis Sci.* 2003;44:1492–1500.

24. Gwiazda JE, Hyman L, Norton TT, et al. Accommodation and related risk factors associated with myopia progression and their interaction with treatment in COMET children. *Invest Ophthalmol Vis Sci.* 2004;45:2143–2151.

25. Scheiman M, and the COMET Group. Pals for children: can they slow myopia. *Rev Optom.* 2008;79:55–59.

26. Ciner EB. Management of refractive error in infants, toddlers, and preschool children. In: Scheiman M, ed. *Pediatric Optometry.* Philadelphia, PA: JB Lippincott; 1990.

27. Gwiazda J, Scheiman M, Mohindra I, Held R. Astigmatism in children: changes in axis and amount from birth to six years. *Invest Ophthalmol Vis Sci.* 1984;25:88–92.

28. Dobson V, Fulton AB, Sebris SL. Cycloplegic refractions of infants and young children: the axis of astigmatism. *Invest Ophthalmol Vis Sci.* 1984;25:83–87.

29. Mohindra I, Held R, Gwiazda J, Brill J. Astigmatism in infants. *Science.* 1978;202:329–331.

30. Mohindra I, Held R. Refraction in humans from birth to five years. *Doc Ophthalmol Proc Ser.* 1981;28:19–27.

31. Ingram RM, Barr A. Changes in refraction between the ages of 1 and 3 1/2 years. *Br J Ophthalmol.* 1979;63:339–342.

32. Baldwin WR. Refractive status of infants and children. In: Rosenbloom AA, Morgan MW, eds. *Principles and Practice of Pediatric Optometry.* Philadelphia, PA: JB Lippincott; 1990:104–112.

33. Gianutsos R, Ramsey G. Enabling survivors of brain injury to receive rehabilitative optometric services. *J Vis Rehab.* 1988;2:37–58.

34. Zost M. Diagnosis and management of visual dysfunction in cerebral injury. In: Maino D, ed. *Diagnosis and Management of Special Populations.* New York, NY: CV Mosby; 1995:75–134.

35. Scheiman M. *Assessment and Management of the Exceptional Child.* Philadelphia, PA: JB Lippincott; 1990.

36. Poe GS. Eye care visits and use of eyeglasses or contact lenses: United States, 1979 and 1980. In: *Vital Health Statistics.* Hyattsville, MD: Department of Health and Human Services; 1984. Publication PHS 84–1573. Series 10, No. 45.

37. Bader D, Woodruff ME. The effects of corrective lenses on various behaviors of mentally retarded persons. *Am J Optom Physiol Opt.* 1980;57:447–459.

38. Rosner J, Rosner J. Comparison of visual characteristics in children with and without learning difficulties. *Am J Optom Physiol Opt.* 1987;64:531–533.

39. Young FA. Reading, measures of intelligence and refractive errors. *Am J Optom Arch Am Acad Optom.* 1963;40:257–264.

40. Eames TH. The influence of hypermetropia and myopia on reading achievement. *Am J Ophthalmol.* 1955;39:375–377.

41. Larson JS. The sagittal growth of the eye. IV. Ultrasonic measurement of the axial length of the eye from birth to puberty. *Acta Ophthalmol.* 1971;49:872–878.

42. Boothe RG, Dobson V, Teller DY. Postnatal development of vision in human and nonhuman primates. *Ann Rev Neurosci.* 1985;8:495–545.

43. Maggon EH, Robb RM. Development of myelin in human optic nerve and tract. *Arch Ophthalmol.* 1981;99:655–661.

44. Beauchamp R. Normal development of the neural pathway. In: Rosenbloom AA, Morgan MW, eds. *Pediatric Optometry.* Philadelphia, PA: JB Lippincott; 1990:46–65.

45. Klein BE, Klein R, Linton KL. Prevalence of age-related lens opacities in a population. The Beaver Dam Eye Study. *Ophthalmology.* 1992;99:546–552.

46. Hyman LG, Lilienfeld AM, Ferris FL, 3rd, Fine SL. Senile macular degeneration: a case-control study. *Am J Epidemiol.* 1983;118:213–227.

47. Murphy RP. Age-related macular degeneration. *Ophthalmology.* 1986;93:969–971.

48. Ferris FL, 3rd, Fine SL, Hyman L. Age-related macular degeneration and blindness due to neovascular maculopathy. *Arch Ophthalmol.* 1984;102:1640–1642.

49. Fine AM, Elman MJ, Ebert JE, et al. Earliest symptoms caused by neovascular membranes in the macula. *Arch Ophthalmol.* 1986;104:513–514.

50. Hirvela H, Luukinen H, Laara E, et al. Risk factors of age-related maculopathy in a population 70 years of age or older. *Ophthalmology.* 1996;103:871–877.

51. Klaver CC, Wolfs RC, Assink JJ, et al. Genetic risk of age-related maculopathy. *Arch Ophthalmol.* 1998;116:1646–1651.

52. Klein R, Klein BE, Franke T. The relationship of cardiovascular disease and its risk factors to age-related maculopathy. The Beaver Dam Eye Study. *Ophthalmology.* 1993;100:406–414.

53. Newsome D. Medical treatment of macular diseases. *Ophthalmol Clin North Am.* 1993;6:307–314.

54. Cho E, Hung S, Willett WC, et al. Prospective study of dietary fat and the risk of age-related macular degeneration. *Am J Clin Nutr.* 2001;73:209–218.

55. Seddon JM, Rosner B, Sperduto RD, et al. Dietary fat and risk for advanced age-related macular degeneration. *Arch Ophthalmol.* 2001;119:1191–1199.

56. Seddon JM, Cote J, Rosner B. Progression of age-related macular degeneration: association with dietary fat, transunsaturated fat, nuts, and fish intake. *Arch Ophthalmol.* 2003;121:1728–1737.

57. Age-Related Eye Disease Study Research Group. A randomized, placebo-controlled, clinical trial of high-dose supplementation with vitamins C and E, beta carotene, and zinc for age-related macular degeneration and vision loss: AREDS report no. 8. *Arch Ophthalmol.* 2001;119:1417–1436.

58. Azab M, Benchaboune M, Blinder KJ, et al. Verteporfin therapy of subfoveal choroidal neovascularization in age-related macular degeneration: meta-analysis of 2-year safety results in three randomized clinical trials: treatment of age-related macular degeneration with photodynamic therapy and verteporfin in photodynamic therapy study report no. 4. *Retina.* 2004;24:1–12.

59. Scheiman M, Scheiman M, Whittaker SG. *Low Vision Rehabilitation: A Practical Guide for Occupational Therapists.* Thorofare, NJ: SLACK Incorporated; 2007.

60. Hollows FC, Graham PA. Intra-ocular pressure, glaucoma, and glaucoma suspects in a defined population. *Br J Ophthalmol.* 1966;50:570–586.

61. Tielsch JM, Sommer A, Katz J, et al. Racial variations in the prevalence of primary open-angle glaucoma. The Baltimore Eye Survey. *JAMA.* 1991;266:369–374.

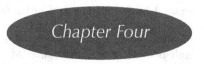
Chapter Four

Three Component Model of Vision, Part Two
Visual Efficiency Skills

Mitchell Scheiman

Visual Efficiency Skills

Definition and Classification of Visual Efficiency Disorders

Visual efficiency refers to the effectiveness of the visual system to clearly, efficiently, and comfortably allow an individual to gather visual information at school, work, or play. The various component skills that are important in this process are called visual efficiency skills and include the subcategories of accommodation, binocular vision, and ocular motility. Table 4.1 illustrates a classification system of visual efficiency disorders.

Accommodation Disorders

Definition and Description

Assuming that any refractive error has been corrected with eyeglasses, the normal human visual system is physiologically focused for objects at distances of 20 feet and greater. If an object is brought closer than 20 feet, a focusing adjustment must be made or the object will appear blurred. This focusing adjustment is referred to as accommodation. Accommodation is the ability to change the focus of the eye so that objects at different distances can be seen clearly. The accommodative system of the human eye generally works so well that most people are totally unaware that they even have a focusing system until about the age of 40 to 45 when there is a natural decline in accommodative ability that begins to cause blurred vision when reading.

Accommodation occurs by stimulating the smooth muscle of the ciliary body in the eye to contract, thereby enabling the lens to change its shape. Figure 4.1a is a cross-section of the human eye showing the lens and the ciliary muscle in its relaxed state. The light rays entering the eye are focused behind the retina, which would cause blurred vision. In Figure 4.1b, the ciliary muscle has contracted and allows the light rays to focus on the retina.

A blurred image on the fovea of the eye is the stimulus for accommodation and initiates a signal that is received at area 17 of the occipital cortex and continues to area 19. This acts as a stimulus for motor signals that will cause contraction of the ciliary muscle. The projection from area 19 to

DOI: 10.4324/9781003526841-4

Figure 4.1a. A cross-section of the human eye showing the lens and the ciliary muscle in its relaxed state with the light rays focused behind the retina. (Reprinted with permission from Scheiman M, Scheiman M, Whittaker SG. *Low Vision Rehabilitation: A Practical Guide for Occupational Therapists*. Thorofare, NJ: SLACK Incorporated; 2007.)

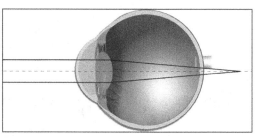

Figure 4.1b. The ciliary muscle has contracted and allows the light rays to focus on the retina. (Reprinted with permission from Scheiman M, Scheiman M, Whittaker SG. *Low Vision Rehabilitation: A Practical Guide for Occupational Therapists*. Thorofare, NJ: SLACK Incorporated; 2007.)

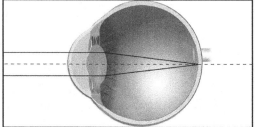

the midbrain complex is not well established. The actual innervation of the ciliary muscle is carried in the autonomic fibers of the third cranial nerve. These are axons of neurons originating in the Edinger-Westphal nuclei of the oculomotor complex. During accommodation, not only does the lens focus, but the pupil constricts as well. Both of these actions are mediated by parasympathetic components of the third cranial nerve.

The accommodative ability of an individual is inversely related to age. We use the term *accommodative amplitude* to refer to the total amount of accommodation available for a particular patient. Young children have very large amplitudes of accommodation, and this declines with age. This relationship between age and accommodative amplitude is so consistent across the population that it is possible for an optometrist to predict a patient's age within several years simply by measuring the amplitude of accommodation. The accommodative amplitude declines gradually with age, and by 40 to 45 years of age, the decline is significant enough to interfere with the ability to see small print held at reading distance. This is why most people begin wearing reading glasses or bifocals once they reach about 40 to 45 years of age. This is referred to as presbyopia and is described later in the chapter.

Clinically, we are not only interested in the amount of accommodation available, but also in the facility and sustaining ability of the accommodative response. This is called accommodative facility. Facility testing is designed to assess a number of key factors. The first is referred to as the latency of the accommodative response and relates to the amount of time it takes for the accommodative system to begin to respond once a stimulus is presented. The second factor is the velocity of the response or how fast the system can fully accommodate to the demand presented. The final factor assessed during accommodative facility testing is the ability to change accommodation over time or sustaining ability. The reason for the interest in accommodative facility is that studies have shown that there is a significant relationship between patient symptoms and problems with accommodative facility.

Accommodative disorders are commonly encountered in the general population. A recent study found that approximately 6% of children between 6 and 18 years old had clinically significant accommodative problems.[1] Accommodative problems are more common in physically, mentally, and developmentally delayed children, learning disabled children and adults, and children who have had cerebrovascular accident or traumatic brain injury. The presence and nature of accommodative problems in these populations are discussed in detail in Chapters Eight, Nine, and Eleven.

Classification of Accommodative Disorders

There are four primary types of accommodative disorders (see Table 4.1).[1] Accommodative insufficiency is a condition in which the amount of accommodation available (amplitude of accommodation) is less than expected for the individual's age. The result is that when a child attempts to accommodate when reading, for example, they experience intermittent blurred vision. In an attempt to regain clear vision, the child exerts extra effort to stimulate additional accommodation. This effort may lead to the signs and symptoms listed in Table 4.2.

Presbyopia is a condition in which near visual acuity is decreased because of an age-related decline in accommodative ability. There is a universal decline in the amplitude of accommodation with age. For instance, at 10 years of age, the normal amplitude of accommodation is about 20 D. This declines to 10 D at age 20, 7 D by age 30, and 4 to 5 D by age 40. As accommodative ability declines with age, it eventually becomes difficult to read and perform other close work. This is the reason why most adults need to use reading glasses or bifocals at around 40 to 45 years of age. All adults after the age of 45 or so have the condition called presbyopia and require reading glasses or some modification of their eyeglasses to account for this condition. Both presbyopia and accommodative insufficiency are problems in which the amplitude of accommodation is reduced, but presbyopia is an age-related disorder with an onset around 40 to 45 years of age, whereas

---

Table 4.1

Classification of Visual Efficiency Disorders

Accommodative Disorders

- Accommodative insufficiency
- Accommodative excess
- Accommodative infacility
- Presbyopia

Amblyopia

- Strabismic amblyopia
- Anisometropic amblyopia
- Isometropic amblyopia
- Stimulus deprivation amblyopia
- Hysterical amblyopia

Binocular Vision Disorders

Strabismic Binocular Vision Disorders

- Esotropia
- Exotropia
- Hypertropia
- Noncomitant strabismus

Nonstrabismic Binocular Vision Disorders

- Esophoria
- Exophoria
- Hyperphoria

Ocular Motility Disorders

- Saccadic dysfunction
- Pursuit dysfunction
- Disorders of fixation (nystagmus)

Table 4.2

Accommodative Disorders: Symptoms and Effects on Performance

Accommodative Infacility

These symptoms are generally related to the use of the eyes for reading or other near tasks:

- Blurred vision particularly when looking from near to far or far to near
- Headaches
- Eyestrain
- Reading problems
- Fatigue and sleepiness
- Loss of comprehension over time
- A pulling sensation around the eyes
- Movement of the print
- Avoidance of reading and other close work
- Difficulty with activities of daily living that require sustained close work

Accommodative Insufficiency and Presbyopia

These symptoms are generally related to the use of the eyes for reading or other near tasks:

- Blurred vision
- Headaches
- Eyestrain
- Reading problems
- Fatigue and sleepiness
- Loss of comprehension over time
- A pulling sensation around the eyes
- Movement of the print
- Avoidance of reading and other close work
- Difficulty with activities of daily living that require sustained close work

Accommodative Excess

These symptoms are generally related to the use of the eyes for reading or other near tasks:

- Blurred vision, worse after reading or other close work
- Headaches
- Eyestrain
- Difficulty focusing from far to near
- Sensitivity to light
- Difficulty with activities of daily living that require sustained close work

---

accommodative insufficiency generally affects children and young adults. The signs and symptoms of presbyopia are identical to those of accommodative insufficiency.

Another common accommodative disorder is called accommodative excess. This is a condition in which the amplitude of accommodation is normal, but the ciliary muscle has a tendency to spasm. Typically, the problem is intermittent and variable. The individual may report that after reading for a period of time, they experience blurred vision when looking at a distant object. They may also experience some of the other symptoms listed in Table 4.2.

The fourth accommodative problem is called accommodative infacility. This is a condition in which the amplitude of accommodation is normal, but the speed of the response is reduced. The most common complaint associated with accommodative facility is blurred vision when looking from near to far or far to near.

Clinical Assessment

While accommodative testing is routinely performed by most eye care professionals, there is a great deal of variability in the extent of testing performed from one doctor to another. The test performed by most eye doctors is measurement of the amplitude of accommodation. This is a very simple and quick test to perform and is described in Chapter Six as one of the standard screening tests for occupational therapists. Evaluation of accommodative amplitude can generally be performed from about 2 to 3 years of age. The unit of measure used for accommodative amplitude is the diopter (D). A natural decline in the amplitude of accommodation occurs with age.

Too many eye doctors limit their evaluation of accommodation to this one measure. However, of the four accommodative disorders described previously, only accommodative insufficiency and presbyopia can be detected using accommodative amplitude testing alone. The other two conditions cannot be diagnosed unless additional testing is performed. Two additional tests are very important to enable the doctor to adequately evaluate accommodation.

To evaluate accommodative speed and sustaining ability, optometrists perform a test called accommodative facility testing. The test probes the individual's ability to change accommodation rapidly and for a sustained period of time. It is considered a key test, is very sensitive to mild to moderate accommodative problems, and is the only method of detecting the condition called accommodative infacility.

Another important method of evaluating accommodation is called near point retinoscopy. Using an instrument called the retinoscope, the clinician is able to objectively evaluate the accommodative system. This test allows us to determine how accurately the patient accommodates and is an important test for detecting the condition called accommodative excess.

Development of Accommodation

Accommodation is very poorly developed at birth. Newborns are unable to accommodate, and their focus appears to be set at about 30 cm from their eyes. Like visual acuity, however, there is a very rapid development, and by 6 months of age, accommodation appears to reach adult levels.[2]

As described above, an interesting fact about accommodation is the natural and expected decline that occurs with age. At about the age of 40 to 45 years, accommodation has declined to the point that reading becomes difficult and uncomfortable. This condition is called presbyopia. By the age of about 65 years, accommodation is virtually absent, and we become dependent on eyeglasses to help us focus.

Significance of Accommodative Disorders for Occupational Therapy

Table 4.2 lists the symptoms of accommodative problems. Accommodative disorders will interfere whenever an occupational therapist asks a patient to engage in an activity that requires visual concentration on small objects or print at a close distance.

Binocular Vision Disorders

Definition and Description

The human visual system works so well and reliably that most people take it for granted that when we look at the world with two eyes, we receive one single impression of the external world. When a problem is encountered, however, it becomes apparent that the system that allows single vision to occur is very elaborate, requiring a delicate balance of neural and muscular processes. Binocular vision is the ability of the visual system to fuse or combine the information from the right and left eyes into one image. Visual information that enters the right and left eyes remains monocular as it passes from the optic nerve through the chiasm, the optic tract, the lateral geniculate body, and the optic radiation. At the level of the visual cortex (area 17), the information finally reaches cortical cells capable of binocular processing.

For binocular vision to occur, the information arriving from each eye must be identical and approximately equal in clarity and size. To satisfy these requirements, the two eyes must be aligned so that they point at the same object at all times, and the optics or refractive error of the two eyes must be approximately equal. Problems with either alignment or refractive equality will cause binocular vision disorders. The hallmark symptom of a binocular vision disorder is double vision (diplopia).

When the two eyes actually lose alignment, it is referred to as strabismus. When strabismus occurs and the eyes drift in, out, up, or down, each eye views a different part of the environment and sends different information to the visual cortex. The result is the perception of diplopia. Because diplopia is intolerable, the visual system attempts to eliminate the problem through one of two mechanisms: by trying to overcome the problem and restore normal alignment using muscular effort or by adapting to the misalignment of the eyes. In some cases, the tendency for the eye to turn can be overcome with muscular effort. In such cases, patients often successfully eliminate double vision and experience binocular vision, but may be uncomfortable. They report eyestrain, headaches, the inability to sustain attention for long periods of time, intermittent blurred vision, and occasional diplopia. The other option is to allow the eye to turn but to eliminate diplopia by either ignoring the information coming from the eye that turns (suppression) or by altering the neurophysiology of the eye (anomalous correspondence). Until the age of about 6 years, the human visual system has been shown to have an extraordinary plasticity and ability to adapt to strabismus. Age affects adaptation; generally, younger children adapt more quickly than older children and adults. It is also more likely to occur if the eye turn is a constant, rather than an intermittent, problem.

The human visual system has two modes of adaptation. The first is called suppression and, in such cases, the information entering the eye that turns is ignored at the cortical level. Suppression eliminates diplopia, but as a result of this adaptation, normal visual development does not occur, leading to a loss of vision called amblyopia. The second mode of adaptation demonstrates the high level of plasticity of the human visual system during the sensitive period and is called anomalous

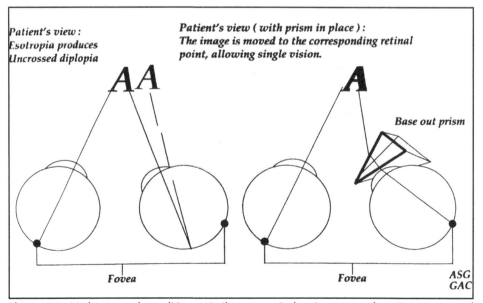

Figure 4.2. Under normal conditions, similar anatomical points on each retina correspond neurophysiologically with the retina of the fellow eye. In this figure, the corresponding points illustrated are the foveas of the two eyes.

correspondence. Under normal conditions, similar anatomical points on each retina correspond neurophysiologically with the retina of the fellow eye (Figure 4.2). When these two "corresponding" retinal points are stimulated, the brain experiences single vision. The visual system is born with this normal correspondence between similar points on the retinas of the two eyes. As long as visual experience is normal, this correspondence remains stable throughout life. However, if strabismus occurs during the first 5 to 6 years of life, resulting in diplopia, the visual system must make a choice to overcome the eye turn with muscular effort or to allow the eye turn to exist and to try to adapt to it. The second possible adaptation is for the normal correspondence to be altered. In such cases, the neurophysiology of the visual system makes an adjustment to the new alignment of the eyes, and the corresponding points of the two retinas are altered to allow single vision to occur in spite of the strabismus. This is called anomalous correspondence and only occurs if the eye turn develops early, is small to moderate in size, is stable and constant, and is present for a long period of time.

If the individual overcomes the eye turn by adapting either with suppression or anomalous correspondence, the strabismus becomes more difficult to eliminate with treatment, and additional problems such as loss of vision in the eye that turns (amblyopia) and several other significant secondary conditions may occur.

If a strabismus develops after the age of 6 years or so, the option of adaptation is no longer viable. The age of 6 is an approximation, and there is certainly individual variation in the end of the period of visual plasticity. The important concept, however, is that the visual system is incapable of adapting to a strabismus that develops in older children or adults. Thus, late-onset strabismus will generally result in either constant or intermittent double vision. This is the reason why adults experiencing strabismus after traumatic head injury will have double vision.

Prevalence of Binocular Vision Disorders

Other than refractive error, the most common vision problems encountered in clinical practice are binocular vision disorders. In a study of a clinical pediatric population, Scheiman et al.[3] found that about 25% of children from 6 months to 18 years old had significant binocular vision disorders. Similar prevalence data have been found in adult populations.[4] Binocular vision problems are more common in physically, mentally, and developmentally delayed children; learning disabled children; and adults who have had a cerebrovascular accident or traumatic brain injury.[5-9] These studies have shown that convergence insufficiency (a binocular vision problem) is the most common vision disorder after acquired brain injury on both the civilian population[5,9] and soldiers returning from the wars in Iraq and Afghanistan.[6,7,10]

Classification of Binocular Vision Disorders

There are two main types of binocular vision disorders: strabismic and nonstrabismic binocular disorders (Tables 4.3 and 4.4).

STRABISMUS

Strabismus is a condition in which the eyes are misaligned. It occurs in about 3% to 5% of the general population and is often very obvious cosmetically. Other terms used to describe strabismus include *heterotropia*, *tropia*, *squint*, *cross-eyed*, and *wall-eyed*. Strabismus can also be categorized based on four characteristics:

1. Direction: Whether the eyes turn in, out, or up.
2. Frequency: The percentage of time the eye is misaligned.
3. Laterality: Whether one eye always turns or if the two eyes alternate.
4. Comitancy: Whether the magnitude of the eye turn is the same in all positions of gaze.

Table 4.3

Classification of Strabismic Binocular Vision Disorders

Direction
- Esotropia: Eyes turn in
- Exotropia: Eyes turn out
- Hypertropia: One eye turns up

Each of these conditions is also classified based on the following characteristics.

Frequency
- Intermittent esotropia or constant esotropia
- Intermittent exotropia or constant exotropia
- Intermittent hypertropia or constant hypertropia

Laterality
- Right esotropia, left esotropia, or alternating esotropia
- Right exotropia, left exotropia, or alternating exotropia
- Right hypertropia, left hypertropia, or alternating hypertropia

Comitancy
- Comitant or noncomitant esotropia
- Comitant or noncomitant exotropia
- Comitant or noncomitant hypertropia

Table 4.4

Classification of Nonstrabismic Binocular Vision Disorders

Direction
- Esophoria: Eyes have a tendency to turn in
- Exophoria: Eyes have a tendency to turn out
- Hyperphoria: One eye has a tendency to turn up
- Nonstrabismic binocular vision disorders can also be classified based on the relationship between the magnitude of the phoria at distance and the magnitude of the phoria at near.

Distance to Near Relationship
- Magnitude equal at distance and near: Basic esophoria
                                             Basic exophoria
- Magnitude greater at distance: Divergence excess (exophoria)
                                     Divergence insufficiency (esophoria)
- Magnitude greater at near: Convergence insufficiency (exophoria)
                                  Convergence excess (esophoria)

Direction

The three most common types of strabismus are esotropia (eyes turn in), exotropia (eyes turn out), and hypertropia (one eye turns up). Combinations of these are possible and often occur. For example, the right eye could turn up and out or down and in. The direction of the strabismus has some significance in terms of prognosis for treatment using different treatment modalities. For example, the prognosis for the treatment of exotropia using vision therapy is good to excellent, while with esotropia it is only fair.

Frequency

Strabismus can be classified according to the percentage of time it is present. Strabismus present 100% of the time is called constant strabismus, while strabismus present less than 100% of the time is referred to as intermittent strabismus. This characteristic has very significant clinical implications. If the strabismus is intermittent, it means that binocular vision is still present at least some of the time. Rehabilitation using vision therapy is considerably easier and more effective if binocular vision has been present even part of the time. The prognosis, therefore, is excellent for elimination of an intermittent strabismus using vision therapy. If the strabismus is constant and has been present for a long period of time, normal binocular vision will be absent, and adaptations such as suppression and anomalous correspondence, described above, may have developed. These adaptations make it considerably more difficult to restore normal binocular vision and reduce the prognosis for vision therapy.

Laterality

Another important characteristic is called laterality and refers to whether the same eye always turns or whether the two eyes alternately turn. A strabismus in which the right or left turns all of the time is called a unilateral strabismus. If the right eye and left eye turn alternately, it is called an alternating strabismus. The laterality of the strabismus also has significant clinical implications. A unilateral, constant strabismus will generally cause the development of amblyopia or loss of vision in the eye that turns. If the strabismus is alternating, amblyopia does not develop, and the visual acuity remains normal in each eye because each eye continues to receive normal stimulation.

Comitancy

Figure 4.3 illustrates the nine positions of gaze that are generally tested in a clinical evaluation. A strabismus is referred to as comitant if the size of the strabismus remains relatively constant in all nine positions of gaze. It is important to understand that comitancy testing takes place at a constant working distance from the patient. For example, a clinician measures the size of the strabismus in the nine positions of gaze at 40 cm or at 6 m. The size of the strabismus is not compared from one distance to another, only from one position of gaze to another at the same distance. Thus, if the strabismus is 20 prism D (prism D is the unit of measurement for strabismus) at 6 m and 60 prism D at 40 cm, this is not an indication of noncomitancy. However, if the strabismus is 20 prism D in right gaze and 60 prism D in left gaze, with both measurements taken at 40 cm from the patient, the strabismus is noncomitant. The three most common causes of adult-onset noncomitant strabismus are trauma, vascular problems, and neoplasm. In children, the three most common causes

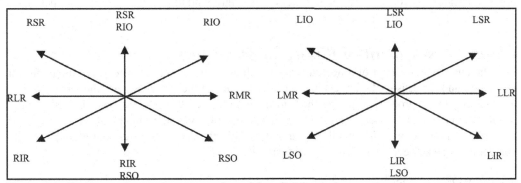

Figure 4.3. Positions of gaze that are evaluated by clinicians when testing the extraocular muscles. (RSR=right superior rectus, RLR=right lateral rectus, RIR=right inferior rectus, RSO=right superior oblique, RMR=right medial rectus, RIO=right inferior oblique, LSR=left superior rectus, LLR=left lateral rectus, LIR=left inferior rectus, LSO=left superior oblique, LMR=left medial rectus, LIO=left inferior oblique.)

are congenital, trauma, and acute viral infection.[10] Occupational therapists frequently encounter noncomitant strabismus in patients with traumatic brain injury and stroke.

NONSTRABISMIC BINOCULAR VISION DISORDERS

Remember that strabismus is a condition in which the eyes are actually misaligned at least 1% of the time. If the eyes have a tendency to turn in, out, or up but this tendency is controlled at all times, the deviation is categorized as a nonstrabismic binocular vision disorder. Other frequently used terms to describe this condition are *heterophoria* and *phoria*. The tendency for the eyes to misalign in cases of heterophoria can vary from very slight to very large. In fact, in the average person, a slight tendency for the eyes to drift outward is expected. We become concerned about heterophoria when the tendency becomes moderate to large and, in addition, the patient's ability to compensate is inadequate. For example, if the individual's eyes have a tendency to drift out, we are clinically interested in their ability to converge or pull the eyes in. If the ability to converge is not sufficient to comfortably control the tendency for the eyes to drift outward, symptoms occur.

The most common method of categorizing heterophoria is by direction of the deviation. The three most common types of heterophoria according to this classification are exophoria (the eyes have a tendency to turn out), esophoria (the eyes have a tendency to turn in), and hyperphoria (one eye has a tendency to turn up).

Another popular way of classifying nonstrabismic binocular vision disorders is by comparing the size of the problem at 6 m to the size of the disorder at 40 cm. This system only applies to esophoria or exophoria, not hyperphoria. The phoria may be equal at distance and at near, or the problem may be greater at near than at distance or greater at distance than at near. This leads to six different possibilities listed in Table 4.4. The two most common types of heterophoria according to this classification system are convergence insufficiency and convergence excess.

Convergence insufficiency is probably the most common nonstrabismic binocular vision disorder that occupational therapists will encounter. It is a condition in which the eyes have a tendency to drift outward when being used for near work such as reading, while at a far distance the eyes work well together. This is one of the leading causes of eyestrain and discomfort. In the general population, convergence insufficiency is present in about 5% of the population, while in the populations managed by occupational therapists the prevalence is considerably greater. Convergence insufficiency is one of the most common vision problems that occurs after cerebrovascular accident or traumatic brain injury in both civilian[5,9,11–15] and military populations.[6–8]

Convergence excess also affects close vision, but in this case the eyes have a tendency to turn inward rather than outward. Again, if the patient can control this tendency all of the time, the problem is called a phoria. Convergence excess has been found to be slightly more prevalent than convergence insufficiency in a clinical population.

Clinical Assessment of Binocular Disorders

The clinical assessment of binocular vision is divided into two major areas: the motor fusion evaluation and the sensory fusion evaluation. In reference to the visual system, the term *fusion* is used to refer to the process of uniting the information received from the two eyes into one single image. The neural and muscular mechanism that brings the eyes into alignment on the object of interest is called motor fusion, while the activity within the cerebral cortex that allows a single perception to be achieved is called sensory fusion.[16]

MOTOR FUSION EVALUATION

Several tests are used to evaluate the neural and muscular mechanism that brings the eyes into alignment on the object of interest. While the equipment used for this part of the evaluation is simple and inexpensive, advanced clinical skills and significant clinical experience are required to interpret the patient's responses. At least the five tests listed in Table 4.5 must be performed to properly assess motor fusion. Many clinicians consider the cover test to be the most important test in this group. This test is illustrated in Figure 4.4 and involves the use of a plastic cover paddle and a fixation target. Using this simple equipment, the clinician is able to determine many key binocular vision characteristics, including the magnitude, direction, frequency, laterality, and comitancy of the deviation. The cover test is an objective test and can, therefore, be effectively used with patients of any age including infants and patients who are nonverbal, mentally disabled, and autistic.

A test that many occupational therapists may already be aware of is the measurement of the near point of convergence. This procedure is illustrated in Figure 4.5 and only requires the use of a small penlight target. This test probes the ability of the individual to converge the eyes and to maintain their alignment as an object is brought closer and closer to the eyes. This is one of the key tests used to reach the diagnosis of convergence insufficiency. The normal response is to be able to converge to about 2 to 4 inches from the eyes. This test is part of the vision screening described in detail in Chapter Six.

Comitancy is evaluated by asking the patient to follow a light as it is moved in the nine diagnostic positions of gaze illustrated in Figure 4.3. The clinician observes the relationship of the eyes as in the various positions of gaze. Ruling out a noncomitant strabismus is a critical part of the examination because such a condition may suggest a serious underlying etiology for the binocular vision disorder.

The final two critical tests are used to assess the ability of the patient to compensate for the strabismus or heterophoria that is present. This characteristic is called fusional vergence, and the

---

Table 4.5

Tests Used to Evaluate Motor and Sensory Fusion

Motor Fusion Testing
- Cover test
- Near point of convergence
- Comitancy testing
- Fusional vergence amplitude testing
- Fusional vergence facility testing

Sensory Fusion Testing
- Stereopsis testing
- Suppression testing (Worth 4 Dot)
- Anomalous correspondence testing (Bagolini Striated Lenses, After Image Test)

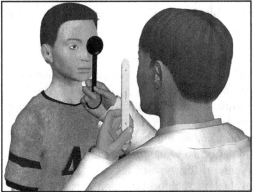

Figure 4.4. The cover test using a plastic cover paddle and a fixation target.

Figure 4.5. Measurement of the near point of convergence using a small penlight target.

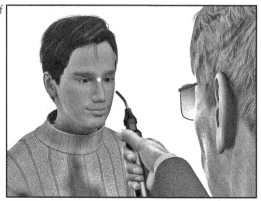

Figure 4.6. Fusional vergence testing using a prism bar.

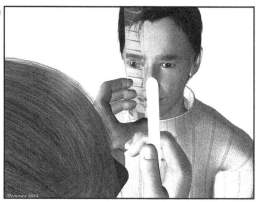

testing is referred to as fusional vergence testing. As a general rule, if the problem is an esodeviation (the eyes tend to turn in), clinicians are most interested in the ability of the patient to diverge or move the eyes outward, whereas if the problem is an exodeviation, clinicians are most interested in the ability of the patient to converge or move the eyes inward. Again, very simple equipment is required as illustrated in Figure 4.6. Two measurements are important: the fusional vergence amplitude and fusional vergence facility. This is comparable to the assessment of accommodation in which we are also interested in both amplitude and facility.

While some binocular vision testing is routinely performed by most eye care professionals, there is a great deal of variability in the extent of testing performed from one doctor to another. If an occupational therapist is looking to develop a referral relationship with an optometrist, it is critical to determine the type and extent of the evaluation they perform. An incomplete evaluation will often result in a lack of identification of important binocular vision problems. Table 4.5 can be used by occupational therapists to evaluate the type of testing performed by the optometrist.

Sensory Fusion Evaluation

The evaluation of the activity within the cerebral cortex that allows a single perception to be achieved is called sensory fusion. The tests listed in Table 4.5 are often performed to assess this function. While the evaluation of motor fusion requires advanced clinical training to properly interpret patient responses, the same is not true of all aspects of the evaluation of sensory fusion. In addition, good sensory fusion is one indication of adequate motor fusion. These two points have great significance for professionals who want to perform a visual screening. Because sensory fusion is dependent on motor fusion and because some of this type of testing is rather easy to interpret, it becomes an ideal screening test for the evaluation of binocular vision. It is important to

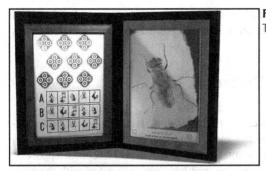

Figure 4.7a. Stereopsis testing equipment (Stereofly Test).

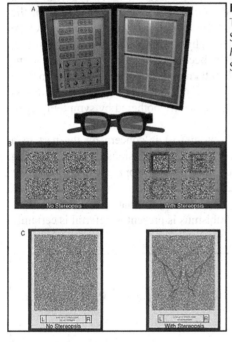

Figure 4.7b. Stereopsis testing equipment (Randot Stereo Test). (Reprinted with permission from Scheiman M, Scheiman M, Whittaker SG. *Low Vision Rehabilitation: A Practical Guide for Occupational Therapists.* Thorofare, NJ: SLACK Incorporated; 2007.)

understand, however, that it is possible to have normal sensory fusion and still have a significant binocular vision disorder. For example, sensory fusion testing may be very close to normal in cases of significant heterophoria.

A very popular probe of sensory fusion is stereopsis testing. Several different tests are illustrated in Figures 4.7a and 4.7b. These tests are inexpensive, simple to administer, and easy to interpret, making them excellent screening tests. Stereopsis testing will be described in detail in Chapter Six.

Other tests are used to probe for suppression (Worth 4 Dot) and anomalous correspondence (Bagolini Striated Lenses, After Image Test).

Development of Binocular Vision

Although the neurophysiology for binocular vision is present at birth, it is not fully developed and requires normal stimulation for proper development to occur. For the first month of life, alignment of the eyes may be variable with occasional strabismus occurring. By 1 month, however, alignment should be normal. Strabismus occurring after the age of 1 month is considered to be a problem. Stereopsis (3-D vision) is the ability to appreciate depth based on binocular input. It is one of the most important clinical indications of normal binocular vision. Stereopsis can be measured in very young infants, and researchers have found that it is absent at birth but reaches adult levels by about 16 to 20 weeks of age.[17]

Significance of Binocular Vision Disorders for Occupational Therapy

Table 4.6 provides a summary of the significance of binocular vision disorders for occupational therapy. If we consider strabismus to be the most extreme or severe binocular vision problem and heterophoria to be the least severe, an interesting phenomenon becomes apparent. The most significant symptoms related to binocular vision problems are associated with the least severe binocular vision problems. Strabismus is the most severe binocular vision problem, yet it has the fewest and least significant symptoms associated with it in all populations except for the traumatic brain injury/cerebrovascular accident population. Heterophoria, which is the least severe binocular vision problem, at least from a standpoint of neurophysiology and cosmetic appearance, may be associated with the most severe symptoms. This is because children develop adaptations to long-standing, early-onset strabismus that eliminate all bothersome symptoms. Adults who have experienced traumatic brain injury or cerebrovascular accident and have developed strabismus as a result cannot make these adaptations and are, therefore, frequently bothered by symptoms associated with strabismus and heterophoria.

A common misconception that I often hear as an optometrist is concern on the part of a referring occupational therapist that the presence of a very obvious strabismus must be affecting a child's performance and ability to learn. A strabismus may be very apparent to the observer who sees a very obvious crossed eye, for example. The adaptations that occur after the onset of strabismus, however, eliminate any symptoms and any impact on performance or learning. This does not mean that the child should not be referred if a strabismus is present. A referral is certainly

---

Table 4.6

Binocular Vision Disorders: Symptoms and Effect on Performance

Strabismic

Cosmetic problem, the eyes look crossed or "wall-eyed"

If intermittent, may cause double vision that can interfere with eye-hand and mobility tasks

If intermittent, may cause eyestrain

Loss of vision if left untreated and the strabismus is unilateral

Nonstrabismic

These symptoms are generally related to the use of the eyes for reading or other near tasks:

Blurred vision

Headaches

Eyestrain

Reading problems

Fatigue and sleepiness

Loss of comprehension over time

A pulling sensation around the eyes

Movement of the print

Avoidance of reading and other close work

Difficulty with activities of daily living that require stereopsis (driving, near tasks involving reaching for objects, pouring liquids)

appropriate in such cases. However, the concern is related to the negative effects of the strabismus on the development of the visual system and not to performance or learning. In many cases, children with strabismus may also have a number of other vision anomalies that do have a negative effect on performance and function, such as ocular motility and accommodative and visual perceptual problems.

Nonstrabismic binocular vision problems, which are the less severe form of binocular vision disorder, are related to the most significant symptoms. Because patients can overcome a phoria using neuromuscular effort, the eyes never appear misaligned in such cases. Thus, the child's visual cosmetic appearance is normal. The neuromuscular effort required to overcome the phoria, however, causes a host of symptoms that can have a very severe impact on function and performance.

Amblyopia

Definition and Description

Amblyopia is a condition in which the visual acuity is less than 20/20, and this loss of visual acuity cannot be attributed to refractive error or observable eye disease. This means that even after prescribing the best possible eyeglasses, the patient has reduced vision in one or both eyes. Amblyopia is not an optical problem but rather a neurophysiological problem in which the visual pathway from the eye to the visual cortex does not develop normally or deteriorates due to some type of interference during the sensitive period.

Most people are familiar with amblyopia, which is commonly called "lazy eye" by the public. The term *lazy eye* is a misnomer and does not really describe the condition well. The eye is not lazy; it simply has not received proper stimulation for one of several reasons described next. The classic treatment is use of an eye patch to force the child to use the weaker eye.

Classification of Amblyopia

The classifications of amblyopia are listed in Table 4.1. The most common type of amblyopia is caused by refractive error problems. There are two types of refractive error problems that can cause amblyopia. The most common of these is called anisometropic amblyopia. This problem, which is described in Chapter Three, is a condition in which the prescription in one eye is considerably stronger than the prescription in the fellow eye. The inequality in vision and size of the images in the two eyes creates difficulty for the visual cortex in its attempt to fuse the two images. Because the two images are incompatible, the brain cannot fuse them and tends to ignore the input from the eye with the more significant refractive error. If this occurs before 5 to 6 years of age or so, visual development does not proceed normally. The result is reduced visual acuity, which we call amblyopia.

Another refractive disorder that can lead to the development of amblyopia is called isometropic amblyopia. This is a condition in which there is a very high refractive error in both eyes. For example, both eyes may have a very high degree of astigmatism, hyperopia, or myopia. If left uncorrected during the first 5 to 6 years of life, amblyopia can occur.

Another common form of amblyopia is caused by strabismus. If one eye always turns in, out, or up and the problem begins during the first 5 to 6 years of life, amblyopia will occur. When one eye turns at all times during the sensitive period of development, the child will initially experience double vision because of the misalignment of the eyes. Because double vision is intolerable, the child's visual system will make one or more adaptations to eliminate this double vision. These adaptations are generally successful in eliminating the double vision. However, they lead to deterioration or lack of development of visual acuity.

Two other forms of amblyopia are considerably less common. The first is called stimulus deprivation amblyopia and occurs when a very young infant has a problem, such as a congenital cataract or some type of corneal scar, that interferes with the ability of visual information to enter one eye. The second unusual form is called hysterical amblyopia. This type of amblyopia is caused by emotional factors, and there are no actual physical or physiological changes. Generally, patients with this type of amblyopia present with poor vision, and the eye doctor is unable to find a cause during the examination. Often in such cases, the child is under a great deal of emotional stress because of personal or family problems.

Clinical Assessment

Amblyopia is detected during the course of any traditional eye examination using visual acuity testing. The cause of the amblyopia must then be determined using tests designed to evaluate refraction, binocular vision, and eye health.

Significance of Amblyopia for Occupational Therapy

Unless the amblyopia is present in both eyes, the condition has little significance for occupational therapists. If the visual acuity is reduced in one eye, the other eye still sees well, and the patient generally does not experience any functional deficits.

Ocular Motility Disorders

Definition and Description

We use the term *ocular motility disorders* to refer to eye movement problems in any one or more of the following areas: fixation, saccades, and pursuits (see Table 4.1). Other terms used to describe ocular motility disorders are *eye movement disorders*, *tracking problems*, and *visual scanning problems*. Visual scanning is particularly popular in the rehabilitation and occupational therapy literature. Warren[18] stresses the importance of identifying visual scanning deficits in adults after acquired brain injury. She defines visual scanning as one of the primary means by which the central nervous system obtains visual information from the environment and describes scanning as a function that involves both eye movements and fixation. The optometric literature, on the other hand, stresses the three component model of eye movements, and authors generally refer to disorders of fixation, saccades, and pursuits.[1]

Eye movement disorders are an important diagnostic and management concern because of the effect such problems may have on the functional capability of an individual. Much of the emphasis of both researchers and clinicians has been on the relationship between eye movements and reading. During reading, the three important components of eye movements are saccades, fixations, and regressions. Saccades take up approximately 10% of the reading time. The average saccade is about eight to nine character spaces.[19] The duration of the saccade is a function of the distance covered. For instance, a 2 degree saccade takes about 25 to 30 msec, and a 5 degree saccade takes about 35 to 40 msec.[19] Between saccades, the eye is relatively still in a fixational pause. For normal readers, the average duration of the fixation is 200 to 250 msec. The third important characteristic of reading eye movements is the regression. A regression is a right to left movement and occurs 10% to 20% of the time in skilled readers. Regressions occur when the reader overshoots the target, misinterprets the text, or has difficulty understanding the text.

Because eye movement deficiencies intuitively seem to be so closely linked with reading, numerous studies have investigated this relationship. Two basic viewpoints have evolved about the relationship between eye movements and reading. The first suggests that eye movement disorders can cause below-average reading ability.[20–29] Investigators using a variety of methods to assess eye movements have found that poor readers tend to make more fixations and regressions than normal readers. The second position is that the random and unskilled eye movement skills observed with poor readers are secondary to deficient language skills that cause reading disorders. Thus, the reading difficulty itself leads to erratic and inconsistent eye movements.[30-34] A third perspective is probably most likely to be correct and is essentially a combination of the first two viewpoints. This alternative suggests that, in some cases, problems with fixation and saccadic abilities may be a primary interference in a patient's ability to read quickly, comfortably, and with adequate comprehension.[35] In other cases, the eye movement deficiencies observed during reading may simply be a reflection of poor reading ability.

Another important background issue is that during reading, eye movements are integrated with higher cognitive processes including attention, memory, and the utilization of the perceived visual information.[36-38] Some optometrists believe that there is a relationship between poor ocular motor skills and attention problems.[39-41] When such a relationship exists, treatment of eye movement disorders may lead to improvement in attention and concentration.

Eye movement problems have also been reported to be one of the more common and problematic vision problems secondary to acquired brain injury.[18,42-45] Problems with saccades after head trauma can interfere with occupational therapy. Warren[18] suggests that visual scanning deficits contribute to the failure of some adults to regain independence in many daily activities including self-care, reading, arithmetic, and driving. Strano[46] also describes the importance of saccades for driving and suggests that abnormal saccades greatly affect quick and accurate fixation on a target in the periphery and ability to return to the traffic ahead.

There have been several studies of the prevalence of eye movement disorders in children with learning and reading disabilities. In a sample of 50 children with learning disabilities between the ages of 6 and 13 years old, Sherma[47] found that 96% had problems with ocular motor inefficiency (saccadic and pursuit problems). Hoffman[48] reported on a larger sample of 107 children with learning problems. The children's ages ranged from 5 to 14 years old. His results revealed that 95% of the sample had ocular motor problems. It is interesting to note that both Sherman and Hoffman found that ocular motor dysfunction was the most prevalent vision disorder in their samples of learning disabled children.

In my experience, and in the studies described above, eye movement disorders are rarely present in isolation. Rather, they are generally found associated with accommodative, binocular, and visual information processing dysfunctions. As a result, treatment of eye movement deficiencies should not occur in isolation, instead such treatment should take place within the context of an overall treatment approach designed to deal with other problems as well.

Classification of Ocular Motility Disorders

Ocular motility disorders can be divided into three distinct areas: fixation stability, saccadic function, and pursuit function. Ocular motility disorders can reflect serious underlying central nervous system disease or functional/developmental problems. It is always important to consider the possibility that abnormalities in fixation stability, saccades, and pursuits may require additional consultation.

Assessment of fixation is an important part of the routine examination. An individual with inadequate fixation ability may look away from the task more often than other children. This "off-task" behavior may give the impression that the person is inattentive or impulsive. Asking the patient to fixate on a target during the initial evaluation is sufficient to evaluate fixation status. All patients, except the very young, anxious, hyperactive, or inattentive, should be able to sustain precise fixation with no observable movement of the eyes for 10 seconds.[38,49] A variety of disorders of fixation can occur and may represent organic or functional anomalies. A very significant disorder of fixation commonly seen by occupational therapists is nystagmus.

Nystagmus is a condition in which there are involuntary, rhythmic oscillations of one or both eyes. It may be a sensory problem due to very poor visual acuity or a disorder of ocular motor control. Nystagmus can be thought of as a disorder of the mechanisms that keep fixation stable. The pursuit, optokinetic, and vestibular systems act to maintain a steady image on the retina. Any lesion that

---

Table 4.7

Ocular Motility Disorders: Symptoms and Effect on Performance

- Excessive head movement
- Frequent loss of place
- Skips lines
- Poor attention span
- Copying is slow and coloring and drawing results are poor
- Difficulty with activities of daily living that require frequent change in fixation and accurate eye movements (driving, reading, writing)

---

creates an imbalance in these neurological systems can cause nystagmus by making the eyes drift off target. Nystagmus affects about one in every 5,000 to 10,000 people. It is much more prevalent in patients who have certain ocular and/or systemic health conditions. For example, a large percentage of people with cerebral palsy have nystagmus, and approximately 10% to 15% of visually impaired school-age children have nystagmus. Nystagmus will be discussed in detail in Chapter Eleven.

Saccadic dysfunction is a condition in which the accuracy and speed of saccadic eye movements are reduced relative to expected findings for the individual's age. Saccades are eye movements that enable us to rapidly redirect our line of sight so that the point of interest stimulates the fovea. Saccades are the fastest eye movement with velocities as high as 700 degrees per second.[50] The ideal saccade is a single eye movement that rapidly reaches and abruptly stops at the target of interest. Saccades may be inaccurate, however, in two ways. The most common inaccuracy is a slight undershoot. In most cases, the saccade is slightly short of the target, and the eye "glides" to alignment but, in more extreme cases, a second, smaller saccade is made to reach the target. A less common inaccuracy is an overshoot of the target.

Saccadic fixation problems can lead to the signs and symptoms listed in Table 4.7. Problems with fixation and saccadic abilities may be a primary factor interfering with a child's ability to read quickly, comfortably, and with adequate comprehension. As described above, there may be a relationship between poor saccadic ability and attention problems. Saccadic problems have also been reported to be one of the more common and problematic vision problems secondary to acquired brain injury.

Pursuit dysfunction is a condition in which the individual is unable to accurately follow a moving object. Pursuit eye movements enable continuous clear vision of moving objects. This visual following reflex ideally produces eye movements that ensure continuous foveal fixation of objects moving in space. Pursuit movements are affected by age, attention, and motivation. Because pursuit eye movements are only involved when a target is moving, they are more difficult to relate to reading and school performance than saccades. However, pursuits may play a more significant role in other activities of daily living, such as driving and sports, and any other activities in which the individual is moving or the object of regard is moving.

Clinical Assessment

Examination of eye movements involves three distinct steps: Assessment of stability of fixation, saccadic function, and pursuit function. To evaluate fixation stability, we simply ask the patient to fixate on a target during the initial evaluation. All patients, except the very young, anxious, hyperactive, or inattentive, should be able to sustain precise fixation with no observable movement of the eyes for 10 seconds.

The purpose of saccadic testing is to assess the quality and accuracy of saccadic function. A variety of assessment procedures have been developed to evaluate saccades. Tests may involve direct observation by the clinician, timed or standardized tests involving a visual-verbal format, and objective eye movement recording using electro-oculographic instruments. There are problems associated with all of these methods, however. Electro-oculographic procedures are expensive, time-consuming, and difficult to use with young elementary school children and patients with cognitive or attention problems. Subjective techniques involving observation of the patient's eye movements have been developed along with rating scales. These rating scales are highly subjective, and inexperienced clinicians may have difficulty learning to effectively use them. A study by Maples and Ficklin[51] did show that the rating scale used in their study was reliable and repeatable. An important advantage of subjective rating scales is that they can be used with some of the more challenging populations managed by occupational therapists. This method of evaluating eye movement can be used with nonverbal, intellectually challenged, autistic, and low-functioning adults after acquired brain injury.

Direct observation tests require the subject to look from one object to another while the clinician observes the patient's saccades. Several rating scales have been developed to create better uniformity in observation. One of these rating scales is described in detail in Chapter Six.

Another alternative is the use of tests using a visual-verbal format. These tests are inexpensive, easily administered, and provide a quantitative evaluation of eye movements in a simulated reading environment.[52] They assess ocular motor function on the basis of the speed in which a series of numbers can be seen, recognized, and verbalized with accuracy. The most popular test of this type is the Developmental Eye Movement (DEM) test. This test requires the subject to be functioning at a 6-year-old level at least.

The second method described above is the use of timed and standardized tests. The most widely used test today is the DEM test. The patient is asked to call off a series of numbers as quickly as possible without using a finger or pointer as a guide. The response times and number of errors are then compared to tables of expecteds. This test is also described in detail in Chapter Six.

The third approach to the assessment of saccades is objective eye movement recording. Currently, the clinical device available for this purpose is the Visagraph ([Figure 4.8] Stockholm, Sweden). This system consists of a computer unit and goggles. Objective eye movement recording has several advantages over direct observation and timed or standardized tests. The Visagraph system provides a permanent recording of the evaluation, is an objective procedure, and does not depend on the skill of the examiner. The information gained from objective recording is also more sophisticated. It provides information about number of fixations, regressions, duration of fixations, reading rate, relative efficiency, and grade equivalence. All of this information can be compared to established norms for elementary school children through adulthood. The disadvantage of the Visagraph is the expense of the instrument. It is also difficult to use with patients who are inattentive or hyperactive or who have poor fixation. Most clinicians use a combination of direct observation using rating scales like those described in Chapter Six along with the DEM test.

The purpose of pursuit testing is to assess the quality and accuracy of pursuit function. There are not as many testing alternatives for pursuits as there are for saccades. Direct observation of

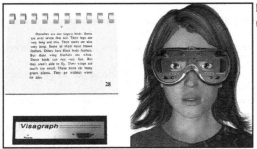

Figure 4.8. The Visagraph used for objective eye movement recording.

the patient following a moving target is the most commonly used clinical technique. Several rating scales have been developed for direct observation of pursuit movements. We suggest using the one described in Chapter Six.

Development of Ocular Motility

Unlike visual acuity, accommodative, and binocular vision skills that reach adult levels of development very early in infancy, clinical assessment indicates that eye movement development is considerably slower, continuing through the early elementary school years.[53,54] Because of the long developmental process for eye movement control, slow development can leave a child with inadequate skills to meet the demands of the classroom.

Significance of Ocular Motility Disorders for Occupational Therapy

Table 4.7 provides a summary of the symptoms of ocular motility disorders and their effect on performance. Problems with fixation and saccadic abilities may be a primary factor interfering with a patient's ability to read quickly, comfortably, and with adequate comprehension. There may be a relationship between poor saccadic ability and attention problems. Eye movement disorders may even interfere with the ability of the patient to perform well during vision information processing testing. Pursuit problems may play a significant role in activities of daily living such as driving and sports and any other activities in which the individual is moving or the object of regard is moving.

Summary

Visual efficiency problems are highly prevalent in the populations served by occupational therapists. The possible effects on a patient's performance are very significant, and if left uncorrected, visual efficiency problems will interfere with progress in occupational therapy. In spite of the significance of visual efficiency problems, they are often undetected even after a professional eye examination. If these problems are suspected, it is incumbent upon occupational therapists to make a referral to an eye care professional who will perform the type of testing battery that can detect these disorders.

References

1. Scheiman M, Wick B. *Clinical Management of Binocular Vision: Heterophoric, Accommodative and Eye Movement Disorders.* 5th ed. Philadelphia, PA: Wolters-Kluwer; 2019.
2. Brookman KE. Ocular Accommodation in human infants. *Am J Optom Physiol Opt.* 1980;60:91–95.
3. Scheiman M, Gallaway M, Coulter R, et al. Prevalence of vision and ocular disease conditions in a clinical pediatric population. *J Am Optom Assoc.* 1996;67:193–202.
4. Hokoda SC. General binocular dysfunctions in an urban optometry clinic. *J Am Optom Assoc.* 1985;56:560–562.
5. Suchoff IB, Kapoor N, Waxman R, Ference W. The occurrence of ocular and visual dysfunctions in an acquired brain-injured patient sample. *J Am Optom Assoc.* 1999;70:301–308.
6. Goodrich GL, Kirby J, Cockerham G, et al. Visual function in patients of a polytrauma rehabilitation center: a descriptive study. *J Rehabil Res Dev.* 2007;44:929–936.
7. Brahm KD, Wilgenburg HM, Kirby J, et al. Visual impairment and dysfunction in combat-injured servicemembers with traumatic brain injury. *Optom Vis Sci.* 2009;86:817–825.
8. Stelmack JA, Frith T, Van Koevering D, et al. Visual function in patients followed at a veterans affairs polytrauma network site: an electronic medical record review. *Optometry* 2009;80:419–424.
9. Ciuffreda KJ, Kapoor N, Rutner D, et al. Occurrence of oculomotor dysfunctions in acquired brain injury: a retrospective analysis. *Optometry.* 2007;78:155–161.
10. Capo-Aponte JE, Jorgensen-Wagers KL, Sosa JA, et al. Visual dysfunctions at different stages after blast and non-blast mild traumatic brain injury. *Optom Vis Sci.* 2017;94:7–15.

11. Krohel GB, Kristan RW, Simon KW, Barrows N. Posttraumatic convergence insufficiency. *Ann Ophthalmol.* 1986;18:101–104.

12. Pratt-Johnson JA, Tillson G. Acquired central disruption of fusional amplitude. *Ophthalmol.* 1979;86:2140.

13. Padula WV, Shapiro JB, Jasin P. Head injury causing post trauma vision syndrome. *New Eng J Optom.* 1988:16–21.

14. Harrison RJ. Loss of fusional vergence with partial loss of accommodative convergence and accommodation following head injury. *Bin Vis.* 1987;2:93–100.

15. Cohen M, Groswasser Z, Barchadski R, Appel A. Convergence insufficiency in brain-injured patients. *Brain Injury.* 1989;3:187–191.

16. Solomons H. *Binocular Vision. A Programmed Text.* London: Heinemann; 1978.

17. Birch EE, Gwiazda J, Held R. Stereoacuity development for crossed and uncrossed disparities in human infants. *Vision Res.* 1982;22:507–513.

18. Warren M. Identification of visual scanning deficits in adults after cerebrovascular accident. *Am J Occup Ther.* 1990;44:391–399.

19. Rayner K. Eye movements in reading and information processing. *Psych Bull.* 1978;85:618–660.

20. Zangwill OL, Blakewell C. Dyslexia: reversal of eye movements during reading. *Neuropsychologica* 1972;10:371–373.

21. Rubino CA, Minden H. An analysis of eye movements in children with a reading disability. *Cortex.* 1973;9:217–220.

22. Griffin DC. Saccades as Related to reading disorders. *J Learn Disab.* 1974;7:50–58.

23. Goldrich SG, Sedgwick H. An objective comparison of oculomotor functioning in reading disabled and normal children. *Am J Optom Physiol Optics.* 1982;59:82P.

24. Raymond JE, Ogden NA, Fagan JE, et al. Fixational stability in dyslexic children. *Am J Optom Physiol Opt.* 1982;65:174–179.

25. Jones A, Stark L. Abnormal patterns of normal eye movements in specific dyslexia. In: Rayner K, ed. *Eye Movements in Reading: Perceptual and Language Processes.* New York, NY: Academic Press; 1983:481–498.

26. Pavlidis GT. Eye movement differences between dyslexics, normal, and retarded readers while sequentially fixating digits. *Am J Optom Physiol Optics.* 1985;62:820–832.

27. Pavlidis GT. Eye movements in dyslexia: diagnostic significance. *J Learn Disabil.* 1985;18:42.

28. Flax N. Problems in relating visual function to reading disorder. *Am J Optom Arch Am Acad Optom.* 1970;47:366–372.

29. Ludlam WM, Twarowsk IC, Ludlam DP. Optometric visual training for reading disability – a case report. *Am J Optom Arch Am Acad Optom.* 1973;50:58–66.

30. Heath EJ, Cook P, O'Dell N. Eye exercises and reading efficiency. *Acad Ther.* 1976;11:435–445.

31. Pierce JR. Is there a relationship between vision therapy and academic achievement? *Rev Optom.* 1977;114:48–63.

32. Getz D. Learning enhancement through vision therapy. *Acad Ther.* 1980;15(4):457–466.

33. Adler-Grinberg D, Stark L. Eye movements, scanpaths, and dyslexia. *Am J Optom Physiol Optics.* 1978; 55:557–570.

34. Brown B, Haegerstrom Portney G, Adams A, et al. Predictive eye movements do not discriminate between dyslexic and control children. *Neuropsychologica.* 1983;21:121–128.

35. Olson RK, Kliegl R, Davidson BJ. Dyslexic and normal readers eye movements. *J Exp Psychol Hum Percep Perform.* 1983;9:816–825.

36. Stanley G, Smith GA, Howell EA. Eye movements and sequential tracking in dyslexic and control children. *Brit J Psych.* 1983;74:181–187.

37. Black JL, Collins DWK, De Roach JN, Zubrick SR. A detailed study of sequential eye movements for normal and poor reading children. *Percept Motor Skills.* 1984;59:423–434.

38. Grisham D, Simons H. Perspectives on reading disabilities. In: Rosenbloom AA, Morgan MW, ed. *Pediatric Optometry.* Philadelphia, PA: Lippincott; 1990:518–559.

39. Garzia RP, Richman JE, Nicholson SB, Gaines CS. A new visual verbal saccade test: the Developmental Eye Movement test (DEM). *J Am Optom Assoc.* 1990;61:124–135.

40. Richman JE. Use of a sustained visual attention task to determine children at risk for learning problems. *J Am Optom Assoc.* 1986;57:20–27.

41. Simon MJ. Use of a vigilance task to determine school readiness in preschool children. *Percept Motor Skills.* 1982;54:1020–1022.

42. Warren M. A hierarchical model for evaluation and treatment of visual perceptual dysfunction in adult acquired brain injury, part 2. *Am J Occup Ther.* 1993;47:55–66.

43. Schlageter K, Gray B, Hall K, et al. Incidence and treatment of visual dysfunction in traumatic brain injury. *Brain Inj.* 1993;7:439–448.

44. Bouska MJ, Gallaway M. Primary visual field deficits in adults with brain damage: management in occupational therapy. *Occup Ther Pract.* 1991;3:1–11.

45. Baker RS, Epstein AD. Ocular motor abnormalities from head trauma. *Surv Ophthalmol.* 1991;35:245–267.

46. Strano CM. Effects of visual deficits on ability to drive in traumatically brain injured population. *J Head Trauma Rehabil.* 1989;4:35–43.

47. Sherman A. Relating vision disorder's to learning disability. *J Am Optom Assoc.* 1973; 44:140–141.

48. Hoffman LG. Incidence of vision difficulties in children with learning disabilities. *J Am Optom Assoc.* 1980;51:447–451.

49. Higgins JD. Oculomotor system. In: Barresi B, ed. *Ocular Assessment.* Boston, MA: Butterworth; 1984.

50. Leigh RJ, Zee DS. *The Neurology of Eye Movement.* Philadelphia, PA: FA Davis Co; 1983.

51. Maples WC, Ficklin TW. Interrater and test retest reliability of pursuits and saccades. *J Am Optom Assoc.* 1988;59:549–552.

52. Richman JE, Walker AJ, Garzia RP. The impact of automatic digit naming ability on a clinical test of eye movement functioning. *J Am Optom Assoc.* 1983;54:617–622.

53. Benjamin WJ, Borish IM. *Borish's Clinical Refraction.* St. Louis, MO: WB Saunders; 1998.

54. Rouse MW, Ryan J. Clinical examination in children. In: Rosenbloom AA, Morgan MW, eds. *Pediatric Optometry.* Philadelphia, PA: Lippincott; 1990.

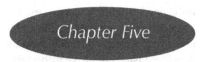

Chapter Five

Three Component Model of Vision, Part Three
Visual Information Processing Skills

Mitchell Scheiman

Visual Information Processing Skills

Visual information processing, or visual perception, is an area in which both occupational therapy and optometry are actively involved. The goal of this chapter, therefore, is not to teach occupational therapists how to evaluate visual information processing skills. Most occupational therapists already evaluate and treat such problems. Rather, this chapter is designed to help the occupational therapist better understand the way optometrists think about and evaluate visual information processing skills. I believe that most occupational therapists will recognize some differences as well as similarities between the approach presented in this chapter and their own clinical practice. As we learn more about these differences and similarities, we will be able to work together more effectively for the benefit of our patients.

Definition and General Concepts

A vision problem could still be present even if an individual has good visual acuity; no refractive error or eye health disorder; and normal accommodation, binocular vision, and ocular motility. Vision is more than just seeing clearly and comfortably. An individual must also be able to analyze, interpret, and make use of the incoming visual information in order to interact with the environment. We refer to this final aspect of our three-part model as visual information processing. Visual information processing refers to a group of visual cognitive skills used for extracting and organizing visual information from the environment and integrating this information with other sensory modalities and higher cognitive functions.[1] Other terms such as *visual perception*, *visual perceptual-motor*, and *visual processing* have been used to describe similar skills.

Visual processing involves the ability to extract and select information from the environment. So much information reaches the visual system that a selection process must occur. The person must select the incoming information that is most relevant to the task they are performing. This selection is dependent on prior experience and development.[2] Once information is extracted or selected from the environment, meaning has to be attached to the visual stimuli. This process involves a complex interaction between visual processing and cognitive factors that are

DOI: 10.4324/9781003526841-5

influenced by past experiences, motivation, and development.[1] In the model presented in this chapter, perception and cognition are considered overlapping concepts that influence each other in the processing of visual information and are not seen as distinct entities. Essentially, perception provides visual cognitive information that is used in higher-order cognitive functions. As a result, the term *visual information processing* is used to describe the visual processing skills evaluated by optometrists.[1]

The model presented in this book is based on an approach recommended by Scheiman and Rouse.[3] This model divides visual information processing into three components: visual spatial, visual analysis, and visual motor. Each of these components relates to specific skills an individual could perform.

VISUAL SPATIAL SKILLS: DEFINITION AND DESCRIPTION

These skills allow the individual to develop normal internal and external spatial concepts and are used to interact with and organize the environment. They allow the individual to make judgments about location of objects in visual space in reference to other objects and to the individual's own body. Visual spatial skills develop from an awareness within the individual's body of concepts such as left and right, up and down, and front and back. Visual spatial skills are important for the development of good motor coordination, balance, and directional senses when reading and writing. Component skills include bilateral integration, laterality, and directionality.

Bilateral Integration

Bilateral integration is the ability to be aware of and use both sides of the body separately and simultaneously.

Laterality

Laterality is the ability to be internally aware of and identify right and left on one's self.

Directionality

Directionality is the ability of the individual to interpret right and left directions in three separate components of external space.

VISUAL ANALYSIS SKILLS: DEFINITION AND DESCRIPTION

These skills contribute to the individual's ability to analyze and discriminate visually presented information, to determine the whole without seeing all of the parts, to identify more important features and ignore extraneous details, and to use visual imagery to recall past visual information. Visual analysis skills include the ability of the child to be aware of the distinctive features of visual forms, including shape, size, color, and orientation. Early in life, a child uses visual analysis skills to recognize familiar faces, toys, or objects in the house. As the child approaches preschool age, they begin using visual analysis skills to analyze and comprehend more abstract shapes, such as the visual symbols we use to represent sounds and quantities. These analysis skills represent one of the basic foundational skills that enable a child to learn to recognize letters, numbers, and eventually whole words. These skills are also important for the development of math concepts.

Clinically, we subclassify visual spatial dysfunction into four categories: visual discrimination, visual figure ground, visual closure, and visual memory and visualization.

Visual Discrimination

This is the ability of the child to be aware of the distinctive features of forms, including shape, orientation, size, and color.

Visual Figure Ground

This is the ability of the child to attend to a specific feature or form while maintaining an awareness of the relationship of this form to the background information.

Visual Closure

This is the ability of the child to be aware of clues in the visual stimulus that allow them to determine the final percept without the necessity of having all the details present. In reading, for example, visual closure allows us to perceive an entire word accurately when we may only have seen part of the word.

Visual Memory and Visualization

This is the ability of the child to recognize and recall visually presented information. Spelling requires recall of visual information, as does word recognition in reading when we try to match the word on the page with an image that is stored in the brain. Visualization, or the ability to mentally manipulate a visual image, is important in reading comprehension and math.

VISUAL MOTOR SKILLS: DEFINITION AND DESCRIPTION

These skills are related to the individual's ability to integrate visual information processing skills with fine motor movement. Another term for visual motor integration is eye-hand coordination. A very concrete example of a task requiring eye-hand coordination is catching a ball. A child must make a number of visual judgments about the ball, including speed and direction, and then translate the visual judgments into appropriate motor responses of their hand and body. If the visual motor integration is accurate, the child will catch the ball.

Handwriting is a more abstract and higher-level example of visual motor integration. As a child begins to write a letter, no external stimulus guides their hand. Rather, they must use their "mind's eye" to guide their hand in the desired direction and pattern. As the written product emerges, the child must continuously use visual analysis skills to judge whether the shape or size of the letter is appropriate. They must also use fine motor skills to manipulate the pencil. If they can accurately integrate (or combine) their visual analysis skills and fine motor skills, the desired letter will be successfully completed. Thus, visual motor skills are a necessary prerequisite for learning good handwriting and keyboard skills as well as throwing and catching a ball.

The two subskills in this category are visual motor integration and fine motor coordination.

Visual Motor Integration Skills

These skills are related to the individual's ability to integrate visual information processing skills with fine motor movement.

Fine Motor Coordination Skills

These skills are related to the ability to manipulate small objects or a pencil or pen.

Clinical Assessment of Visual Information Processing Skills

The assessment battery includes tests to evaluate the three diagnostic categories described above and is based on the testing approach recommended by Scheiman and Rouse.[3] Although this is a popular approach used by many optometrists, it is important to understand that visual information processing or visual perceptual motor anomalies can be assessed and subclassified in many ways. If the reader is interested in full details about these tests, references and addresses are provided in Appendix A.

The testing approach described below makes extensive use of standardized objective tests. Standardized objective testing has several important characteristics:

* Subjective judgments by the clinician are minimized, although not excluded.
* Testing is performed in a uniform way, and theoretically every trained observer would achieve the same result.
* Scoring follows specific rules, and performance is compared to normative data.

Using standardized testing, we can more confidently know what we are measuring, and we are better able to communicate our results to other professionals. For the less experienced clinician or for students learning to evaluate visual information processing for the first time, these characteristics are highly desirable. While experienced clinicians can sometimes make meaningful decisions about visual information processing simply by watching the patient in an unstructured task, less experienced clinicians are unable to do so.

There is evidence that even an experienced clinician's subjective and intuitive judgments may not always be reliable or valid.[4] Solan and Groffman[4] state, "There will always be some persons whose quality of judgment enables them to make more accurate estimates than others. Unfortunately, there are also persons who tend to utilize intuitive judgments based on inadequate data and whose conclusions are not accurate." The use of standardized objective testing eliminates this problem.

The case history helps direct the evaluation of the child with learning problems. Children with visual information processing disorders present with a characteristic case history. Specific signs and symptoms also suggest problems in certain aspects of visual information processing. Table 5.1 lists the various diagnostic categories along with their characteristic signs and symptoms. If a patient presents with a chief complaint of difficulty with handwriting and copying skills, for

---

Table 5.1

Visual Information Processing Problems:
Symptoms and Effect on Performance

Visual Spatial Dysfunction

- Poor athletic performance
- Difficulty with rhythmic activities
- Lack of coordination and balance
- Clumsy, falls and bumps into things often
- Tendency to work with one side of the body while the other side does not participate
- Difficulty learning left and right
- Reverses letters and numbers when writing or copying
- Writes from right to left

Visual Analysis Dysfunction

- Has trouble learning the alphabet, recognizing words, and learning basic math concepts of size, magnitude, and position
- Confuses likenesses and minor differences
- Mistakes words with similar beginnings
- Cannot recognize the same word repeated on a page
- Cannot recognize letters or simple forms
- Cannot distinguish the main idea from insignificant details
- Overgeneralizes when classifying objects
- Has trouble writing and remembering letters and numbers

Visual Motor Dysfunction

- Difficulty copying from the board
- Sloppy drawing or writing skills
- Poor spacing and inability to stay on lines
- Erases excessively
- Can respond orally but not produce answers in writing
- Difficulty completing written assignments in allotted period of time
- Seems to know the material but does poorly on tests
- Difficulty writing numbers in columns for math problems

example, the most likely clinical hypothesis would be a visual motor integration problem as indicated in Table 5.1. A problem with reversals and learning left and right would suggest a clinical hypothesis of a visual spatial problem. Although knowledge of the symptoms and signs of the various diagnostic categories may allow the clinician to predict the results of the evaluation, we still recommend evaluation of all three areas discussed below.

VISUAL SPATIAL SKILLS

Component skills in this category include bilateral integration, laterality, and directionality. Tests are used to probe each one of these areas.

Evaluation of Bilateral Integration

Standing Angels in the Snow (for 3- to 8-year-olds). This test probes the child's ability to be aware of and use both sides of the body separately and simultaneously. The examiner sits and the child stands directly in front of the examiner. The examiner's legs should be separated so that the child is standing midway between them (Figure 5.1). The examiner asks the child to make a very specific series of arm and leg movements. The movements range from very simple to complex. It is important for the examiner to not only observe if the correct movements are made, but also to watch for motor overflow, inappropriate movement, and other indications of performance breakdowns.

Evaluation of Laterality

Piaget Test of Left-Right Concepts (for 5- to 11-year-olds). This test evaluates the child's ability to differentiate right from left on their own body (laterality), on another person, and on the location of objects in space (directionality). The examiner and child sit in chairs facing each other, and the examiner asks the child a series of questions designed to probe their knowledge of right and left. The questions asked are listed in Table 5.2.

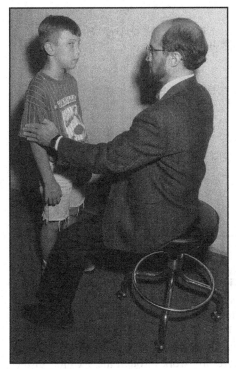

Figure 5.1. For the Standing Angels in the Snow test, the examiner sits, and the child stands directly in front of the examiner.

Table 5.2

Piaget Test of Left-Right Concepts: Questions Asked

Section A

Subject's body parts: Ask the child the following questions and record the responses:
- Show me your right hand.
- Show me your left leg.
- Touch your left ear.
- Show me your left hand.
- Show me your right leg.
- Point to your right eye.

Section B

Examiner's body parts: Sit opposite the child.
- Show me my left hand.
- Point to my right ear.
- Show me my left leg.
- Show me my right hand.
- Point to my left ear.
- Show me my right leg.

Section C

Place a coin on the table to the left of a pencil in relation to the child.
- Is the pencil to the right or to the left of the coin?
- Is the coin to the right or to the left of the pencil?

Now have the child walk around to the opposite side of the table.
- Is the pencil to the right or to the left of the coin?
- Is the coin to the right or to the left of the pencil?

Section D

Sit opposite the child with a coin in your right hand and a watch or bracelet on your left arm.
- Do you see this coin? Do I have it in my right hand or my left hand?
- Is this bracelet on my right arm or my left arm?

Section E

Place three objects in front of the child: A pencil to the left, a key in the middle, and a penny to the right.
- Is the pencil to the left or to the right of the key?
- Is the pencil to the left or to the right of the penny?
- Is the key to the left or to the right of the penny?
- Is the key to the left or to the right of the pencil?
- Is the penny to the left or to the right of the pencil?
- Is the penny to the left or to the right of the key?

Evaluation of Directionality

The Gardner Reversal Frequency Test: Recognition Subtest (for 5- to 15-year-olds). This test consists of three subtests that assess different aspects of directionality. We include two of the three tests in our test battery. This test evaluates the existence, nature, and frequency of occurrence of receptive letter and number reversals (reversals that the patient can recognize). In this test, the patient is asked to mark off those letters and numbers that are written backward or reversed (Figure 5.2). Once seated properly, the patient is asked to carefully work through the six lines of the

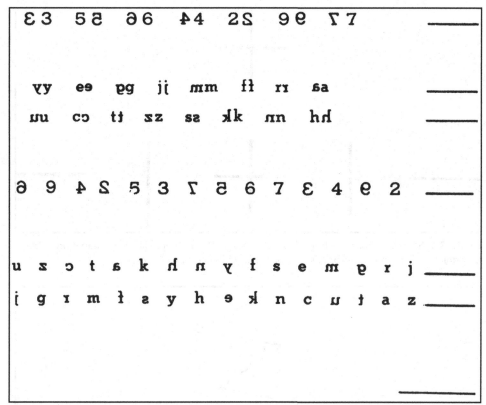

Figure 5.2. For the Gardner Reversal Frequency Test: Recognition Subtest, the child is asked to mark off those letters and numbers that are written backward or reversed.

test worksheet and cross out the numbers or letters that appear backward. The test is untimed, and the patient is allowed to erase. Nevertheless, it is important for the examiner to observe and take into consideration the amount of time it takes and the ease with which the patient completes this task. For example, if one 7-year-old patient completes the test in 2 minutes with five errors and a second patient completes the test in 8 minutes with five errors, certainly the qualitative difference in performance must be noted.

Gardner Reversal Frequency Test: Execution Subtest (for 5- to 15-year-olds). This test evaluates the existence, nature, and frequency of occurrence of expressive letter and number reversals (reversals that the patient actually makes during a writing task). In this test, the patient is asked to write letters and numbers as they are dictated. As with the recognition subtest, it is important to seat the patient so that they cannot observe books and other written material that may provide information about letter and number orientation. Give the patient a pencil with an eraser, place the test sheet in front of them, and ask them to print the numbers and letters you dictate. These numbers and letters are dictated one by one, and there is no time limit to this test. The letters must be reproduced as lowercase letters.

As with the recognition subtest, it is important to remember that although the test is untimed, the amount of time and ease with which the patient performs this task may suggest qualitative differences in performance that are important in diagnosis and treatment.

VISUAL ANALYSIS SKILLS

Clinically, we subclassify visual analysis dysfunction into four categories: visual discrimination, visual closure, visual figure ground, and visual memory.

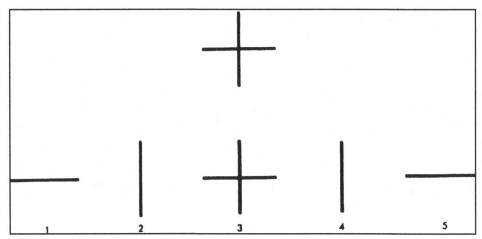

Figure 5.3. Sample of stimulus from the Test of Visual Perceptual Skills: Discrimination Subtest. (Reprinted with permission from Psychological and Educational Publications Inc.)

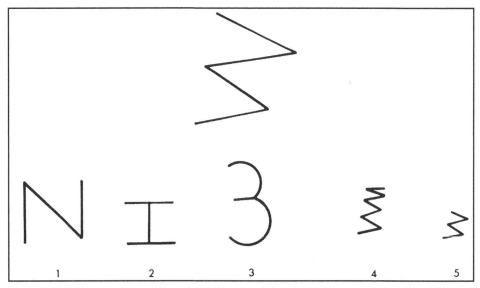

Figure 5.4. Sample of stimulus from the Test of Visual Perceptual Skills: Form Constancy Subtest. (Reprinted with permission from Psychological and Educational Publications Inc.)

Evaluation of Visual Discrimination

Test of Visual Perceptual Skills: Discrimination, Form Constancy, and Spatial Relationships (for 4-year-old to adult level). These three subtests evaluate the ability of the patient to be aware of the distinctive features of forms, including shape, orientation, and size. The three subtests are identical in their construction, administration, and scoring. Each test is made up of 16 different plates with stimuli that become more complex. Figures 5.3 through 5.5 are illustrations of one of the early stimuli used in each of these tests. The patient must choose the matching figure from among five choices.

Evaluation of Visual Closure

Test of Visual Perceptual Skills: Visual Closure (for 4-year-old to adult level). This subtest evaluates the ability of the patient to be aware of clues in the visual stimulus that allow them to

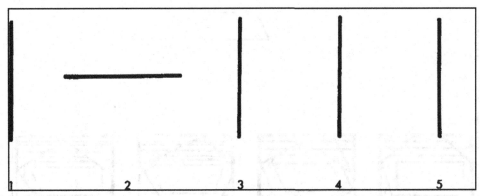

Figure 5.5. Sample of stimulus from the Test of Visual Perceptual Skills: Spatial Relationships Subtest. (Reprinted with permission from Psychological and Educational Publications Inc.)

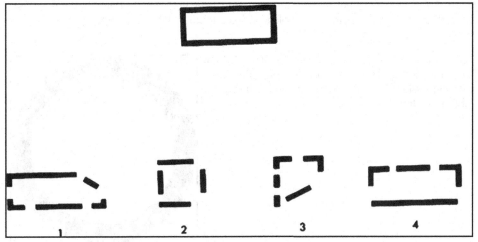

Figure 5.6. Sample of stimulus from the Test of Visual Perceptual Skills: Visual Closure Subtest. (Reprinted with permission from Psychological and Educational Publications Inc.)

determine the final percept without the necessity of having all the details present. The test is made up of 16 different plates with stimuli that become more complex. Figure 5.6 is an illustration of one of the early stimuli used in this test. The patient is asked to look at the picture on top and to find the one that would look like the top form if the lines were connected or completed.

Evaluation of Visual Figure Ground

Test of Visual Perceptual Skills: Figure Ground (for 4-year-old to adult level). This subtest evaluates the ability of the patient to attend to a specific feature or form while maintaining an awareness of the relationship of this form to the background information. The test is made up of 16 different plates with stimuli that become more complex. Figure 5.7 is an illustration of one of the early stimuli used in this test. The patient is asked to look at the picture on top and to find the exact form from among the forms below.

Evaluation of Visual Memory

Test of Visual Perceptual Skills: Visual Memory (for 4-year-old to adult level). This subtest evaluates the ability of the patient to recognize and recall visually presented information. The test is made up of 16 different plates with stimuli that become more complex. Figure 5.8a is an

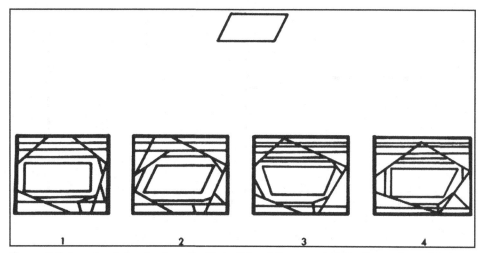

Figure 5.7. Sample of stimulus from the Test of Visual Perceptual Skills: Figure Ground Subtest. (Reprinted with permission from Psychological and Educational Publications Inc.)

Figure 5.8a. Sample of stimulus from the Test of Visual Perceptual Skills: Visual Memory Subtest. (Reprinted with permission from Psychological and Educational Publications Inc.)

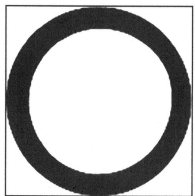

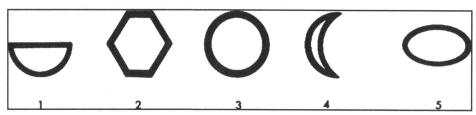

Figure 5.8b. Sample of stimulus from the Test of Visual Perceptual Skills: Visual Memory Subtest. (Reprinted with permission from Psychological and Educational Publications Inc.)

illustration of one of the early stimuli used in this test. The patient is asked to look at an isolated picture for 5 seconds. After the stimulus is removed, they are asked to select the one that looks the same from among five choices (Figure 5.8b).

Test of Visual Perceptual Skills: Visual Sequential Memory (for 4- to 13-year-olds). This subtest evaluates the ability of the patient to recognize and recall visually presented information when sequence is important, such as in spelling. The test is made up of 16 different plates with stimuli that become more complex. Figure 5.9a is an illustration of one of the early stimuli used in this

Figure 5.9a. Sample of stimulus from the Test of Visual Perceptual Skills: Visual Sequential Memory Subtest. (Reprinted with permission from Psychological and Educational Publications Inc.)

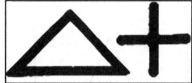

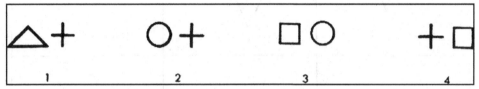

Figure 5.9b. Sample of stimulus from the Test of Visual Perceptual Skills: Visual Sequential Memory Subtest. (Reprinted with permission from Psychological and Educational Publications Inc.)

test. The patient is asked to look at a series of pictures for 5 seconds. After the stimulus is removed, they are asked to select the one that has the same sequence from among four choices (Figure 5.9b).

VISUAL MOTOR INTEGRATION SKILLS

The two subskills in this category are visual motor integration and fine motor coordination.

Evaluation of Visual Motor Integration

Developmental Test of Visual Motor Integration (Beery) (for 4- to 18-year-olds). This test evaluates the patient's ability to integrate visual information processing and fine motor skills by assessing their ability to accurately copy a visual stimulus. The patient is presented with pictures of increasing complexity and is asked to reproduce the pictures as accurately as possible. Figure 5.10 is a sample of some of the forms used in this test. To score the test, clinicians must use the very detailed scoring criteria included in the scoring manual.

Wold Sentence Copy Test (for school-aged children). This test evaluates the patient's fine motor and visual motor integration skills. The Wold Sentence Copy Test is a timed test used to determine a patient's speed and accuracy in copying a sentence from the top to the bottom of a page (Figure 5.11). The test is comparable to a common school task of copying from a book to a notebook and provides the clinician with a sample of the patient's handwriting skill.

To administer this test, the test is placed in front of the patient, and the patient is told to copy the sentence on the blank lines on the bottom of the test sheet. The patient is instructed to go as fast as they can, but to be as neat as possible.

Evaluation of Fine Motor Skills

Grooved Pegboard Test (for kindergarten to fifth-grade children). This test evaluates the patient's fine motor skills. Other skills that are indirectly evaluated are visual attention, concentration, and directionality. The test requires the patient to place pegs in a pegboard as quickly as possible (Figure 5.12). Prior to administration of the test, hand dominance is established by asking questions about how the patient brushes their teeth, hammers a nail, cuts with a pair of scissors, writes with a pencil, and throws a ball. The examiner tries to establish which hand is used for these activities. The dominant hand is the one that is used for the majority of the tasks.

Once the dominant hand is determined, the patient is told to place the pegs in the holes by matching the groove of the peg to the groove of the hole. Let the patient try the first row to demonstrate that they understand the task. Once they understand the task, ask the patient to place all of the pegs in the holes as quickly as possible.

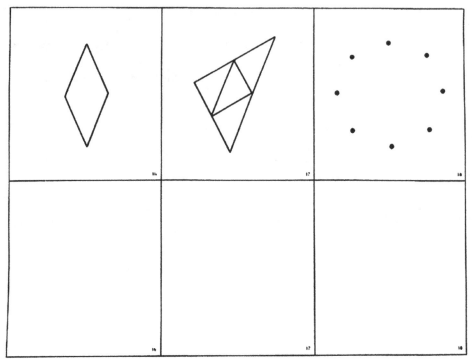

Figure 5.10. Developmental Test of Visual Motor Integration by Keith E. Beery and Norman A. Buktenica. © 1989 Modern Curriculum Press. (Reprinted with permission from Simon and Schuster Elementary.)

Figure 5.11. The Wold Sentence Copy Test is a timed test used to determine a child's speed and accuracy in copying a sentence.

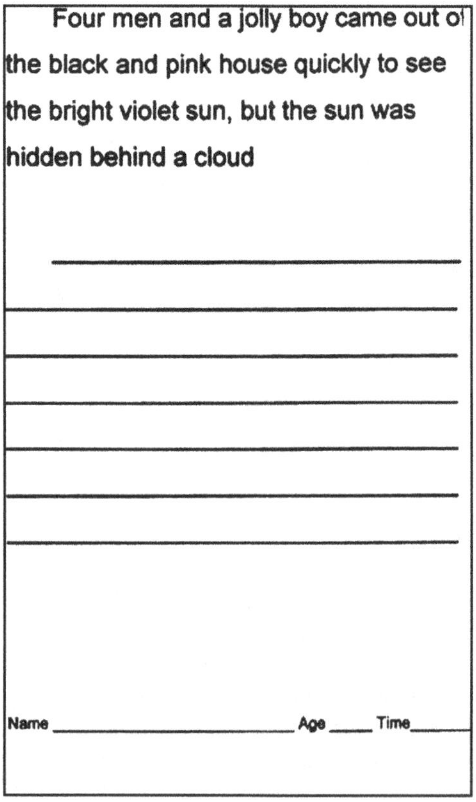

Four men and a jolly boy came out of the black and pink house quickly to see the bright violet sun, but the sun was hidden behind a cloud

Name _____ Age ____ Time____

Figure 5.12. Grooved Pegboard Test used to evaluate a child's fine motor skills.

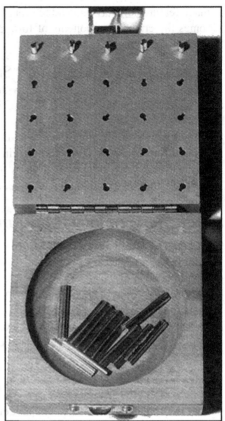

Development of Visual Information Processing Skills

The rate of development of visual processing skills is not uniform during infancy, preschool, and school-aged years. In the early years, the rate of development is more rapid than that seen in the later years. The difference between a 4-year-old child and a 5-year-old child is much greater than the difference between a 12-year-old child and a 13-year-old child.[1] This is important when comparing performance among different age groups, because a 1-year delay at 5 years of age is much more significant than a 1-year delay at 13 years of age.

VISUAL SPATIAL SKILLS

These skills allow the individual to develop normal internal and external spatial concepts and are used to interact with and organize the environment. Preschool children who are 3 to 4 years of age can correctly identify front and back and up and down on themselves and on objects.[5] The correct identification of right and left on self is usually seen at 6 to 7 years of age,[5,6] and identification of right and left directions on objects in space develops between 7 and 12 years of age.[5,6]

Reversal of letters and numbers is a common finding in children just entering school. These errors should decline in frequency, and most reversals should cease by the middle of the second grade.[7]

VISUAL ANALYSIS SKILLS

The development of form perception and discrimination in infants and young children has been extensively studied. Research indicates that face recognition, size, and shape consistency are present by 6 months.[8–10] Even though infants possess many of the basic form perception skills, they are unable to use them efficiently. During the preschool- and school-aged years, the ability to make feature comparisons and to search and explore patterns in a complete and systematic way becomes the crucial components of form perception development.[1] The ability to efficiently use these form perception skills probably does not reach adult levels until early adolescence.[1]

VISUAL MOTOR INTEGRATION SKILLS

These skills are related to the individual's ability to integrate visual information processing skills with fine motor movement. These skills begin in early infancy. White and Held[11] found that infants begin swiping with a closed fist at objects at about 2 to 3 months of age. By 5 months, the infant is able to integrate the eye and the hand. During the preschool years, the use of visual motor skills to reproduce visual form begins to develop. The first attempts at drawing usually occur around 1½ to 2 years of age. At 3 years of age, a child can draw a circle; at 4½ years of age, a square; at 5 to 5½ years of age, a triangle; and at 8 years of age, a diamond.[12]

Significance of Visual Information Processing Skills for Occupational Therapy

Table 5.1 provides a summary of the significance of visual information processing skills for occupational therapy. The effect of these problems on occupational therapy will obviously be directly related to the demand the activity places on visual information processing skills. Visual information processing problems will have the greatest effect when the patient must make decisions about directional orientation, if the task involves symbol and word recognition, matching of shapes, visual memory, visualization, and copying of visual stimuli.

Summary

Of the three components in our model of vision, visual information processing disorders are the most likely to be neglected by eye care professionals. In my experience, these problems are rarely found in isolation. It is more common for there to be a combination of visual efficiency and visual information processing disorders. It is important for occupational therapists to realize that normal visual information processing or visual perceptual function depends on normal visual acuity and visual efficiency. This hierarchical relationship has been discussed in both the optometric[3] and occupational therapy literature.[13,14] Warren[13] and Bouska et al.[14] have developed models that emphasize this point. They discuss the importance of detecting and treating ocular motor, accommodative, and binocular vision disorders before the management of visual processing disorders. This is why it is so critical that occupational therapists have a comprehensive understanding of all aspects of all three components of the model of vision presented in this book.

References

1. Borsting E. Overview of visual and visual processing development. In: Scheiman M, Rouse MW, eds. *Optometric Management of Learning Related Vision Problems*. 2nd ed. St. Louis, MO: CV Mosby; 2006:35–68.
2. Blankenship E. A first primer in visual perception. *J Learn Disabil*. 1971;10:39–42.
3. Scheiman M, Rouse MW. *Optometric Management of Learning Related Vision Problems*. 2nd ed. St. Louis, MO: CV Mosby; 2006.
4. Solan HA, Groffman S. Understanding and treating developmental and perceptual motor disabilities. In: Solan HA, ed. *The Treatment and Management of Children With Learning Disabilities*. Springfield, IL: Charles C. Thomas; 1982.
5. Ilg FL, Ames LB. *School Readiness*. New York, NY: Harper & Row; 1972:159–189.
6. Laurendeau M, Pinard A. *The Development of the Concept of Space in the Child*. New York, NY: International Universities Press; 1970:278–309.
7. Gardner RA. *The Objective Diagnosis of Minimal Brain Dysfunction*. Cresskill, NJ: Creative Therapeutics; 1979.
8. Fantz RL, Fagen JF, Miranda SB. Early visual selectivity. In: Cohen LB, Salapatek P, eds. *Infant Perception: From Sensation to Cognition*. New York, NY: Academic Press; 1975.

9. Fagen JF. Infant's recognition of invariant features of faces. *Child Dev.* 1976;47:627–638.
10. Goldstein EB. *Sensation and Perception.* Belmont, CA: Wadsworth Publishing; 1989:333–337.
11. White BL, Held R. Observations on the development of visually directed reaching. In: Hellmuth J, ed. *Exceptional Infant.* Seattle, WA: Special Child Publications; 1967.
12. Beery KE. *The Developmental Test of Visual Motor Integration.* Cleveland, OH: Modern Curriculum Press; 1982.
13. Warren M. Identification of visual scanning deficits in adults after cerebrovascular accident. *Am J Occup Ther.* 1990;44:391–399.
14. Bouska MJ, Kauffman NA, Marcus SE. Disorders of the visual perceptual system. In: Umphred DA, Jewell MJ, eds. *Neurological Rehabilitation.* St. Louis, MO: CV Mosby; 1985:552–585.

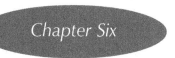

Chapter Six

Screening for Visual Acuity, Visual Efficiency, and Visual Information Processing Problems

Mitchell Scheiman

In the first five chapters, I have tried to establish the importance of vision and the various ways in which vision can possibly interfere with occupational therapy progress. It is critical that an occupational therapist be aware of the characteristics of the visual system of any patient they are treating. Ideally, this information should be readily available before treatment begins. In most cases, however, no information or very limited information will be available. In a school system, the child may have been screened in the past by the school nurse. School screenings generally consist of only a test to screen for visual acuity problems, myopia, and high degrees of hyperopia and astigmatism. Early day care centers will often have medical records available that may include a screening performed by the pediatrician. This will most often consist of only an evaluation of eye health. In a hospital setting, an ophthalmological consultation may occur before the occupational therapist treats a patient. Even if this has been done, it is very likely that the only aspects of the visual system that will have been tested will be visual acuity, refractive error, and eye health. Very little attention is paid to binocular vision, accommodation, eye movements, and visual fields in acute care or rehabilitation hospitals.[1–4] Gianutsos,[2] a well-respected researcher and clinician in the area of rehabilitation of acquired brain injury, states:

> *Generally, after brain injury, the visual system is not comprehensively evaluated, sometimes because there is a lack of articulated complaints due to impaired subjective experience or reduced cognition. Visual system evaluations are frequently neglected. Often referrals, if they are made at all, are made to ophthalmologists, reflecting the medical orientation of the delivery system. Ophthalmologists, however, are primarily concerned with the physiologic health of the eye. Important as this is for the survivor of brain trauma, further issues of concern for visual information processing pertain to the function of the full visual system.*

Thus, information about vision will be limited and, when available, may be incomplete. It is advantageous for an occupational therapist to be able to gather information about the three different aspects of vision covered in our model. This can be accomplished using a series of simple screening tests. While such a screening is not a substitute for a comprehensive examination by an

DOI: 10.4324/9781003526841-6

> **Table 6.1**
>
> ## Questions to Ask the Eye Doctor Before Referring a Patient
>
> - Do you have experience working with learning disabled children?
> - Do you have experience working with developmentally delayed, autistic, and physically impaired children?
> - Do you have experience working with patients with acquired brain injury?
> - Do you test accommodative amplitude and facility?
> - Do you evaluate fusional vergence amplitude and facility?
> - Do you evaluate visual information processing skills?
> - Do you offer vision therapy as a service in your practice?

---

optometrist, it can be helpful in establishing the need for such an examination. It also helps the therapist to plan their therapy program, taking vision into consideration. Because the prevalence of vision disorders is so high in the types of patients seen by occupational therapists, all patients should have a full vision examination before therapy begins. Remember that the absence of symptoms should not be the criterion for deciding whether or not to refer a patient for a vision evaluation. It is well established that patients who have experienced changes in their functional skills have difficulty accepting or acknowledging new and unwanted vision deficits or may actually be totally unaware of these changes. For example, partial visual field loss is rarely experienced for what it is by the patient. This failure to experience partial visual field loss has been termed the *completion effect*.[2]

When a referral for a comprehensive vision examination is made, it is critical that the doctor to whom the referral is made practices with a full appreciation of the complexity of vision. I suggest that therapists call eye doctors in their area and determine if the model of vision is comparable to that described in this book. Table 6.1 is a series of questions the therapist can ask the doctor before making a referral. If the eye doctor does not answer yes to each of these questions, I suggest looking elsewhere. Using this system, you will invariably find that the eye doctor to whom you refer patients will be an optometrist with some advanced education in vision therapy. A good resource is the College of Optometrists in Vision Development (COVD) directory of fellow and associate members. The address and phone number for the COVD are provided in Appendix A. COVD members are more likely than others to practice in a manner consistent with the philosophy described in this book.

Preliminary Issues

Age and Developmental Level of the Patient

A comprehensive vision evaluation can be successfully performed by an experienced optometrist regardless of the age, verbal skills, or cognitive level of the patient. To be successful, however, the examiner must have a great deal of experience with objective testing and specialized equipment. The screening battery described in this chapter will only be useful with patients functioning at about a 3-year-old level and above. The patient will have to interact with the therapist either verbally or nonverbally and will have to be able to attend for short periods of time. If the patient is unresponsive or inattentive, a vision screening may not be possible. That does not mean, however, that vision testing cannot be performed by an experienced optometrist. In virtually all cases, testing can be successfully accomplished. If you are unable to successfully perform a vision screening, it is wise to refer for a comprehensive vision evaluation.

Lighting

The room lighting is very important in all visual testing. The lighting does not have to be excessively bright, but the room should be well illuminated. It is important to eliminate glare and reflections off the stimuli that are being used.

Positioning

The posture of the patient during the screening is very important, and the therapist should ensure that patients with poor head, neck, or trunk control have appropriate support. For the visual screening, the patient should be positioned so that the head is vertically erect, if possible.

Glasses

If the patient wears glasses, the glasses should be used for the screening. When glasses are worn full-time by the patient, they should be used for all screening tasks. If the glasses are used only for a specific distance, such as near or far, they should be used for tests administered at the same distance. When a patient is wearing bifocal glasses, make sure that they look through the top portion for all distance testing and the bottom portion for all near testing.

Symptom Questionnaire

An important part of the screening is completion of the symptom questionnaire. Two sample questionnaires are included in this chapter. The first (Table 6.2) is useful for preschool- and school-aged children, and the second (Table 6.3) is designed for adults after acquired brain injury. In some cases, the patient can complete these questionnaires. In most situations, the therapist will

---

Table 6.2

Symptom Questionnaire: Children

Patient's full name: _____

Birthdate __/__/__ Date __/__/__   Age: _____

Please place a check mark next to any problem that seems to occur often for this child.

Signs of Tracking Problems

Loses place often
Must use finger or guide to keep place
Skips lines and words often
Poor reading comprehension
Short attention span

Signs of Eye Teaming Problems

Covers or closes one eye when reading
Rubs eyes
Child complains of eyestrain
Child complains of headaches
Child complains of double vision
Child complains of words moving on the page
Inattentive
Poor reading comprehension
Loses place

(continued)

Signs of Visual Processing Disorders
Trouble learning left from right
Reverses letters and numbers
Mistakes words with similar beginnings
Cannot recognize the same word repeated on a page
Trouble learning basic math concepts of size, magnitude
Poor reading comprehension
Poor recall of visually presented material
Trouble with spelling and sight vocabulary
Sloppy writing skills
Trouble copying from board to book
Erases excessively
Can respond orally but not in writing
Seems to know material but does poorly on written tests

Signs of Focusing Problems
Child complains of blurred vision
Child complains of blurred vision when looking from desk to board
Child complains of eyestrain
Child complains of headaches
Rubs eyes
Inattentive
Poor reading comprehension
Is tired at the end of the day
Holds things very close

Table 6.3

Symptom Questionnaire: Acquired Brain Injury

Patient's name _____

Date_____

General
- Do you wear glasses? Bifocals? Trifocals?
- Do your glasses work as well now as before the trauma, stroke?
- Do you have blurry vision? Is the difficulty at far or near?

Binocular Vision
- Do you ever see double? See overlapping or shadow images?
- Do you ever have to close one eye?
- Do you experience eyestrain, headaches when using your eyes?
- Do you have difficulty concentrating on tasks?

Accommodation
- Do you have trouble focusing from one distance to another?
- Do your eyes burn or water?
- Do you have difficulty concentrating on tasks?

Ocular Motility
- Do you find yourself losing your place or skipping words or lines when reading?
- Do you have difficulty following moving objects?
- Do letters jump around on the page while you are reading?

(continued)

Visual Fields
- Do you bump into chairs, objects?
- Do you have any difficulty seeing at night?
- Do you need to hold onto walls, objects, or people when walking?
- Do you ever find that when you reach for an object that you knock it over or your hand misses?
- Are portions of a page or any objects missing?
- Do people or things suddenly appear from one side that you didn't see approaching?

---

have to complete the questionnaire by talking with the patient, parent, and/or spouse; by observing the patient; and by reviewing the questions with others. Occasionally, a screening may not be possible due to age, attention, or cognitive problems. In such cases, the therapist can base their decision about referral for a comprehensive vision evaluation on the results of the symptom questionnaire.

Visual Acuity

Visual acuity is an important screening test. Reduced visual acuity may suggest the presence of significant degrees of myopia, astigmatism, or hyperopia and can help detect amblyopia. Near visual acuity testing is an indirect method of assessing accommodation. Visual acuity testing is particularly important in patients with acquired brain injury.

Distance Visual Acuity for Preverbal Children, Nonverbal Adults

Standard visual acuity testing with a letter or number eye chart cannot be used with this population. Instead, it is important to have a technique that does not require any verbal response from the patient. A number of tests have been developed that simply require a matching response. The test that I have found most useful for this population is the Lea Symbols Test. As illustrated in Figures 6.1a and 6.1b, the test consists of four easily recognizable symbols: a square, circle, house, and apple.

EQUIPMENT NEEDED
- #A2506 Single Symbol Book

   Vision Associates

   Phone: 815-669-0261

   https://visionkits.com/products/lea-products/lea-symbols/low-vision-book-2/

Figure 6.1a. Lea Symbols Book used to test preverbal children and nonverbal adults.

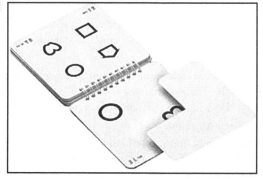

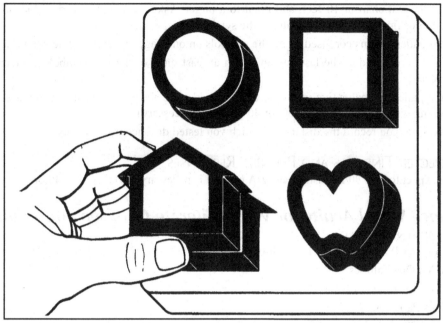

Figure 6.1b. Three-dimensional Lea Symbols Blocks used by a patient to match symbols on the test chart. (Reprinted with permission from Vision Associates, www.visionkits.com.)

SETUP AND TESTING STRATEGY

Typically when an optometrist assesses visual acuity, each eye is tested individually. In a routine optometric examination it is important to know if there is a difference between the two eyes. However, the purpose of visual acuity screening for an occupational therapist is different. The goal is to determine if there is a visual acuity problem with both eyes open that might be affecting the patient's ability to engage in various activities of daily living. It is not important to know if one eye is worse than the other. This will have minimal impact on activities of daily living. What is of primary importance is the visual acuity with both eyes together. Thus, for all of the following visual acuity tests the recommendation is to test with both eyes open.

When testing children or adults with cognitive and perceptual problems, it is wise to test at near before distance. It is easier to hold the patient's attention and teach the procedure at near than at far. It is helpful to create a play- or game-like situation with children. Before testing begins, it is also important to determine the best method of communication with the patient. Some patients will be able to verbally name the object, while others may have to find or point to the matching block. Once the patient has demonstrated an understanding of the procedure, you can begin the actual testing. Positioning is important, and the occupational therapist should try to find the best positioning that permits the patient to attend and concentrate on the task.

PROCEDURE

1. With a patient, create a pleasant play situation.
2. Establish the best method of communication.
3. Before beginning the actual testing procedure, make sure that the patient understands the task and can either verbally identify all four test objects when held at a close distance or can successfully match all four symbols on a consistent basis.
4. Test with both eyes open.
5. Place the 3-D blocks on the patient's lap.

6. Hold the test chart at 10 feet, and point to a target. Ask the patient to verbally identify the symbol or find the block that matches the symbol.

7. If the patient seems confused by all the symbols on one page, isolate one line at a time.

8. Acuity is recorded as the last line on which at least three of the five symbols are identified correctly.

9. If the patient is inattentive when the chart is held at 10 feet, perform the testing at a closer working distance (move to 80, 60, or 40 inches, if necessary).

10. Make sure you record the distance at which you tested distance visual acuity.

EXPECTED FINDINGS AND POSSIBLE RESPONSES
We expect to find 20/20 visual acuity. A referral is necessary if vision is 20/40 or worse.

Distance Visual Acuity for Verbal/Literate Children and Adults
EQUIPMENT NEEDED
- Chronister Portable Acuity Test (CPAC Test)

  Gulden Ophthalmics

  225 Cadwalader Ave

  Elkins Park, PA 19027

  Phone: 800-659-2250

  https://guldenophthalmics.com/product/pediatric-chronister-pocket-acuity-chart/

SETUP AND TESTING STRATEGY
Test with both eyes open.

PROCEDURE
1. Hold the CPAC at 20 feet (Figure 6.2) and ask the patient to verbally identify the letter on the 20/40 line.

2. If the patient has trouble with letters, attempt to test visual acuity using the Lea Symbols Test.

3. Continue until the patient misses more than 50% of the letters at any size.

4. Record acuity as the last line in which the patient can successfully identify more than 50% of the letters.

EXPECTED FINDINGS AND POSSIBLE RESPONSES
We expect to find 20/20 visual acuity. A referral is necessary if vision is 20/40 or worse.

Binocular Vision

To screen for binocular vision problems, it is important to test for both eye alignment and sensory fusion. The screening tests described below will enable the occupational therapist to detect a large phoria, poor convergence, and suppression.

Alignment of the Eyes
EQUIPMENT NEEDED
- Binocular Vision Screening Software (BVA)

  (www.bernell.com/product/HTSBSP/Software)
- Computer (PC)

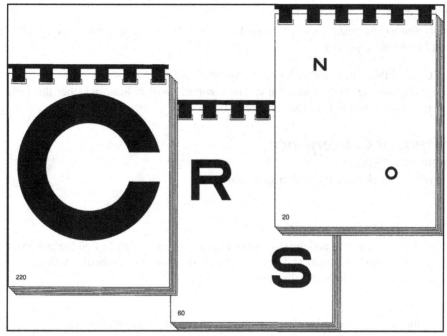

Figure 6.2. The Chronister Portable Acuity Test used to test distance visual acuity in verbal and literate children and adults. (Reprinted with permission of Gulden Ophthalmics.)

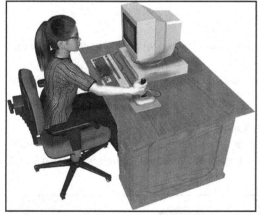

Figure 6.3. BVA binocular vision screening software.

SETUP AND TESTING STRATEGY

Positioning is important, and the occupational therapist should try to find the positioning that best permits the patient to attend and concentrate on the task. For binocular vision testing, the patient's head should be vertically erect.

The software is loaded onto the computer that will be used for the vision screening (Figure 6.3). Once it is loaded you select "NEW TEST," enter the patient's name, and begin the screening. The initial screen will allow you to select various testing procedures. The recommended tests for this screening are:

- Worth 4 Dot
- Phoria
- Fusional vergence

PROCEDURE

Simply follow the onscreen instructions for each of the three screening tests (Worth 4 Dot, phoria, and fusional vergence).

EXPECTED FINDINGS AND POSSIBLE RESPONSES

The scoring on the BVA is automatic. The computer will indicate whether the patient has passed or failed the screening for each area tested.

Near Point of Convergence

EQUIPMENT NEEDED

- Thin pick-up stick or pencil with a sharp point
- Ruler

SETUP AND TESTING STRATEGY

Positioning is important, and the occupational therapist should try to find the best positioning that permits the patient to attend and concentrate on the task. For binocular vision testing, the patient's head will ideally be vertically erect.

PROCEDURE

1. Slowly move the pencil toward the patient at eye level and between the two eyes (Figure 6.4).
2. Ask the patient to keep the pencil tip single for as long as possible.
3. Ask the patient to tell you when they see two pencil tips.
4. Once diplopia occurs, move the pencil in another inch or two and then begin to move it away from the patient.
5. Ask the patient to try to see "one" again.
6. Also watch the eyes carefully, and observe whether the eyes stop working together as a team. One eye will usually drift out (Figure 6.5).
7. Record the distance at which the patient reports double vision and when the patient reports recovery of single vision.

EXPECTED FINDINGS AND POSSIBLE RESPONSES

We expect the patient to report double vision or for the eyes to lose alignment when the pencil comes within 2 inches of their eyes. This is called the break, and a normal finding is between 2 and

Figure 6.4. Near Point of Convergence Test.

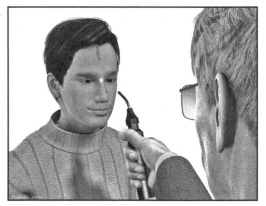

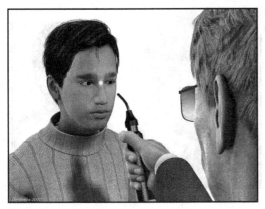

Figure 6.5. The patient's left eye has turned out during the Near Point of Convergence Test.

4 inches. After the patient experiences double vision, we expect a recovery of fusion (single vision) from 4 to 6 inches. If a patient has a long-standing, significant binocular vision problem, they may not report double vision because they are suppressing the eye that turns out. That is why it is so important for the therapist to watch the patient's eyes to make an objective assessment of when the break and recovery occur. When a break occurs, you should be able to observe one eye drift out, and when the patient recovers fusion, you should be able to see the eyes move back into alignment.

Accommodative Testing

Accommodative problems are prevalent in school-aged children with learning problems and in patients with acquired brain injury. As discussed in Chapter Four, in a comprehensive evaluation, it is important to evaluate both accommodative amplitude and accommodative facility. In a screening, however, we generally only evaluate amplitude directly, and we try to gather information about facility from the symptom questionnaire. If we find a low amplitude of accommodation, we can predict that accommodative facility will also be abnormal. A normal amplitude of accommodation, however, does not necessarily mean that accommodative facility would be normal as well. The questionnaire in Appendix B can help you identify an accommodative facility problem. If the patient complains of several of the symptoms in the "Signs of Focusing Problems" section, a facility problem should be considered. One symptom that is particularly characteristic of a facility problem is that the patient complains of blurred vision when looking from far to near or near to far. If amplitude testing is normal and you are suspicious, it is best to refer for a comprehensive evaluation.

Amplitude of Accommodation
Equipment Needed
* 20/30 letter on the Gulden Fixation Stick (Figure 6.6)
  (https://guldenophthalmics.com/product/fixation-sticks/)
* An eye patch

Setup and Testing Strategy
It is important to position the patient so that they are able to maximally attend and concentrate. Vertical positioning of the head is not as important with accommodation as it is with binocular vision testing. If the patient normally reads with glasses, they must be used for this task.

Figure 6.6. Tongue depressor target used to test amplitude of accommodation.

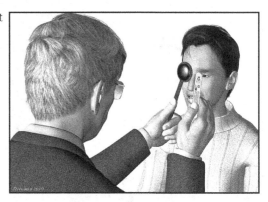

Table 6.4

Expected Amplitude of Accommodation by Age

Age	Expected Number	Age	Expected Number
3	17 D	30	8 D
6	16 D	33	7 D
9	15 D	36	6 D
12	14 D	39	5 D
15	13 D	42	4 D
18	12 D	45	3 D
21	11 D	48	2 D
24	10 D	51	1 D
27	9 D	54	0 D

PROCEDURE

1. Patch the left eye.
2. It is important that the patient does not know the letter on the Gulden Fixation Stick before the test begins.
3. Hold the Gulden Fixation Stick with the 20/30 target about 1 inch in front of the right eye. The patient will be unable to identify the stimulus on the Gulden Fixation Stick at this distance.
4. Slowly move the target away from the patient's eye, and ask the patient to report as soon as they can identify the target.
5. Using a ruler, measure the distance from the eye to the Gulden Fixation Stick at which the patient was able to identify the stimulus. Record this measurement.
6. Divide 40 by the measurement found in Step 5 to determine the amplitude of accommodation. For example, say the patient is able to identify the target at 8 inches. To find the amplitude, divide 40 by 8, which equals 5 D.
7. Compare the patient's amplitude of accommodation to the expected amplitude for the patient's age (Table 6.4).

EXPECTED FINDINGS AND POSSIBLE RESPONSES

The amplitude of accommodation should be within 2 D of the expected finding to pass this screening test.

Ocular Motility (Saccades and Pursuits)

There are several methods of evaluating ocular motility function. These include direct observation, visual-verbal format tests, and objective tests. The objective tests require expensive equipment and are, therefore, not suitable for a screening. The first two methods, however, require only minimal equipment and are appropriate for a screening. The direct observation tests described below can be used for patients from the age of 5 years old through adulthood. Although there are several direct observation methods available, I have chosen a system that has received the most critical research scrutiny. The direct observation method described below was developed at the Northeastern State University College of Optometry (NSUCO).[5] Some experience is required to become comfortable with the test, and therapists should first perform the test with children and adults without vision problems before attempting to screen a patient with a potential problem. The advantage of direct observation tests is that only limited verbal interaction is required, and the examiner can make objective observations.

The other testing approach is called a visual-verbal format because the patient has to look at numbers and say the numbers out loud. This test is valuable with school-aged children and adults, and the results can be compared to normative data. This test is valuable when a child or adult is experiencing difficulty with reading, loss of place, skipping words, difficulty scanning the environment, and localizing objects. It requires good attention and expressive language skills. If there is an expressive language problem and difficulty with number recall, the test cannot be administered. A reliable and valid visual-verbal format test is only available for saccades, not pursuits.

Saccades: Direct Observation Method

EQUIPMENT NEEDED
- Two Gulden Fixation Sticks (https://guldenophthalmics.com/product/fixation-sticks/)
- Place a red circular sticker on one and a blue circular sticker on the other

SETUP AND TESTING STRATEGY
If possible, the patient should be standing with their feet shoulder-width apart directly in front of the examiner. If the patient cannot stand, try to position the patient so that the head is erect and not supported in any way. If this is not possible, it is best to position the head vertically erect with support. The test is performed binocularly and is appropriate for patients at least 5 years of age.

PROCEDURE
1. Hold two different Gulden Fixation Sticks, 16 inches from the patient's face with each target about 4 inches from the patient's midline. The total horizontal separation of the targets should be about 8 inches (Figure 6.7).
2. No instructions are given to the patient to move or not to move their head.

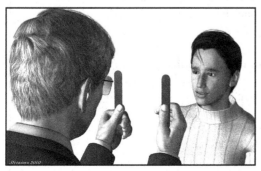

Figure 6.7. Saccades testing: Direct observation method using two different targets 16 inches from the patient's face with each target about 4 inches from the patient's midline.

3. Use the following instructional set: "When I say red, look at the red target. When I say blue, look at the blue target. Remember, do not look until I tell you."

4. Ask the patient to look from one target to the other for five round trips or a total of ten fixations.

5. Determine if the patient can keep their attention under control to complete five round trips for saccades. Assign a score of 1 through 5 based on the scoring criteria in Table 6.5.

6. Observe the accuracy of the eye movement. Does it take one eye movement to reach the target or multiple saccades? Assign a score of 1 through 5 based on the scoring criteria in Table 6.5.

7. Observe if the patient moves their head or body. Assign a score of 1 through 5 based on the scoring criteria in Table 6.5.

8. Compare the patient's score to the failure criteria in Table 6.6.

EXPECTED FINDINGS AND POSSIBLE RESPONSES

Table 6.5 lists the scoring criteria for direct observation of saccades, and Table 6.6 lists the failure criteria. Any score below the minimal levels listed in Table 6.6 would be reason for referral.

Pursuits: Direct Observation Method

EQUIPMENT NEEDED

*   One Gulden Fixation Stick with a red circular sticker (https://guldenophthalmics.com/product/fixation-sticks/)

Table 6.5

NSUCO Scoring Criteria for Direct Observation of Saccades

Ability

Points	Observation
1	Completes less than two round trips
2	Completes two round trips
3	Completes three round trips
4	Completes four round trips
5	Completes five round trips

Accuracy
(Can the patient accurately and consistently fixate so that no noticeable correction is needed?)

Points	Observation
1	Large over- or undershooting is noted one or more times
2	Moderate over- or undershooting is noted one or more times
3	Constant slight over- or undershooting is noted (>50% of time)
4	Intermittent slight over- or undershooting is noted (<50% of time)
5	No over- or undershooting noted

Head and Body Movement
(Can the patient accomplish the saccade without moving their head?)

Points	Observation
1	Large movement of the head or body at any time
2	Moderate movement of the head or body at any time
3	Slight movement of the head or body (>50% of time)
4	Slight movement of the head or body (<50% of time)
5	No movement of the head or body

Table 6.6

NSUCO Saccade Test Referral Criteria by Age and Sex

Sex	Ability	Accuracy	Head Movement
Boys	Less than 5	Less than 3	5 to 6 years: less than 2
			All other ages: less than 3
Girls	Less than 5	Less than 3	5 years: less than 2
			6 to 9 years: less than 3
			All other ages: less than 4

SETUP AND TESTING STRATEGY

If possible, the patient should be standing with feet shoulder-width apart directly in front of the examiner. If the patient cannot stand, try to position the patient so that the head is erect and not supported in any way. If this is not possible, it is best to position the head vertically erect with support. The test is performed binocularly and is appropriate for patients who are at least 5 years of age.

PROCEDURE

1. Hold one Gulden Fixation Stick 16 inches from the patient's face.
2. No instructions are given to the patient to move or not to move their head.
3. Use the following instructional set: "Watch the red circle as it goes around. Don't take your eyes off the red circle."
4. Move the target clockwise for two rotations and counterclockwise for two rotations.
5. Determine if the patient can keep their attention under control to complete four rotations. Assign a score of 1 through 5 based on the scoring criteria in Table 6.7.
6. Observe the accuracy of the pursuit eye movements. Assign a score of 1 through 5 based on the scoring criteria in Table 6.7.
7. Observe if the patient moves their head or body. Assign a score of 1 through 5 based on the scoring criteria in Table 6.7.

EXPECTED FINDINGS AND POSSIBLE RESPONSES

Table 6.7 lists the scoring criteria for direct observation of pursuits, and Table 6.8 lists the failure criteria findings.

Saccades: Visual-Verbal Format

This test is less dependent on the skill of the examiner than the direct observation method of screening saccades. The test has also been normed for children 6 to 13 years old. After age 13, only limited additional improvement can be expected in performance on this test. Therefore, even though norms are only available for children, the test can be used with adults with acquired brain injury. In such cases, the expectation is that the patient should at least perform as well as the top level norms provided in the manual. Therapists interested in using this test should purchase the test and study the manual to gain maximum insight about administration and scoring.

EQUIPMENT NEEDED

- Developmental Eye Movement (DEM) Test (www.bernell.com/product/DEM/Visual_Non-Visual)

> ### Table 6.7
>
> # NSUCO Oculomotor Test Scoring Criteria for Direct Observation of Pursuits
>
> *Ability*
>
> | Points | Observation |
> |---|---|
> | 1 | Cannot complete half rotation in either clockwise or counterclockwise direction |
> | 2 | Completes half rotation in either direction |
> | 3 | Completes one rotation in either direction but not two rotations |
> | 4 | Completes two rotations in one direction but less than two rotations in the other direction |
> | 5 | Completes two rotations in each direction |
>
> *Accuracy*
> (Can the patient accurately and consistently fixate so that no noticeable refixation is needed when doing pursuits?)
>
> | Points | Observation |
> |---|---|
> | 1 | No attempt to follow the target or requires greater than ten refixations |
> | 2 | Refixes five to ten times |
> | 3 | Refixes three to four times |
> | 4 | Refixes two times or less |
> | 5 | No refixations |
>
> *Head and Body Movement*
> (Can the patient accomplish the pursuit without moving their head?)
>
> | Points | Observation |
> |---|---|
> | 1 | Large movement of the head or body at any time |
> | 2 | Moderate movement of the head or body at any time |
> | 3 | Slight movement of the head or body (>50% of time) |
> | 4 | Slight movement of the head or body (<50% of time) |
> | 5 | No movement of the head or body |

> ### Table 6.8
>
> # NSUCO Pursuit Test Referral Criteria by Age and Sex
>
> | Sex | Ability | Accuracy | Head Movement |
> |---|---|---|---|
> | Boys | Less than 5 | 5 to 6 years: less than 2 | 5 to 6 years: less than 2 |
> | | | 7 to 9 years: less than 3 | 7 to 9 years: less than 3 |
> | | | 10 years and older: less than 4 | 10 years and older: less than 4 |
> | Girls | Less than 5 | 5 to 8 years: less than 3 | 5 to 9 years: less than 3 |
> | | | 9 years and older: less than 4 | All other ages: less than 4 |

SETUP AND TESTING

The patient should be seated, and it is helpful to use a slantboard for the testplates. The test is performed binocularly.

PROCEDURE

1. Ask the patient to call out the numbers on Tests A and B as quickly as possible from top to bottom without using their finger (Figure 6.8).

Figure 6.8. The student must call out the numbers going down the columns on Test A (Developmental Eye Movement Test).

2. Record time and any errors. There are a variety of errors the patient can make, including errors of addition, omission, and substitution. It is important to consult the testing manual about types of errors and recording procedures.

3. Ask the patient to call out the numbers on Test C (Figure 6.9) as quickly as possible without using their finger. This time, the patient must call out the numbers going across the page.

4. Record time and any errors. There are a variety of errors the patient can make, including errors of addition, omission, and substitution. It is important to consult the testing manual about types of errors and recording procedures.

5. Determine the adjusted time by taking errors into consideration (consult manual for details).

6. Determine the ratio score (horizontal adjusted time/vertical adjusted time), and convert this raw score into a percentile based on the patient's age. This score gives us an assessment of the saccadic speed.

7. Determine the number of errors, and convert this raw score into a percentile based on the patient's age. This score gives us an assessment of accuracy.

EXPECTED FINDINGS AND POSSIBLE RESPONSES

A score at the 50th percentile is considered average. Both errors and ratio (speed) are scored separately. For screening purposes, a score below the 15th percentile on either errors or ratio is considered significantly low and requires a referral.

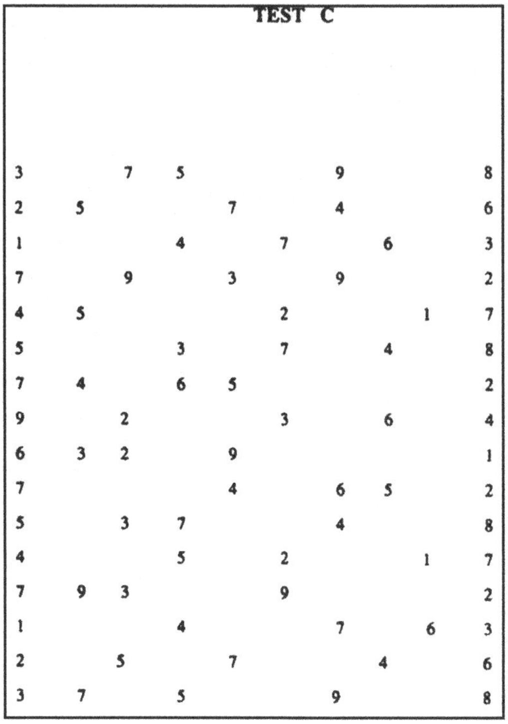

Figure 6.9. This time, the patient must call out the numbers going across the page on Test C as quickly as possible (Developmental Eye Movement Test).

				TEST C				
3		7	5			9		8
2	5			7		4		6
1			4		7		6	3
7		9		3		9		2
4	5				2		1	7
5			3		7	4		8
7	4		6	5				2
9		2			3		6	4
6	3	2		9				1
7				4		6	5	2
5		3	7			4		8
4			5		2		1	7
7	9	3			9			2
1			4			7	6	3
2		5		7			4	6
3	7		5			9		8

Visual Fields

Confrontation Fields

One of the more common vision problems associated with acquired brain injury is a visual field defect. Confrontation field testing is a method of screening for such deficits. It allows the therapist to screen for gross, peripheral vision field loss. It is important to realize that this screening procedure may be insensitive with some patients, and it is possible to miss a significant visual field loss using this procedure.[6,7] Therefore, it must be viewed as a screening test only. If the results of the screening are negative yet the patient displays behavior indicative of a field loss, a referral is still necessary.

EQUIPMENT NEEDED
- None

SETUP AND TESTING STRATEGY

Typically when an optometrist assesses visual fields, each eye is tested individually. In a routine optometric examination it is important to know if there is a difference between the two eyes. However, the purpose of visual field screening for an occupational therapist is different. The goal is to determine if there is a visual field problem with both eyes open that might be affecting the patient's ability to engage in various activities of daily living. It is not important to know if there is a significant visual field loss in just one eye. This will have minimal impact on activities of daily living. What is of primary importance is the visual field with both eyes together. Thus, the recommendation is to test with both eyes open.

The patient must be seated opposite the examiner, and it is important to position the patient so that the head is vertical. Confrontation field testing is not necessary in children who have not experienced head trauma. I suggest that it be reserved for adults and children with acquired brain injury. Although this is a significant test to attempt when dealing with such patients, it is important to remember that good fixation ability and a high level of concentration and attention are necessary. If these skills are not present, this testing will not be possible.

The underlying concept when doing confrontation field testing is that you compare your own visual field to the patient's visual field. Specifically, if you can see the target that you are presenting, then the patient should be able to see it.

PROCEDURE

1. Sit directly opposite the patient. You should be about 20 inches from the patient. It is preferable that the background for the patient be dark and uniform.

2. Explain that you will be moving the target from the side, and the patient should report as soon as they see it while looking directly at your finger which you hold between your eyes.

3. Begin at the 12 o'clock position, and slowly move the target down until the patient first reports seeing it. Compare the patient's response to yours. If the patient cannot see the target as soon as you can, it is an indication of a possible problem.

4. Move clockwise to the 2, 4, 6, 8, and 10 o'clock positions, and repeat Step 3.

5. Record approximately where the patient reports seeing the target in each orientation tested.

Visual Inattention/Neglect

Confrontation field testing described above is designed to detect a left or right hemianopia or quadrant defect. However, it is also necessary to screen for visual inattention or visual neglect. A standardized test is available for this purpose called the Behavioural Inattention Test (BIT). The BIT is an objective behavioral test of everyday skills relevant to visual neglect, aimed at increasing the understanding of specific difficulties patients experience.

EQUIPMENT NEEDED
*   Behavioural Inattention Test
    Pearson
    Phone: 800-627-7271
    www.pearsonassessments.com

SETUP AND TESTING STRATEGY
Testing is performed with both eyes open. The patient and examiner are seated at a table.

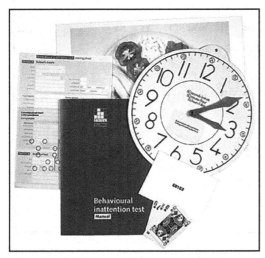

Figure 6.10. Behavioural Inattention Test (BIT).

PROCEDURE

Follow the instructional set of the BIT. There are two parallel versions, each comprising six "conventional" subtests and nine behavioral subtests (Figure 6.10). Short and easy to understand and interpret, the BIT is applicable to a wide range of environmental settings. The BIT has been validated against conventional tests of neglect and therapists' reports. It also has excellent inter-rater, test retest, and alternate form reliability.

Visual Information Processing Screening

Visual Spatial Skills

The test described below evaluates the existence, nature, and frequency of occurrence of receptive letter and number reversals (reversals that the patient can recognize). In this test, the patient is asked to mark off those letters and numbers that are written backward or reversed (Figure 6.11). This test gives us information about the patient's development of normal internal and external spatial concepts.

EQUIPMENT NEEDED

• Gardner Reversal Frequent Test: Recognition Subtest (www.bernell.com/product/GRFT/ Perceptual_Skills)
• A pencil

SETUP AND TESTING STRATEGY

This test is appropriate for children 5 to 15 years old. After age 15, only limited additional improvement can be expected in performance on this test. Therefore, even though norms are only available for children 5 to 15 years old, the test can be used with adults with acquired brain injury. In such cases, the expectation is that the patient should at least perform as well as the top level norms provided in the manual. When administering this test, it is important to seat the patient so that they cannot observe books and other written material that may provide information about letter and number orientation. This is an untimed test, and patients who have difficulty in this area may become frustrated by this task and take excessively long periods of time to complete the test.

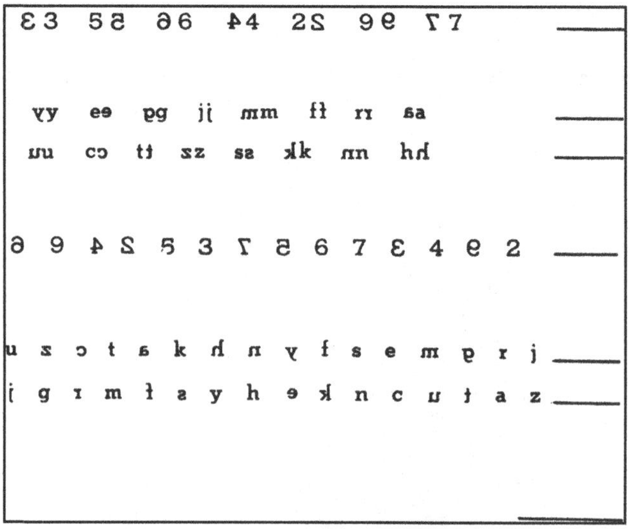

Figure 6.11. In the Gardner Reversal Frequent Test: Recognition Subtest, the child is asked to mark off those letters and numbers that are written backward or reversed.

Because we are performing this test as a screening, I recommend that you discontinue the test if it becomes clear after a short period of time that the patient is struggling.

PROCEDURE

1. Give the patient a pencil with an eraser and the examination sheet, and say the following: "In this first row, there are pairs of numbers. In each pair, one of the numbers is pointing in the right direction, and one is pointing in the wrong direction. Draw an X over the number pointing in the wrong direction."

2. Use similar instructions for the next two lines of letters.

3. For rows 4 through 6, use the following instructions: "In this row, some of the numbers are pointing in the right direction and some are pointing in the wrong direction. Draw an X over all of the numbers pointing in the wrong direction."

4. The test is scored by counting the total number of errors. Two types of errors can occur: errors of omission and errors of commission. Errors of omission refer to mistakes in which the patient fails to cross out a letter or number that is printed backward. Errors of commission refer to errors in which the patient crosses out a letter or number that is actually correct.

5. The total of the two types of errors is the raw score, which can then be converted to a percentile score by using the tables supplied in the test manual.

EXPECTED FINDINGS AND POSSIBLE RESPONSES

For screening purposes, a score falling one standard deviation from normal (below the 15th percentile) is considered significant and requires referral or a complete visual information processing evaluation.

Visual Analysis Skills

To screen this area, I suggest using the Test of Visual Perceptual Skills (TVPS): Form Constancy Subtest illustrated in Figure 6.12.

EQUIPMENT NEEDED

*   Test of Visual Perceptual Skills: Form Constancy Subtest
    Bernell Corp
    Phone: 800-348-2225
    www.bernell.com/category/s?keyword=TVPS

SETUP AND TESTING STRATEGY

This test probes the patient's ability to be aware of the distinctive features of forms including shape, orientation, and size without the need for motor involvement. It is made up of 16 different plates with stimuli that become more complex. It can be used between the ages of 4 and adult.

PROCEDURE

1. Introduce the test by telling the patient that they may not be able to answer all of the items correctly and that the pictures become more and more difficult.

2. Once you have the patient's attention, say the following: "Look at the picture" (point to the picture on top). "Now, find the one picture from these five that looks the same even though it may be bigger, smaller, darker, turned around, or upside down."

3. If the patient correctly determines the answer to plate A, continue with the rest of the items until the patient misses four of five consecutive items.

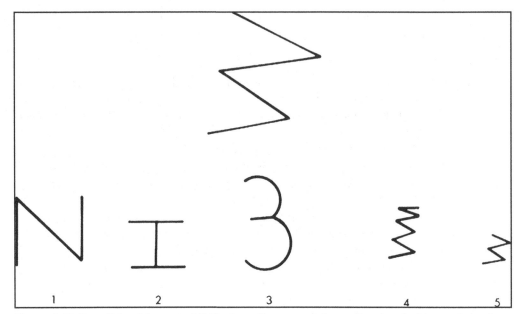

Figure 6.12. Test of Visual Perceptual Skills: Form Constancy Subtest. (Reprinted with permission from Psychological and Educational Publications Inc.)

4. If the patient cannot determine the answer to plate A, point out and explain the correct response, then proceed once the patient seems to understand.

5. Discontinue when the patient fails four of five consecutive items.

6. It is important to prompt the patient to try even if they are unsure.

7. Record the patient's responses on the scoring sheet.

8. The raw score equals the number of correct responses up to the point where the patient misses four of five consecutive stimuli.

9. Refer to the test manual to convert the raw score to a percentile rank.

EXPECTED FINDINGS AND POSSIBLE RESPONSES
For screening purposes, a score falling one standard deviation from normal (below the 15th percentile) is considered significant and requires referral or a complete visual information processing evaluation.

Visual Motor Integration Skills
A well-known and accepted method of assessing visual motor integration skills is the Developmental Test of Visual Motor Integration. This test has well-developed normative data and can be used from age 3 years old through adulthood.

EQUIPMENT NEEDED
• Developmental Test of Visual Motor Integration (Beery and Buktenica) (www. pearsonassessments.com)

SETUP AND TESTING STRATEGY
This test evaluates the patient's ability to integrate visual information processing and fine motor skills by assessing their ability to accurately copy a visual stimulus. The patient is presented

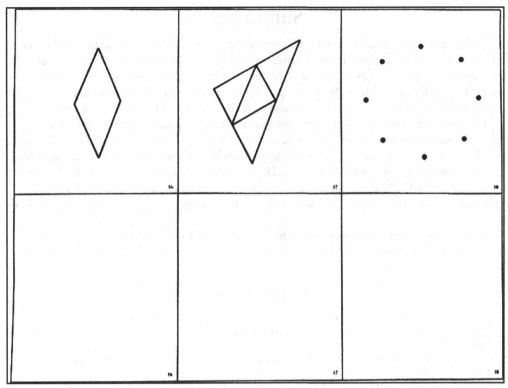

Figure 6.13. Developmental Test of Visual Motor Integration by Keith E. Beery and Norman A. Buktenica. © 1989 Modern Curriculum Press. (Reprinted with permission from Simon and Schuster Elementary.)

with pictures of increasing complexity and is asked to reproduce the pictures as accurately as possible. Figure 6.13 is a sample of some of the forms used in this test.

When administering this test, it is important to have the test booklet and the patient's body centered with the desk and the booklet throughout the testing. Do not let the patient trace the picture, and erasures or second tries are not allowed.

PROCEDURE
1. Place the test form in front of the patient with the first three patterns to be copied and say, "These forms are to be copied in order. Give each space only one try."
2. Point to the first form and say, "Can you make one just like this? You make yours right here" (point to the space in which the patient is to draw the form). "Go ahead now and do the rest of them. There is no erasing allowed."
3. To score the test, use the very detailed scoring criteria included in the scoring manual.
4. Testing should be discontinued after three consecutive incorrect responses.
5. The raw score is the total of all correct forms, and this score can be converted to a percentile score using the tables in the scoring manual that comes with the test.

EXPECTED FINDINGS AND POSSIBLE RESPONSES
For screening purposes, a score falling one standard deviation from normal (below the 15th percentile) is considered significant and requires referral or a complete visual information processing evaluation.

Summary

The screening tests described in this chapter can be used by an occupational therapist to screen for vision problems in the three important areas of vision described earlier in this book. Tests that allow detection of problems in visual acuity, refraction, visual field, binocular vision, accommodation, ocular motility, and visual information processing are included. The screening form included in Appendix B can be used to record results and includes referral guidelines for each screening test.

If a problem is detected, referral for a comprehensive vision examination is important. I have stressed the need to make sure that the professional to whom you refer the patient practices using the full model of vision described in this book. Otherwise, you will most likely be disappointed with the information you receive in return. The directories of optometrists who have achieved fellow status in the College of Optometrists in Vision Development and those who have achieved Diplomate status in the American Academy of Optometry are good resources for potential referral sources.

If the screening tests are inconclusive but you continue to observe behavior that suggests a vision problem, you should certainly refer the patient for a comprehensive vision examination.

References

1. Anderson DP, Ford RM. Visual abnormalities after severe head injuries. *Can J Surg.* 1980;23:163–165.
2. Gianutsos R. Rehabilitative optometric services for survivors of acquired brain injury. *Arch Phys Med Rehabil.* 1988;69:573–578.
3. Warren M. Identification of visual scanning deficits in adults after cerebrovascular accident. *Am J Occup Ther.* 1990;44:391–399.
4. Bouska MJ GM. Primary visual field deficits in adults with brain damage: management in occupational therapy. *Occup Ther Pract.* 1991;3:1–11.
5. Maples WC, Atchley J, Ficklin T. Northeastern State University College of Optometry's oculomotor norms. *J Beh Optom.* 1992;3:143–150.
6. Trobe JD, Acosta PC, Krischer JP, Trick GL. Confrontation visual field techniques in detection of anterior visual pathway lesions. *Ann Neurol.* 1981;10:28–34.
7. Harrington DO. *The Visual Fields: A Textbook and Atlas of Clinical Perimetry.* St. Louis, MO: CV Mosby; 1971.

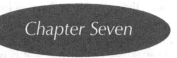

Chapter Seven

Management of Refractive, Visual Efficiency, and Visual Information Processing Disorders

Mitchell Scheiman

Optometric Treatment Methods

This chapter is designed to describe various ways in which an occupational therapist can help in the management of patients with vision disorders. The first goal is to provide information about how optometrists treat various vision disorders using lenses, prism, occlusion, low vision aids, and vision therapy. The second objective is to provide detailed suggestions about how the occupational therapist can work along with the optometrist when managing children who are also being treated for a vision disorder. The final goal is to provide several treatment sequences that can be used by occupational therapists to supplement the vision therapy being performed by an optometrist in the areas of eye movements and visual information processing skills.

This chapter describes treatment for school-aged children and adults with normal cognitive ability. Children with learning disabilities or children and adults with mild cognitive and perceptual problems after acquired brain injury could also be treated according to the guidelines established in this chapter. Chapters Ten and Twelve deal specifically with treatment issues related to children functioning at a lower level and to children and adults with acquired brain injury with moderate to severe sequelae.

The tools that optometrists use to treat vision problems are lenses, prism, occlusion, low vision aids, and vision therapy. These treatment modalities can be used in isolation or in combination.

Use of Lenses

Lenses are effective for the treatment of various forms of refractive error including myopia, hyperopia, and astigmatism. Optometrists are often asked whether the child's nearsightedness or farsightedness will decrease as a result of wearing eyeglasses. The lenses that are prescribed are not intended to remediate or eliminate the refractive disorder. Rather, the eyeglasses are compensatory and allow the individual to see clearly while wearing the glasses.

LENSES FOR MYOPIA

Lenses have a very beneficial effect on myopia—immediately restoring clear vision. The type of lens that is used is called a concave lens or a "minus lens" (Figure 7.1).As described in Chapter

DOI: 10.4324/9781003526841-7

Three, the rays of light focus in front of the retina in myopia, and a concave or minus lens moves the point of focus to the plane of the retina (Figure 7.2). Because myopia is a condition that generally causes reduced vision only at far, a decision has to be made about when the patient should wear the eyeglasses. Sometimes, it is only necessary to have the patient wear glasses for far tasks, such as driving and watching television and movies. When the degree of myopia is high or if in addition to myopia the patient has astigmatism, glasses may be prescribed for full-time wear. In some situations, the prescription that enables the patient to see at far is actually inappropriate for close work and tends to cause esophoria and accommodative problems that lead to eyestrain and discomfort. If this problem is detected during the examination, several options are available. In some cases, we simply ask the patient to remove the glasses for all reading tasks.

In certain situations, however, such as when treating a school-aged child, frequent removal of the glasses would be inconvenient and problematic. If the child is copying from the chalkboard and needs the glasses to see the board but needs to remove the glasses when they look down at the desk, copying will be very difficult. A similar problem might occur with an adult working in an office setting. If this individual needs glasses to see across the room and to walk around but not for the computer terminal or deskwork, they will need to repeatedly remove the glasses. In both situations, we often prescribe a bifocal lens. With this type of lens, we can prescribe the best lens for distance and the best lens for near, allowing the patient to comfortably wear the eyeglasses at all times.

Myopia is a vision problem that in some cases can also be controlled or reduced using special intervention procedures. While some forms of myopia are based on hereditary factors, other forms may be environmental in nature.

Lenses for Hyperopia

The type of lens that is used for hyperopia is called a convex lens or a "plus lens" (Figure 7.3). In hyperopia, the rays of light focus behind the retina. A convex or plus lens moves the point of

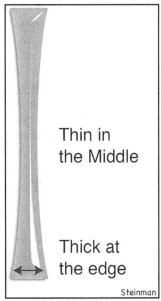

Figure 7.1. A concave lens or a "minus lens" used to treat myopia. (Reprinted with permission from Scheiman M, Scheiman M, Whittaker SG. *Low Vision Rehabilitation: A Practical Guide for Occupational Therapists.* Thorofare, NJ: SLACK Incorporated; 2007.)

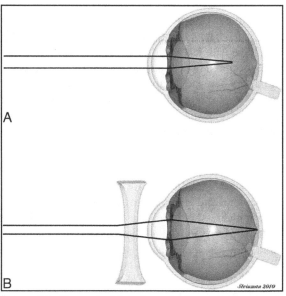

Figure 7.2. The rays of light focus in front of the retina in myopia and a concave or minus lens moves the point of focus to the plane of the retina.

focus to the plane of the retina (Figure 7.4). Most people are slightly hyperopic, and glasses are not prescribed for all degrees of hyperopia. When the amount of hyperopia becomes clinically significant, however, glasses are prescribed because significant uncorrected hyperopia can lead to discomfort, eyestrain, blurred vision, and difficulty with attention and concentration when reading. Eyeglasses may be prescribed just for reading and close work, or if the amount of hyperopia is large enough, glasses may be necessary for full-time wear.

Esophoria, intermittent esotropia, and constant esotropia are conditions that are often associated with hyperopia, and the final eyeglass prescription must take these conditions into account as well. In most cases, prescribing for hyperopia has a beneficial effect on these binocular vision problems as well. Occupational therapists will often have to deal with an important issue when working with patients wearing glasses for hyperopia. If the patient is a child and unless the degree of hyperopia is very large, it is usually possible for the child to see just as clearly without as with the glasses. As discussed in Chapter Four, patients can overcome the blurred vision caused by hyperopia by accommodating. Because children can generally see as well without the glasses, we sometimes encounter problems with compliance. The occupational therapist will experience this when dealing with these children. It is important, therefore, to understand the importance of wearing glasses in cases of hyperopia and to reinforce this message. We usually tell parents that the glasses are not being prescribed to make the child's vision clear; rather, the purpose of the glasses is to make vision comfortable and to allow the child to concentrate more effectively in school.

LENSES FOR ASTIGMATISM

Astigmatism is a condition that can cause reduced visual acuity at both far and close distances. It also has a differential effect, and rather than causing blurred vision of all aspects of the stimulus, it is selective for one orientation over others. For instance, one common type of astigmatism causes blurred vision of vertical lines but leaves horizontal lines unaffected. This is the reason why the

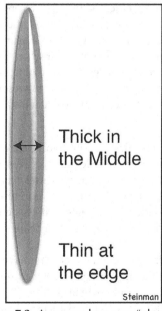

Figure 7.3. A convex lens or a "plus lens" used to treat hyperopia. (Reprinted with permission from Scheiman M, Scheiman M, Whittaker SG. *Low Vision Rehabilitation: A Practical Guide for Occupational Therapists.* Thorofare, NJ: SLACK Incorporated; 2007.)

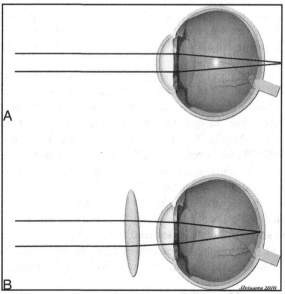

Figure 7.4. In hyperopia, the rays of light focus behind the retina. A convex or plus lens moves the point of focus to the plane of the retina.

lenses used to correct astigmatism are different from those used to treat hyperopia and myopia. The type of lens used to treat astigmatism is called a cylindrical lens and has different powers in different parts of the lens.

If a significant degree of astigmatism is left uncorrected, it can lead to eyestrain, headaches, and difficulty sustaining attention when reading. Thus, astigmatism is more similar to hyperopia than myopia. The human visual system is able to accommodate to overcome the blur caused by hyperopia and astigmatism. Accommodation has no beneficial effect with myopia. In astigmatism, accommodation is only partially effective, unlike in hyperopia in which accommodation can effectively eliminate the blur. Optometrists sometimes prescribe for mild to moderate degrees of astigmatism because the individual complains of discomfort and eyestrain, although the visual acuity may be adequate. The compliance problem mentioned above relative to hyperopia, therefore, applies to astigmatism as well. A young child may say that they see just as well without as with the glasses and may object to wearing them. It is important that the occupational therapist reinforce the need to wear the glasses and that the purpose is not to make things clearer but to make the vision more comfortable.

Lenses for Accommodative Problems

In Chapter Four, I reviewed the four primary types of accommodative disorders: accommodative insufficiency, excess, infacility, and presbyopia. The treatment of choice for two of the four common accommodative problems (accommodative insufficiency and presbyopia) is lenses for reading. In both cases, the individual has lost the ability to effectively focus on objects that are brought close to them, such as reading from a book. The type of lens used is a convex or plus lens, and these lenses actually do some of the focusing for the individual, allowing them to use less effort. This tends to relieve the discomfort and blurred vision associated with accommodative insufficiency and presbyopia.

Because the eyeglasses used to treat these two conditions are only appropriate for close work, the individual will experience blurred vision when looking at a far object if the glasses are not removed. This can be an inconvenience in certain situations. The problem is almost identical to similar issues mention earlier in reference to myopia. For any task requiring viewing, a near and then a far target will create a challenge. In this case, the individual's vision will be clear when viewing the near material through the eyeglasses, but distance vision will be blurred. To overcome these difficulties, we prescribe bifocal lenses. The top of the bifocal in many cases may have no prescription at all, but allows the individual to see clearly when they look at an object located at a distance.

Lenses for Binocular Vision Problems

A number of binocular vision disorders can be treated with eyeglasses. The two broad categories of binocular vision problems are esodeviations (eyes turn in) and exodeviations (eyes turn out). When the eyes turn in (esotropia) or have a tendency to turn in (esophoria), lenses tend to be very helpful. The use of a convex or plus lens will decrease the tendency for the eye to turn in and will have a beneficial effect on esodeviations. If the esodeviation is the same at distance and at far, a regular eyeglass prescription can be used. If the esodeviation is larger at near than at far, a bifocal may be necessary.

In cases of exodeviations in very young children or in children or adults who do not have the attention and cognitive ability necessary to benefit from vision therapy, minus lenses can sometimes help. Minus lenses tend to help the eyes turn inward and assist the patient in trying to use both eyes together. These lenses do not provide a long-term solution, however, and are usually used for short periods of time or as an aid in vision therapy.

Lenses for Amblyopia

Two common forms of amblyopia called anisometropic and isometropic amblyopia are caused by a refractive condition of the eye. An essential part of the treatment program for these conditions is the use of eyeglasses. Eyeglasses are prescribed for full-time wear, and in many cases, additional treatment modalities such as occlusion therapy (patching) and vision therapy are required as well. Success in these cases is very dependent on the use of eyeglasses, and occupational therapists treating children with such problems can play an important role by reinforcing the need to wear the glasses.

LENSES FOR PREVENTION OF VISION PROBLEMS

Optometrists believe that some vision problems develop over time as a result of environmental factors. Myopia and some binocular vision and accommodative disorders fall into this category. In today's society, with the emphasis on reading and computer work, a great deal of stress is placed on the visual system. While some people can effectively deal with this stress, others experience great discomfort and interference with functional performance. Skeffington[1] refers to this as the socially compulsive, biologically unacceptable near point stress and believes this is the etiology of many of the visual problems people experience. According to Skeffington, refractive, binocular, and accommodative disorders are adaptations to the basic problem of excessive stress on the visual system. He developed an approach that includes the use of plus lenses and vision therapy to help prevent and reduce vision problems caused by environmental factors. The use of such lenses is an attempt to decrease the stress on the visual system and help restore the normal equilibrium that should be present. While there is some disagreement in the optometric profession about this theory, it is popular enough that occupational therapists will certainly see many patients who might be wearing lenses for this purpose. It is important, therefore, to understand that glasses may be prescribed for prevention of vision problems and to help reinforce compliance.

SUMMARY

Lenses are used very often in the treatment of refractive, accommodative, and binocular vision disorders, but they generally do not "correct" or eliminate the existing condition. Rather, in most cases, lenses allow the person to compensate and function visually in spite of the presence of an underlying vision disorder. In certain circumstances, optometrists may prescribe lenses to either try to prevent the development of vision problems or to try to reverse some of the adverse adaptations that may have occurred. Compliance with the doctor's wearing instructions is very important, and eye doctors need as much assistance from as many people as possible to ensure that eyeglasses are worn properly. In cases such as hyperopia, binocular vision, and accommodative disorders and amblyopia, poor compliance with the doctor's instructions can lead to decreased functional performance and lack of progress in treatment. Occupational therapists are in an ideal position to help in this way.

While most patients receive single vision lenses, some vision problems require the use of bifocals as described above. Bifocals are, therefore, not just for older adults; many children and young adults require bifocals as well. It is important for occupational therapists to have some insight into the reasons for bifocals to reinforce the need and importance of the eyeglasses in such cases. This means that communication between the optometrist and occupational therapist is important. You should certainly receive a complete report from any eye doctor who examines a patient who is under your care. It is wise to ask the patient or parent to request such a report as soon as you know such an examination will be taking place.

Use of Prism

A prism is a wedge-shaped lens that is thicker on one side than the other. Prisms, unlike lenses used to treat refractive error, do not have any optical power. Rather, the purpose of a prism is to deflect or bend the light rays in such a way so that the eyes can function more effectively as a team. Prism is used for three purposes in optometric care: (1) to treat some binocular vision disorders, (2) to expand visual field in patients with hemianopia, and (3) to modify posture and balance.

Figure 7.5 illustrates the two defining characteristics of any prism: the base and the apex. The base of a prism is the thicker portion. When prescribing prism to compensate for binocular vision problems, we prescribe base-in, base-out, base-down, or base-up prism. This refers to the location of the base of the prism relative to the patient's eye. In Figure 7.6a, the base-in prism is in front of the right eye, and in Figure 7.6b, the base-up prism is in front of the right eye. To treat exophoria, we prescribe base-in prism before both eyes; and for esophoria, we prescribe base-out before both eyes. For a vertical deviation, base-down prism is placed before one eye, and base-up in front of the other.

A less commonly prescribed type of prism is called conjugate, or yoked, prism. A yoked prism prescription differs from the compensatory prism described above because the base of the prism will always be on the same side for each eye. For example, in Figure 7.7, the base of the prism is to the left of the right eye and to the left of the left eye. Compare this to Figure 7.6a, in which compensatory prism to correct for exophoria is placed with the base to the right of the right eye. Yoked prisms have been proposed as a treatment to expand visual field, treat midline shift syndrome, and manage some of the common behaviors present in children with autism such as abnormal eye-gaze direction, head tilts, looking from the corners of eyes.[1-4]

Prisms are available in a variety of forms. In most instances, prism is ground into the optical lens that is used to correct the patient's refractive error. One of the common forms that occupational therapists will see is the Fresnel prism. A Fresnel prism is a flexible, plastic sheet with small ridges (Figure 7.8). This plastic sheet can be cut to the shape of the patient's eyeglass lens and adheres to the back surface of the lens. Fresnel prisms have two advantages over traditional prisms. We are able to try Fresnel prism on a temporary basis, inexpensively, without changing the patient's permanent lenses. Another advantage is that when the amount of prism power required is high, the

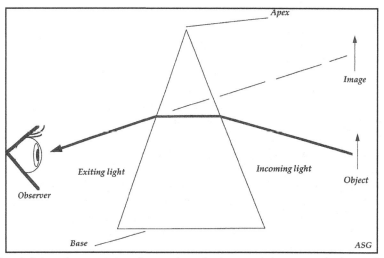

Figure 7.5. Two defining characteristics of any prism: the base and the apex. The base of a prism is the thicker portion.

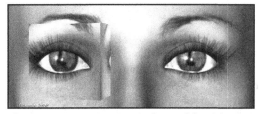

Figure 7.6a. Base-in prism in front of the right eye.

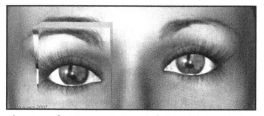

Figure 7.6b. Base-up prism in front of the right eye.

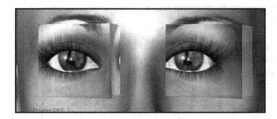

Figure 7.7. Example of yoked prism with the base of the prism to the left of the right eye and to the left of the left eye.

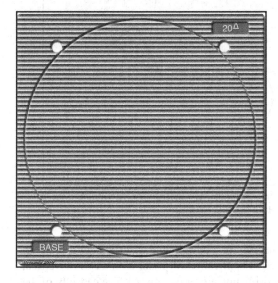

Figure 7.8. A Fresnel prism is a flexible, plastic sheet with small ridges.

traditional optical prism becomes so thick and heavy that it cannot be comfortably worn and is cosmetically unacceptable. Fresnel prism is lighter and less apparent.

PRISMS FOR BINOCULAR VISION DISORDERS

Figure 7.9 illustrates how prism helps a patient with a binocular vision disorder. In Figure 7.9, the eyes turn in (esotropia) as a result of traumatic head injury. If this patient is an adult, they will experience double vision because the light rays are focused on the fovea of the left eye but on a nonfoveal area of the retina on the right eye. If the two foveas are not simultaneously stimulated by similar objects, the perception of double vision occurs. To solve this problem, a prism has been placed in front of the deviated eye. As you can see, the effect of the prism is to bend the light back onto the fovea, restoring single, binocular vision.

Prisms are helpful for certain binocular vision problems because they decrease the demand of the neuromuscular components of the visual system. For example, if a child has an intermittent esotropia (the eyes turn in intermittently), the visual system will have to exert a great deal of neuromuscular effort to pull the eyes outward. This effort can lead to eyestrain, discomfort, and double vision when the effort cannot be sustained. The effect of prism is to simulate a decrease in the magnitude of the intermittent esotropia. This leads to a decrease in the amount of effort required to control the binocular problem. A reasonable analogy is to compare the use of prism for binocular disorders to the use of a cane for a muscle problem in the leg. Neither the prism nor the cane remediates the underlying problem, but while they are being used, the patient can function more effectively with less demand on the affected muscles.

Prisms are an important treatment modality for some binocular vision problems. As a general rule, prism tends to be more effective for esodeviations than for exodeviations.[5] In a recent randomized clinical trial, Scheiman et al.[6] found that prism reading glasses were no more effective than placebo reading glasses for children with the most common exodeviation called convergence

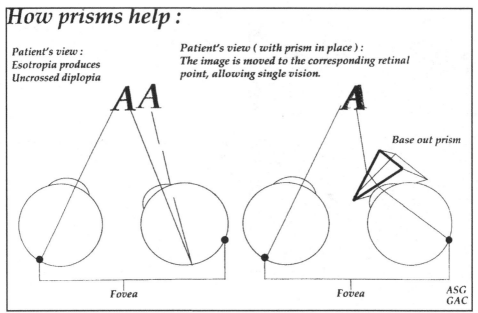

Figure 7.9. Illustration of how prism helps a patient with a binocular vision disorder. The effect of the prism is to bend the light back onto the fovea, restoring single, binocular vision.

insufficiency. In adult patients, prism may be useful for convergence insufficiency based on another randomized clinical trial.[7] The most effective application of prism is in cases of vertical binocular vision disorders. In these cases, one eye drifts upward or downward. The capacity of the visual system to compensate for vertical deviation is very limited, and even the slightest tendency for this to occur is enough to make an individual uncomfortable and to cause significant functional problems in everyday life. The use of prism in such cases is highly effective. Prism is also used to treat certain types of constant strabismus in which the patient has developed very deeply ingrained adaptations, such as anomalous correspondence.

PRISMS FOR VISUAL FIELD DEFICITS

One of the most significant vision problems associated with traumatic brain injury and cerebrovascular accident is visual field loss. One of the treatment modalities available to help a patient compensate for this loss is prism. In recent years, studies[8,9] have demonstrated that a prism field expansion system called the Peli Visual Field Expansion Device for Hemianopia is an effective treatment for patients with hemianopia. As illustrated in Figure 7.10, a small horizontal segment of prism is placed above and below the patient's line of sight. This expands the visual field by as much as 30 to 40 degrees and allows the patient to be aware of potential obstacles in the periphery. Detailed information and a video simulation of this treatment method is available at https://chadwickoptical.com/peli-lens-process/, Chadwick Optical (White River Junction, VT), the company that produces the prism.

PRISMS FOR MODIFICATION OF POSTURE, BALANCE, ATTENTION

Some optometrists use prism to better posture and balance. This is referred to as the use of yoked or ambient prism.[1–3] The two primary uses of yoked prism are to treat patients experiencing visual midline shift syndrome and to treat children with visual and behavioral problems associated with autism.

Focal and Ambient Visual Systems

The visual system is believed to be composed of two separate processes called the focal process and the ambient process. The focal process is related to the central visual function and the

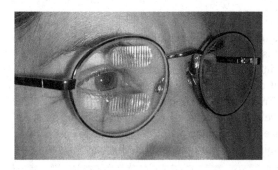

Figure 7.10. Peli Visual Field Expansion Device for Hemianopia is an effective treatment for patients with hemianopia.

macula and provides information about objects at which the patient is looking. The ambient process provides information about location in space, balance, movement, coordination, and posture. After traumatic brain injury, the ambient visual process may lose its ability to match information with other sensory modalities causing difficulty with orientation in space, balance, movement, coordination, and posture.

Yoked or Ambient Prism Lenses for Visual Midline Shift Syndrome

When the prisms' bases face in the same direction in both eyes, they are called yoked. Designed to alter neural organization, yoked or ambient prisms may have an impact on the lives of those with autism and other delays or patients after acquired brain injury. Yoked or ambient prisms address a patient's ability to organize space and create a coherent body schema. These lenses are used therapeutically to change the neuromotor processing of the brain; after rehabilitation occurs, they are no longer needed.

Yoked prisms can cause the environment to appear to be curved up, down, left, or right. Objects may thus appear closer, farther away, or sloped. Prisms are employed in various magnitudes, which are measured in diopters. Altering both the magnitude and the direction of the prism can influence a patient's perception.

Kaplan[4] is the leading advocate of the use of yoked or ambient prism lenses to treat some of the visual and behavioral symptoms of autism. He suggests that yoked prisms deflect the light rays differently through the thin edge at the top and the thick edge at the base, influencing how the brain interprets where the body is in space. These prisms are designed to re-establish normal function of the ambient visual system. Kaplan et al.[2] completed a double-blind crossover design study to assess the efficacy of wearing yoked or ambient lenses to reduce the behavioral symptoms of autism. Eighteen autistic individuals, ranging in age from 7 to 18 years, participated in the study. Behavior, attention, and orientation were evaluated at 1½, 2, 3, and 4 months. Compared to the placebo condition, the results showed a decrease in behavior problems at the 1½- and 2-month assessment periods and a slight loss of these benefits at the 3- and 4-month assessment periods. These findings support the prediction that ambient lenses have positive effects on autistic individuals. More study is necessary to demonstrate the effectiveness of these lenses. However, the treatment is relatively quick and inexpensive.

VISUAL MIDLINE SHIFT SYNDROME

Visual midline shift syndrome is a condition that is sometimes associated with acquired brain injury such as traumatic brain injury or stroke. In this condition the patient's midline shifts away from the center, usually away from the neurologically affected side of the body. Persons with a visual midline shift syndrome may walk as if the plane of the floor is tilted. Some patients report that the floor appears to be tilted. A potential treatment is to utilize yoked prisms before both eyes. The goal of the prism is to cause the midline to shift to a more centered position. This treatment has been popularized by Padula[10] in recent years; however, a randomized clinical trial is required to demonstrate its effectiveness. It is a relatively simple and inexpensive treatment option for such patients and, thus, worth an attempt even though there is limited research at this time.

SUMMARY

Prisms have been used for many years for the treatment of binocular vision disorders. They do not "correct" or eliminate the existing binocular vision condition. Rather, prisms are used to allow the person to compensate and function visually in spite of the presence of an underlying vision disorder. More recent uses of prism have been introduced including expansion of visual field and attempts to modify visual behavior after acquired brain injury and in children with autism and other developmental delays. As with lenses, compliance with the doctor's wearing instructions is very important, and eye doctors need as much assistance from as many people as possible to ensure that eyeglasses are worn properly. Occupational therapists are ideal in helping in this way.

Use of Occlusion

Occlusion is used to actively treat amblyopia and strabismus, and as a last resort for patients with double vision who cannot be successfully treated using lenses, prism, vision therapy, or surgery. When prescribing occlusion, the clinician must make decisions about the type of occlusion, the amount of time to use occlusion, and which eye to occlude.

TYPES OF OCCLUSION

The two types of occlusion are opaque and translucent. A variety of occlusion devices are illustrated in Figures 7.11a and 7.11b. The decision is based on the goal of the occlusion. If the objective is to force the patient to use the amblyopic eye to achieve improvement in acuity, an opaque occluder is most desirable. Opaque occlusion completely eliminates all incoming visual stimulation and, therefore, tends to hasten progress. The disadvantage of opaque occlusion is that it has a poor cosmetic effect. When treating children with amblyopia, an opaque adhesive patch is generally recommended. Because this type of patch completely covers the eye, the child is unable to peek. A patch, such as the one illustrated in Figure 7.11b, although opaque, can easily be displaced by the child, and peeking could occur. This, of course, would prevent any progress.

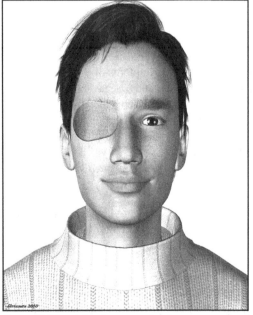

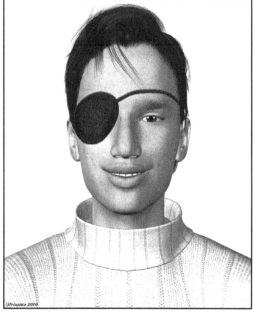

Figure 7.11a. Adhesive eye patch is an example of an opaque occlusion device.

Figure 7.11b. Opaque occluder with elastic cord.

Translucent occlusion is sometimes recommended if cosmesis is an issue. Another situation in which translucent occlusion is indicated for elimination of double vision is in an adult patient. A small, central circular patch using translucent tape is sometimes enough to help a patient avoid double vision (Figure 7.12).

THE AMOUNT OF TIME TO USE OCCLUSION

When treating amblyopia, the amount of time to occlude an eye is an important clinical decision. In children younger than 3 years of age, the visual system is still very plastic and susceptible to interference. Thus, long periods of constant, opaque occlusion can potentially lead to loss of vision in the dominant eye. Clinicians are very careful about the amount of time occlusion is used with infants and young children and re-evaluate often. As the child gets older, however, full-time or constant occlusion for strabismic amblyopia is commonly used.

When visual acuity is very poor, a child may have great difficulty functioning in school. In such cases, clinicians may initially decide to limit the amount of occlusion used. As visual acuity improves in the amblyopic eye, the amount of occlusion time can be increased.

OCCLUSION FOR AMBLYOPIA

Occlusion has been used for amblyopia treatment for more than 200 years. The rationale for using occlusion is that occluding the better eye stimulates the amblyopic eye. This stimulation allows the visual pathway of the amblyopic eye to develop, leading to improved visual acuity and function.

Full-time occlusion is generally recommended for constant strabismus, and part-time occlusion is recommended for intermittent strabismus. Part-time occlusion with an opaque patch is recommended for anisometropic amblyopia. Typically, about 2 to 6 hours of occlusion is recommended. The typical duration for occlusion therapy for strabismic or anisometropic amblyopia is 6 to 11 months with the maximum effect reached in the first 3 to 4 months.

OCCLUSION FOR STRABISMUS

In Chapter Four, I discussed the adaptations that occur in the visual system of a strabismic patient to eliminate double vision. Adaptations such as suppression and anomalous correspondence are common in patients with constant strabismus occurring before the age of 6 years. When both eyes are open, there is an active and constant need for these adaptations. If both eyes are allowed to remain open, these adaptations are constantly being reinforced and strengthened. If the goal of treatment is to restore normal binocular vision, it is important to use occlusion to prevent this reinforcement of suppression and anomalous correspondence. Therefore, even if a strabismic patient does not have amblyopia, occlusion may be used to eliminate binocular vision until the underlying problems are resolved.

OCCLUSION FOR ELIMINATION OF DIPLOPIA

Occlusion can also be used for patients experiencing annoying double vision. Double vision that cannot be eliminated with any form of treatment including lenses, prism, vision therapy, or surgery is referred to as intractable diplopia. This can occur in adults with acquired strabismus secondary to

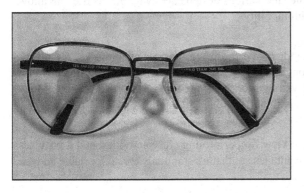

Figure 7.12. A small, central circular patch using translucent tape to help a patient avoid double vision.

head trauma or with neurological disease. It is also a possible complication of strabismus surgery. When all other treatment modalities have failed, occlusion may be recommended as a last resort. When occlusion is used for intractable diplopia, the objective is to use a form of occlusion that has the least effect on cosmetic appearance. Small translucent patches are strategically placed on the patient's glasses. For example, if the double vision occurs when the patient looks down and to the right, the patch would be placed in the lower right-hand section of the right or left lens. In recent years, optometrists have also begun to use specially designed contact lenses that block the vision of one eye.

SUMMARY

Occlusion is an important optometric treatment modality. It is generally considered to be a passive form of therapy in contrast to vision therapy. Occlusion therapy is absolutely essential in the treatment of amblyopia and is an important auxiliary treatment method for strabismus.

Use of Low Vision Aids

Low vision is defined as reduced central visual acuity or visual field loss that even with the best optical correction provided by regular lenses results in visual impairment from a performance standpoint. Although the most important criterion is impairment of performance, for quantification purposes, visual acuity loss is usually used to help define whether a patient may benefit from low vision devices. Visual acuity of 20/70 or less (in the better eye) with best eyeglasses constitutes low vision.

The prevalence of low vision in the populations served by occupational therapists is significant. Visual field loss and decreased visual acuity are common problems associated with acquired brain injury. In the pediatric population, children with multiple impairments may also have either reduced visual acuity or visual field loss. It is likely that occupational therapists will encounter patients who require low vision aids.

TYPES OF AIDS

Low vision aids include a large variety of devices designed to help an individual function as well as possible in spite of visual loss. These aids are compensatory and do not resolve the underlying problem. Aids include specially designed eyeglasses, telescopes, microscopes, magnifiers, closed circuit television systems, contact lenses, reading stands, filters, large-print material, typoscopes, sunglasses, visors, and field expanders.

Telescopes

Telescopes are prescribed to improve performance for distance tasks of 10 feet or greater. Various designs are available, including telescopes that are hand-held and those that can be incorporated into the person's eyeglasses.

Microscopes

Microscopes are used for those tasks that require close work at distances from 2 to 20 cm. These devices usually are mounted in a frame, and various designs are available. Those that allow the largest field of view tend to interfere with mobility.

Magnifiers

Magnifiers are used to improve an individual's performance for near vision tasks. An advantage of a magnifier over a microscope is a longer working distance. As with all low vision devices, however, a longer working distance is achieved by sacrificing the size of the field of view. Many types of magnifiers are available including hand-held, standing, illuminated, and bar magnifiers.

Closed-Circuit Television System

This device provides an excellent field of view for performing close activities, and it provides high contrast and good magnification. Disadvantages are that most models are not portable and the equipment is expensive.

Field Expanders

A number of aids can help individuals with visual field loss. These include lenses, reverse telescopes, and Fresnel prism. Fresnel prism is often used to help people who experience visual field loss after acquired brain injury. This treatment approach is discussed in detail in Chapter Ten.

Other Aids

Other than the optical devices described previously, a number of nonoptical aids can be prescribed. Modification of illumination is very important for patients with low vision. Some patients require high, medium, or low levels of illumination. Large-print materials can be very helpful and include large-print books and large numbers for telephones and playing cards. Because low vision patients may need to hold a magnifier or other devices, stands are often helpful. These include reading stands, table easels, and music stands.

Chapters Thirteen through Fifteen cover the topics of low vision and low vision rehabilitation in detail.

SUMMARY

Individuals who have reduced visual acuity even with best correction or visual field loss may benefit from low vision aids. Prescribing low vision aids requires a great deal of experience. Often, the clinician must make a compromise between the best aid from an optical standpoint and the best aid from a cosmetic standpoint. There is no single aid that is optimal for all patients. Decisions about which aids are most appropriate require a full low vision evaluation by an experienced optometrist or ophthalmologist. Although the prescription of the most appropriate low vision aid is important, the second challenge is to help the patient learn how to use the aid successfully in activities of daily living. This is where the occupational therapist can play a very important role in the care of the patient with low vision. In many cases, co-management of patients with low vision by an optometrist and occupational therapist will lead to the best outcome.

Vision Therapy

WHAT IS VISION THERAPY?

Vision therapy, also known as orthoptics, vision training, visual training, and eye training, is an organized therapeutic regimen used to treat a number of neuromuscular, neurophysiological, and neurosensory conditions that interfere with visual function. Vision therapy encompasses a wide variety of procedures to improve a diagnosed neuromuscular or neurophysiological visual dysfunction. The treatment can be relatively simple, such as patching an eye as part of amblyopia therapy, or it may be complex, involving sophisticated instrumentation and computers.

Vision therapy usually involves a series of treatment visits during which carefully planned functional activities are carried out by the patient under close supervision in order to relieve the visual problem. The specific activities and instrumentation are determined by the nature and severity of the condition. The frequency and duration of treatments are dictated by the individual situation, although established guidelines, suggesting appropriate length of therapy for various diagnoses are available.

WHEN IS VISION THERAPY NECESSARY?

Most vision problems can be very easily corrected with eyeglasses. In fact, about 80% to 85% of the vision problems we detect can be treated with glasses or contact lenses. However, approximately 15% to 20% of the population with symptoms of blurred vision and eyestrain have vision problems that cannot be treated successfully using glasses alone. It is this group of people who need vision therapy. Vision therapy is generally required to treat problems of binocular vision, accommodation, eye movement, amblyopia, strabismus, and visual information processing disorders. Individuals with these problems experience eyestrain when reading or doing other close work, inability to work quickly, sleepiness, inability to attend and concentrate, double vision, and loss of vision. Even more significant, children with amblyopia and strabismus face the possible loss of vision if an appropriate vision therapy program is not initiated in a timely fashion. Children with visual information processing problems may have difficulty learning.

Is Vision Therapy Effective?

In recent years, evidence-based practice has become an important concept in all health care professions, including optometry.[11,12] Evidence-based practice has been defined as the "integration of best research evidence with clinical expertise and patient values."[13] The best evidence is usually found in clinically relevant research that has been conducted using sound methodology.

Clinical research studies can be categorized based on the methodology used and is sometimes referred to as "levels of evidence" and is often portrayed as an evidence pyramid with case studies on the bottom and meta-analysis on top. A clinician may not always find the best level of evidence to answer a clinical question. The base of the pyramid is the weakest level of evidence and usually the most common type of study available. As you move up the pyramid the amount of available literature decreases, but increases in its relevance to the clinical setting. In the absence of the best evidence, the clinician needs to consider moving down the pyramid to other types of studies.

- A meta-analysis examines a number of valid studies on a topic and combines the results using accepted statistical methodology as if they were from one large study.

- Systematic reviews focus on a clinical topic and answer a specific question. An extensive literature search is conducted to identify all studies with sound methodology. The studies are reviewed, assessed, and the results summarized according to the predetermined criteria of the review question.

- Randomized controlled clinical trials are carefully planned projects that study the effect of a therapy on real patients. They include methodologies that reduce the potential for bias (randomization and masking) and that allow for comparison between intervention groups and control groups (no intervention).

- Cohort studies take a large population and follow patients who have a specific condition or receive a particular treatment over time and compare them with another group that has not been affected by the condition or treatment being studied. Cohort studies are observational and not as reliable as randomized controlled studies, since the two groups may differ in ways other than in the variable under study.

- Case series and case reports consist of collections of reports on the treatment of individual patients or a report on a single patient. Because they are reports of cases and use no control groups with which to compare outcomes, they have no statistical validity.

Studies have been performed to evaluate the methodological quality of journal articles in different medical specialties. Based on standardized criteria for the assessment of methodological rigor and clinical relevance of research articles, McKibbon et al. demonstrated that only about 7% of articles published in the top 20 clinical journals in general internal medicine passed the pre-specified criteria as having high methodological quality and clinical relevance.[14] A similar study in physical therapy found only 11% meeting the predefined standard.[15] Lai et al. completed a similarly designed study for the ophthalmology literature and found that only 14.7% of the articles involving treatment passed the methodological assessment.[16]

Although a similar study has not been performed for the optometric literature on vision therapy, the results are likely to be comparable to other professions. Much of the literature on vision therapy effectiveness is based on case reports, case series, cohort studies, and literature reviews.[17–51] There have been some small placebo-controlled studies in the past[27,52–54] and recently a number of randomized clinical trials have been published.[55–61] The weight of the evidence supports the use of vision therapy for most nonstrabismic binocular vision, accommodative, and eye movement problems. Like all health care professions, optometry must strive to plan and implement more studies with rigorous design to investigate the effectiveness of commonly used treatments.

The prognosis for all accommodative and nonstrabismic binocular vision problems is good to excellent.[62] Studies investigating the clinical effectiveness of vision therapy for accommodative dysfunction have shown success in approximately 9 of 10 cases. In a retrospective study of 96 patients, Daum[39] found partial or total relief of both objective and subjective difficulties in 96% of the subjects studied. Hoffman et al.[18] reported a vision therapy success rate of 87.5% in a sample of 80 patients with accommodative problems. Other studies, using objective assessment techniques, have investigated the actual physiological changes that occur due to vision therapy. Liu et al.[24] and Bobier and Sivak[41] found that the speed and velocity of the accommodative response were significantly changed after therapy.

Numerous investigators have shown that vision therapy for nonstrabismic binocular vision disorders leads to improved physiological performance. In both prospective[26] and retrospective studies,[35] Daum showed that relatively short periods of vision therapy can provide long-lasting increases in fusional skills. Other studies have used both experimental and control groups to demonstrate the efficacy of binocular vision therapy.[27,52,63] Daum[27] investigated the effectiveness of vision therapy for improving fusional skills using a double-blind, placebo-controlled experimental design. He found statistically significant changes in the experimental group with no changes in the control group. Vaegan[52] also found large and stable improvement in his experimental group and no changes in the control group. Cooper et al.[54] studied patients with convergence insufficiency using a matched subjects control group crossover design to reduce placebo effects. They found a significant reduction in symptoms and a significant increase in fusional skills after the treatment. During the control phase, significant changes in symptoms and vergence were not found.

Since 2005, the Convergence Insufficiency Treatment Trial Investigator Group has published the results of four randomized clinical trials demonstrating that office-based vision therapy is more effective than home-based vision therapy or a placebo control for the treatment of convergence insufficiency in both children and adults.[6,58,61,64]

In 2005, Scheiman et al.[57] reported the results of a multi-center clinical trial of 47 children aged 9 to 18 years with symptomatic convergence insufficiency who were randomly assigned to receive a 12-week program of home-based pencil push-ups, office-based vision therapy, or office-based placebo therapy. Only patients in the office-based vision therapy group demonstrated both statistically and clinically significant changes in symptoms and clinical findings. In this study, office-based vision therapy was found to be more effective than home-based pencil push-ups or office-based placebo therapy in reducing symptoms and improving signs of convergence insufficiency. Moreover, it was the only treatment that resulted in normalization of convergence insufficiency-related symptoms and signs. Pencil push-up therapy was found to be no more effective than the placebo therapy. Similar results were reported by Scheiman et al. in a study of 46 adult patients (19 to 30 years old) with convergence insufficiency.[58]

In 2008 the same group of investigators reported the results of a large scale multi-center, randomized clinical trial of 221 children aged 9 to 17 years with symptomatic convergence insufficiency who were randomly assigned to receive a 12-week program of home-based pencil push-ups, home-based computer vision therapy and pencil push-ups, office-based vision therapy with home reinforcement, and office-based placebo therapy.[61] The results showed that 12 weeks of office-based vision therapy resulted in a greater percentage of patients reaching predetermined success criteria when compared with home-based pencil push-ups, home-based computer vision therapy and pencil push-ups, and office-based placebo therapy.

Most recently the CITT Investigator group completed another randomized clinical trial.[60] Three hundred and eleven children aged 9 to 14 years with symptomatic convergence insufficiency were randomly assigned to 16 weeks of office-based vergence/accommodative therapy or to placebo therapy. Improvements in (1) near point of convergence (NPC), (2) positive fusional vergence (PFV), and (3) self-reported symptoms (Convergence Insufficiency Symptom Survey [CISS] score) were compared after 16 weeks of treatment. The results demonstrated that office-based vergence/accommodative therapy is effective for improving the NPC and PFV in children with symptomatic convergence insufficiency.

In 2020 Scheiman et al. completed a network meta-analysis of intervention for convergence insufficiency.[59] They included 12 trials (6 in children and 6 in adults) with a total of 1,289 participants. The authors concluded that current research suggests that office-based vergence/accommodative therapy with home reinforcement is more effective than home-based pencil/target push-ups or home-based computer vision therapy.

These recent high-quality studies of the effectiveness of vision therapy for convergence insufficiency indicate that office-based vision therapy is the most effective treatment for the condition and should be the first-line treatment for convergence insufficiency.

Clinical studies have also been performed to investigate the efficacy of treating eye movement dysfunction. Wold et al.[23] reported on a sample of 100 patients who had completed a vision therapy program for a variety of problems including accommodation, binocular vision, pursuits, and saccades. Saccadic and pursuit function was determined using subjective clinical performance scales like those described in Chapter Six. Pre- and post-testing revealed statistically significant changes in both saccadic and pursuit function.

In a more recent clinical study, Rounds et al.[65] used an objective eye movement recording system to assess reading eye movements before and after vision therapy. Although no statistically significant changes were found, the experimental group showed trends toward improving reading eye movement efficiency (less regressions and number of fixations and increased span of recognition) compared to the control group.

Young et al.[66] also used an objective eye movement recording instrument to assess reading eye movements before and after therapy. They studied 13 school children who had failed a vision screening. The children each had three 5-minute vision therapy sessions per day for six weeks. They received a total of 6 hours of eye movement vision therapy. Post-testing revealed a significant decrease in the number of fixations, an increase in reading speed, and a decrease in fixation duration.

Fujimoto et al.[67] investigated the potential for using vision therapy procedures prerecorded on videocassettes for eye movement vision therapy. They had three groups of subjects. The first group of nine subjects received standard eye movement vision therapy. The second group received videocassette-based eye movement therapy, while the third group received no treatment. The results showed that standard eye movement vision therapy and videocassette-based therapy were equally effective in improving saccadic ability.

When evaluating the efficacy of optometric vision therapy as a treatment tool for improving visual information processing skills, it is important to address two separate issues.[68] First, how effective is vision therapy at improving visual information processing skills? For example, when providing a therapy program for visual motor skills, is it likely that this ability will improve? Second, if there are improvements in visual information processing skills, is the child more available or responsive to educational instruction? That is, after remediation of specific visual deficits, will the child respond more appropriately to academic intervention for specific educational deficits?

In addressing the first issue, most studies evaluating the effectiveness of visual therapy have used a broad variety of training procedures in all three areas of visual information processing (visual spatial, visual analysis, and visual motor) at the same time. Academic performance was then re-evaluated following the treatment. Several of these studies have found significant improvements in visual information processing skills following therapy.[69,70] Studies that have concentrated on the treatment of isolated visual perceptual skills have also supported the effectiveness of therapy for visual spatial,[71,72] visual analysis,[73,74] and visual motor skills.[75] For example, Greenspan[72] administered a program of perceptual motor therapy that included therapy for bilaterality and body image development to a group of underachieving children and measured the frequency of reversal errors. The control group received only standard orthoptic therapy. The experimental group showed a statistically significant improvement in directionality and a reduction in the total number of reversal errors following the perceptual therapy. These studies indicate that the level of performance of individual visual information processing skills can be enhanced through an optometric vision therapy program designed to address specific visual information processing deficits.

Improving the ability of the child to benefit from academic instruction has been supported by similar research.[70,74,76,77] These studies have demonstrated statistically significant improvements in standardized tests of academic skills compared to a control group. For example, Seiderman[70] provided visual and perceptual therapy to 18 learning disabled children who were matched with a control group. The experimental group showed an improvement on the Word Reading and Paragraph Meaning subtests of the Stanford Achievement Test.

These studies taken from an interdisciplinary group of researchers provide positive evidence that therapy for visual information processing can be expected to improve specific skills and help the child benefit from academic instruction. In reviewing the literature that addresses therapy for perceptual skills, Solan and Ciner[78] cite several factors that are important for a successful therapy program. First, the patient should have a documented perceptual deficit that is associated with the reading or learning disorder. Broad-based therapy programs to improve readiness skills in normal patients may not be effective. Second, therapy programs should be individualized to address the specific deficits that the patient manifests. Therapy programs should address specific problem areas while taking into account the patient's developmental level, auditory processing, and visual attention and cognitive style. Finally, therapy should complement and not replace reading and other educational instruction. The role of the optometrist in the management of visual information processing deficits is to improve visual spatial, visual analysis, and visual motor skills in those patients who manifest these problems. This should enable the patient to participate more effectively in the classroom and to benefit from other educational therapies.

This research indicates that significant scientific support exists for the effectiveness of vision therapy in modifying and improving ocular motor, accommodative, binocular, and visual information processing disorders.

Influence of Vision Deficits on Occupational Therapy

In Chapters Three through Five, we discussed visual acuity, refractive, eye disease, visual efficiency, and visual information processing problems. In these chapters, we also demonstrated that vision problems can interfere with a person's ability to participate in activities of daily living, such as caring for one's self, working, going to school, playing, and living independently. For occupational therapists to be maximally effective in rehabilitation, they must understand the complexity and importance of vision and take these problems into consideration when planning and implementing occupational therapy.

Occupational Therapy Intervention

Occupational therapy intervention for the various vision problems discussed in this book can take one of three forms: Supportive intervention, compensatory intervention, and direct remediation.

Supportive Intervention

First, the therapist can be supportive of the optometric treatment recommendations and help ensure that the patient follows the treatment recommendations at least during occupational therapy. In most cases, this would involve making sure that the patient wears the prescribed glasses, prisms, or eye patch in the appropriate manner. It is helpful to suggest different frame colors or some other identifying feature for patients who need different glasses for distance and for near.

Compensatory Intervention

The therapist may also be able to modify the task or the environment or help the patient compensate for the vision disorder in question in some other way. The goal should be to manipulate and organize the patient's visual environment so that they receive the highest level of visual processing possible in spite of the deficits. For instance, in situations in which visual acuity is not correctable with lenses, environmental adaptations may be helpful. Examples include enlarging targets, controlling contrast, and lighting. Limitations in eye movements may result in an inability to move the eyes up or down. Management in such cases involves raising or lowering the target or working area to accommodate the patient's needs. Tables 7.1 through 7.5 list the recommended supportive and compensatory interventions for each vision problem discussed in this book.

Table 7.1

Vision Problems: Symptoms, Effect on Function, Occupational Therapy Management Suggestions—Visual Acuity, Refractive Conditions, and Eye Health Problems

Vision Problem	Symptoms and Effect on Function	Supportive and Compensatory Intervention	Direct Remediation
Reduced visual acuity (correctable with lenses)	• Blurred vision • Squinting • Holds objects close or must get close to objects • Avoids visual tasks	• Refer to an optometrist • If glasses are prescribed, support this recommendation and ensure compliance during OT procedures	• If treated early, visual acuity problems generally do not require direct remediation
Low vision: Reduced visual acuity (uncorrectable with lenses)	• Blurred vision • Squinting • Holds objects close or must get close to objects • Avoids visual tasks • Difficulty recognizing faces • Difficulty with mobility • Difficulty with activities of daily living with significant visual requirements (driving, reading, writing, grooming, finances, cooking, cleaning)	• Refer to an optometrist • If glasses or low vision devices are prescribed, support this recommendation and ensure compliance during occupational therapy procedures • Modify working distances for all tasks • Increase lighting • Increase contrast (white plates on dark placemats) • Reduce complexity of task • Enlarge all targets and print • Use visual markers to help patient keep place	• Direct remediation is not effective, only supportive and compensatory procedures are useful
Refractive conditions	• Blurred vision • Excessive effort • Discomfort when involved with any visual task • Squinting • Holds objects close or must get close to objects • Avoids visual tasks	• Refer to an optometrist • Glasses will be necessary • Encourage proper use of glasses • If loss of acuity has occurred, decrease the working distance • If patching is recommended, encourage proper use of the patch	• If treated early, refractive conditions generally do not require direct remediation

> **Table 7.2**
>
> ## Vision Problems: Symptoms, Effect on Function, Occupational Therapy Management Suggestions—Visual Field Deficits
>
> | Symptoms and Effect on Function | Supportive and Compensatory Intervention | Direct Remediation |
> |---|---|---|
> | • Walking: Inferior field loss causes difficulty with mobility; trouble seeing steps or curb; shortened and uncertain stride when walking; poor balance; tendency to trail behind others when walking; walks next to wall and holds onto wall with hands; uncomfortable in middle of room; anchored to ground; does not turn head as much; bumps into things frequently; disoriented when moving whether in car or walking
• Trouble identifying visual landmarks
• Superior field deficit causes difficulty seeing signs, worse if in wheelchair
• Leaves food on half of plate
• Misidentification of details; misreading of long words
• Difficulty with reading; misreads words; poor accuracy; slow reading rate; difficulty with page navigation; cannot stay on line
• Difficulty with writing; cannot stay on line; inaccurate with serious effects on check writing
• Self-grooming: Cannot find necessary items
• Dressing: Cannot find necessary items
• Telephone: Cannot take accurate messages
• Driving: Cannot drive usually
• Shopping: Cannot drive; cannot find items
• Emotional problems: Anxiety; reduced self-confidence; increased passivity; social isolation | • Referral for full vision examination
• Ensure use of appropriate glasses, which may incorporate lenses and prism
• Make patient aware of how visual defect interferes with various activities
• Emphasize conscious attention to detail
• Teach organized scanning techniques into deficient field
• Increase speed and accuracy of eye movements
• Use occlusion to force patient to look into deficient field
• Engage patient in as many real-life activities as possible
• Use ambulation as much as possible
• Use Letter Tracking and Symbol Tracking
• Provide markers to help reading
• When patient is writing, encourage them to look at pen or pencil tip | • Visual field defects cannot be improved through therapy, although supportive and compensatory procedures can have great benefit |

Direct Remediation

A third option in some cases is to attempt to actually eliminate or remediate the underlying vision problem and restore normal visual function. The remainder of this chapter provides detailed information and guidelines for direct remediation in the areas of ocular motor dysfunction and visual information processing disorders and describes a select group of therapy procedures. These procedures are not designed to be used by therapists in isolation of, or instead of, optometric intervention. My goal in this section is to address an issue that occurs virtually every time I co-manage a patient with an occupational therapist. In my clinical experience, the occupational therapist has a number of questions they want me to answer when they refer a patient to me to rule out vision problems that

Table 7.3

Vision Problems: Symptoms, Effect on Function, Occupational Therapy Management Suggestions—Visual Efficiency Problems: Binocular Disorders

Vision Problem	Symptoms and Effect on Function	Supportive and Compensatory Intervention	Direct Remediation
Binocular vision disorders: Strabismic	• Cosmetic problem, the eyes looked crossed or "wall-eyed" • If intermittent, may cause double vision that can interfere with eye-hand and mobility tasks • If intermittent, may cause eyestrain • Loss of vision if left untreated and the strabismus is unilateral	• If strabismus is present, refer to an optometrist • Use eye patch to eliminate double vision during OT activities • Encourage use of an eye patch during OT, if prescribed by the optometrist	• Discuss issue of use of patch during OT procedures • Incorporate motility activities into OT program
Binocular vision disorders: Nonstrabismic	• Intermittent double vision • Discomfort and eyestrain for all visual tasks • Tires easily during occupational therapy session • Inattentive during occupational therapy session • Poor concentration • Loss of place when reading • Difficulty with eye-hand tasks • Difficulty with ADL that require stereopsis (driving, near tasks involving reaching for objects, pouring liquids)	• If symptoms present, refer to optometrist • Glasses and prisms may be necessary—encourage compliance • If bifocals have been prescribed, ensure that the patient does close work while using the bottom of the bifocal • Use of patch may provide relief of symptoms until treatment is complete (consult with optometrist) • Use of guide on page may help decrease loss of place • Take frequent breaks • Reduce emphasis on tasks requiring intense visual attention • Reduce emphasis on tasks requiring stereopsis	• OTs who work with an optometrist in a rehabilitation hospital may be able to perform vision therapy procedures • Under all other conditions, only supportive and compensatory treatment is available
Amblyopia	• If unilateral, generally no symptoms • If bilateral, symptoms will be identical to low vision category although less severe	• Refer to optometrist • If patching is prescribed, ensure that the child uses the patch during OT procedures • During course of active amblyopia treatment, use compensatory approaches listed under "Low Vision" section	• The OT can have the child wear a patch while engaged in any OT procedure • OT may be able to incorporate ocular motility techniques while one eye is patched

Table 7.4

Vision Problems: Symptoms, Effects on Function, Occupational Therapy Management Suggestions—Visual Efficiency Problems: Accommodative and Ocular Motility Disorders

Vision Problem	Symptoms and Effect on Function	Supportive and Compensatory Intervention	Direct Remediation
Accommodative	• Discomfort and eyestrain for all visual tasks • Blurred vision • Rubs eyes • Tires easily during OT session • Inattentive during OT session • Poor concentration • Difficulty with ADL that require sustained close work	• If symptoms present, refer to optometrist • If glasses are prescribed, ensure compliance • If bifocals have been prescribed, ensure that patient does close work while using bottom of bifocal • Use of larger print may help provide relief of symptoms until treatment is complete • Take frequent breaks	• OTs who work with an optometrist in a rehabilitation hospital may be able to perform vision therapy procedures • Under all other conditions, only supportive and compensatory treatment is available
Ocular motility disorders	• Excessive head movement • Frequent loss of place • Skips lines • Poor attention span • Copying is slow and results poor with coloring and drawing • Difficulty with ADL that require frequent change in fixation and accurate eye movements (driving, reading, writing)	• Refer to optometrist for evaluation and treatment recommendations • Use of guide or finger is helpful while treatment is ongoing • De-emphasize tasks requiring precise and frequent eye movement skills	• OTs who work with an optometrist in a rehabilitation hospital may be able to perform vision therapy procedures • OTs in other settings can incorporate eye movement into OT plan with supervision from optometrists; vision therapy suggestions in this book can provide basic guidelines
Nystagmus	• Blurred vision • Squinting • Holds objects close or must get close to objects • Avoids visual tasks • Difficulty recognizing faces • Difficulty with mobility • Difficulty with ADL with significant visual requirements (driving, reading, writing, grooming, finances, cooking, cleaning)	• Refer to optometrist • If glasses are prescribed, support this recommendation and ensure compliance during OT procedures • Modify working distances for all tasks • Increase lighting • Increase contrast (white plates on dark placemats) • Reduce complexity of tasks • Enlarge all targets and print • Use visual markers to help patient keep their place	• Direct remediation is not effective; only supportive and compensatory procedures are useful

---

Table 7.5

Vision Problems: Symptoms, Effect on Function, Occupational Therapy Management Suggestions—Visual Information Processing Problems

Vision Problem	Symptoms and Effect on Function	Supportive and Compensatory Intervention	Direct Remediation
Visual perception disorders	• Confusion of left and right • Confusion of likenesses and differences • Tends to use other senses to make what should be visual discriminations • Unable to selectively attend to appropriate visual stimulus • Performs tasks slowly • Ignores details during visual tasks • Poor recall of visually presented material • Sloppy drawing skills • Difficulty with copying and getting thoughts down on paper • Difficulty with most ADL that have a high demand on visual information processing (driving, reading, writing, sports, mobility)	• Refer to optometrist for consultation to rule out visual acuity, refractive, eye health, and visual efficiency problems • Simplify visual tasks • Careful design of OT program to take attention factors into consideration • Eliminate extraneous distractions • Limit amount of visual stimuli • Use high-contrast stimuli	• OT uses approaches such as sensory motor integration or NDT • OT may prescribe visual perceptual therapy or work together with an optometrist

---

could be affecting occupational therapy. Of course, they want to know if any vision problems are present. If they are present, they want to know how they may be affecting the patient's performance in a variety of functional activities and activities of daily living. Finally, the occupational therapist invariably would like to know how they can intervene to limit the negative effects of the vision problems on performance. They want to know how to be supportive and help the patient compensate and if there is anything they can possibly do to help in the direct remediation of the vision problem.

My approach has always been to encourage therapists to help me with the direct intervention. I believe these patients require as much reinforcement and therapy as possible. If I am seeing the child once or twice a week and vision therapy is reinforced by the occupational therapist at other times, progress is enhanced. It is important to understand that the procedures described below are not a substitute for optometric vision therapy. Rather, the occupational therapist can supplement the work being done in vision therapy. The techniques I describe below can be used by therapists to supplement optometric vision therapy being done in the optometric office. If an occupational therapist uses these procedures, then a very close working relationship with the optometrist and a coordination of techniques are critical.

Another situation in which an occupational therapist may perform vision therapy techniques under the supervision of an optometrist is in a rehabilitation setting. A trend that is growing more common is that optometrists are becoming more directly involved in the care of patients with acquired brain injury within rehabilitation hospitals. In most cases, the optometrist examines the patient within the hospital and prescribes appropriate treatment that may include lenses, prism, occlusion, and vision therapy. The vision therapy is carried out in the hospital by occupational therapists under the supervision of the optometrist (see Chapters Nine and Ten for more detail).

General Principles and Guidelines for Vision Therapy

Before discussing specific vision therapy procedures, it is important to understand that there are general principles and guidelines that apply to all vision therapy techniques. Vision therapy is similar in many ways to other types of therapy that involve learning and education. If we look at other types of learning, it becomes clear that there are specific guidelines to facilitate learning and success. Because vision therapy can be considered a form of learning and education, similar principles and guidelines must be used to achieve success.

The following guidelines have been derived from basic learning theory (Table 7.6):

- Determine a level at which the patient can perform easily. Working on this level makes it easier for the patient to become aware of the important feedback cues, strategies, and objectives involved in vision therapy and also builds confidence and motivation.

- Be aware of the patient's frustration level. Signs of frustration include general nervous and muscular tension, hesitating performance, and possibly a desire to avoid the task.

- Use positive reinforcement. The patient should be rewarded for attempting a task, even if it is not successfully completed. Reinforcers can be verbal praise, tokens that can be exchanged for prizes, or participation in a task that the patient enjoys.

- Maintain an effective training level. Start at the initial level at which the task is easy, and gradually increase the level of difficulty, being very careful to watch for signs of frustration. Vision therapy should be success-oriented (i.e., built on what the patient can do successfully as opposed to giving tasks that are too difficult).

- Make the patient aware of the goals of vision therapy. The patient must know why they are in vision therapy. They should be able to explain what their problem is, how it affects performance, and the goals of vision therapy. This is true for children as well as adults. Even with a young child, the therapist should try to establish some understanding on the part of the child about what is wrong with their eyes and why vision therapy is necessary. For each therapy technique, the child should be able to explain what they need to do to accomplish the desired task.

- Set realistic therapy objectives and maintain flexibility with these objectives or endpoints. With all therapy techniques, we expect to achieve certain general objectives before we proceed to the next procedure. In this text, we call these objectives endpoints. It is important to understand that these endpoints are only guidelines and that flexibility and clinical judgment are ultimately just as important in deciding when to move on to another procedure. The objective of vision therapy is to solve the patient's problems as quickly as possible.

Table 7.6

General Guidelines and Principles for Vision Therapy

- Determine a level at which the patient can perform easily.
- Be aware of the patient's frustration level.
- Use positive reinforcement.
- Maintain an effective training level.
- Make the patient aware of the goals of vision therapy.
- Set realistic therapy objectives and maintain flexibility with these objectives or endpoints.

Computer-Based Versus Non-Computer-Based Vision Therapy

Computers and computer software have become an important component of vision therapy in recent years. Vision therapy can certainly be performed without any computer software, and I have included many non-computer-based techniques in this chapter. However, just as computer software has enhanced many aspects of our lives and the way we function, computer software has become an important element of vision therapy. Today our patients are very comfortable and familiar with computers and almost expect the use of computers in all aspects of their lives.

There are a number of excellent vision therapy software programs available, but most can only be purchased by a licensed optometrist. Occupational therapists do have one vision therapy software program available to them that can be used for both eye movement and visual processing therapy. It is called Tracking and Perceptual Skills for Occupational Therapists (TPOT, www.visionedseminars.com).

TPOT is a software program designed to be used by occupational therapists and other therapists for vision rehabilitation of eye movement and visual processing problems. The software can be used with both children (as young as 6 years old) and adults. TPOT contains 14 different programs that can be used for remediation of eye movement and visual processing problems.

TPOT has procedures for the remediation of the following vision problems:
- Eye movement problems
- Saccadic dysfunction (tracking)
- Visual processing problems
- Visual spatial dysfunction
- Visual analysis dysfunction

The TPOT software can be used with children with developmentally based eye movement and visual processing disorders and adults and children after acquired brain injury with acquired eye movement and visual processing disorders. In both cases the TPOT software can be a useful tool to supplement other therapeutic activities.

The TPOT software can be used in an office or clinic setting as part of an overall therapy program, or the software can be sent home so that the patient can supplement the office-based vision rehabilitation with home-based treatment. We suggest that patients work 5 days per week, 20 minutes per day with the TPOT software at home.

The TPOT software can be ordered at www.visionedseminars.com.

Ocular Motor Therapy: Specific Guidelines

- In all cases of ocular motility dysfunction, consider optical correction of refractive problems before beginning vision therapy. These problems should always be managed in conjunction with an optometrist.
- In all cases of ocular motility dysfunction, consider treatment of accommodative and binocular vision disorders before beginning vision therapy for ocular motor problems.
- Begin working with a technique that is within the capabilities of the patient.
- It is important to achieve some early success.
- Emphasize accuracy first and then speed of either the saccadic or pursuit eye movement.
- Many children with ocular motor dysfunction also have attention problems and impulsive cognitive styles. In fact, sometimes it is not clear if the impulsivity and inattention are the etiology for the poor fixation and ocular motility or whether the motility problems are the basis for the attention and impulsivity problems. To try to slow the child down and work toward

encouraging a more reflective, thoughtful, analytical style, we recommend stressing accuracy of the response at first. As accuracy improves during therapy, speed can then be incorporated as a variable.

- For saccades, go from gross (large) to fine (small) eye movements. For pursuits, the sequence is the opposite, from fine (small) to gross (large) eye movements.
- Begin motility therapy monocularly, and continue until both eyes are approximately equal in ability. Once monocular skills are equal, accurate, and fast, begin binocular ocular motility activities.
- Eliminate head movements during both pursuit and saccadic eye movements that can be reasonably accomplished without head movement.
- Increase the complexity of the task to develop more reflexive, automated pursuits and saccades. This can be accomplished by adding a metronome, a balance board, or simple cognitive tasks during any ocular motility task.

Vision Therapy Techniques for Saccades and Pursuits

The techniques described below should be effective for children and adults functioning at a 5- to 6-year-old level and above (Table 7.7). For patients performing below this level, refer to Chapters Eleven and Twelve.

Non-Computer-Based Therapy Techniques

HART CHART: SACCADIC THERAPY
Objective
The objective of the Hart Chart for saccadic therapy is to increase the speed and accuracy of saccadic fixation.

Equipment Needed
- Large Hart Chart for distance viewing
- Eye patch

Description and Setup
Place the Hart Chart (Figure 7.13) about 5 to 10 feet from the patient. Occlude the patient's left eye with an eye patch, and instruct the patient to call out the first letter in column 1 and then the first letter in column 10, the second letter from the top in column 1 and the second letter from the top in column 10, the third letter from the top in column 1 and the third letter from the top in column 10, and so on. Continue until the patient has called out all letters from columns 1 and 10.

Table 7.7

Ocular Motor Vision Therapy Techniques

- Hart Chart Saccades (1/10)
- Hart Chart Saccades (2/9, 3/8, 4/7, 5/6)
- Symbol Tracking
- Letter Tracking
- Visual Tracing
- Rotator Type Instruments
- Flashlight Tag

```
Y L 4 B E A 8 U M H
K 2 D S U 4 L O F Z
H C 7 A E T 3 1 Y R
P B 9 G N O 5 R V T
L 2 K G B 5 U T 3 D
A W E S 8 R O X N 1
7 A P T 6 E N U R Z
V 4 R 9 S M X 2 J T
S O 2 N 6 E H U 5 W
L 8 V S P D 1 N G 7
```

Figure 7.13. The Hart Chart used to increase the speed and accuracy of saccadic fixation.

As the patient calls out the letters, write down their responses, and when the task is completed, have the patient check their accuracy. Requiring the patient to check for errors is in itself another saccadic therapy technique. Now, the patient will have to make saccades from far to near to check for errors.

Once this task can be completed in about 15 seconds without any errors, you can increase the level of difficulty in several ways. Ask the patient to continue calling out letters in the other columns. Specifically, after completing columns 1 and 10, have the patient call out columns 2 and 9, 3 and 8, 4 and 7, and 5 and 6. The inner columns are more difficult because they are surrounded by other targets.

An even greater level of difficulty can be achieved by requiring saccades from the top of one column to the bottom of another. Instead of a left to right and right to left saccade, the patient will have to make an oblique saccade. For example, ask the patient to call out the top letter in column 1 and then the bottom letter in column 10, the second letter from the top in column 1 and the second letter from the bottom in column 10. Continue this pattern through the entire chart.

Other variations to increase the level of difficulty are possible, including incorporating the beat of a metronome and requiring the patient to maintain balance on a balance board while engaged in the task.

Endpoint
Discontinue this technique when the patient can complete columns 1 and 10 in 15 seconds with no errors, and all of the internal columns in 2 minutes with no errors.

ANN ARBOR LETTER AND SYMBOL TRACKING
Objective
The objective of the Letter and Symbol Tracking is to increase the speed and accuracy of saccadic fixation.

Equipment Needed
* Ann Arbor Letter and Symbol Tracking workbooks
* Plastic sheet, 8½ × 11 inches
* Paper clip
* Pen used for overhead transparencies (washable type)
* Eye patch

Description and Setup
Figures 7.14 and 7.15 illustrate the two workbooks. Both are designed to improve saccadic accuracy and speed. To permit the repeated use of the workbooks, I suggest that you cover the page being used with a plastic sheet and secure the plastic with a paper clip. I use overhead transparency sheets for this purpose.

As you can see in Figure 7.14, each page of Letter Tracking has two or more paragraphs of what appears to be random letters. Occlude one of the patient's eyes, and tell the patient to begin at the upper right and scan from left to right to find the first letter "A" and then make a line through it. Ask the patient to then find the very first "B" and cross it out, and continue through the entire paragraph finding the letters of the alphabet in order. The goal is to complete this task as quickly as possible. The therapist should time the therapy procedure. The patient's accuracy can also be evaluated. If the patient is scanning for the very first letter "D" for instance and inadvertently misses it and finds a "D" later in the paragraph, they will be unable to find the entire alphabet sequence in the paragraph. The workbook has five different size letters, creating another level of difficulty.

I suggest that after the patient finds and marks a specific letter, the pen be lifted off the page so that the patient will have to use saccades to find the next letter.

If the patient experiences difficulty with this task, Symbol Tracking (see Figure 7.15) can be used. Children in first grade will sometimes have difficulty because of lack of familiarity with the alphabet. This can cause great frustration and make the therapy technique very unpleasant for the patient. In such cases, use Symbol Tracking, which uses large pictures, symbols, numbers, and fewer letters. The task is, therefore, considerably easier and is very useful with younger children or those with very severe ocular motility disorders.

ABCDEFGHIJKLMNOPQRSTUVWXYZ
abcdefghijklmnopqrstuvwxyz   19

Iln chako evi nomd zeby thipg nare.
Zuth pirm nuroc dif stok. Nileg myt
lolf. Tixs nom raus zab tuin lugah.
Marb sewt rotsir puje. Yonak nesud
voz alee. Xart chod bugm turh sref
trea gen foru. Vab reps tique kowj.
Dagh meulb fwer ilg sida. Ubc they
bouf yed neoph vaik. Wolen kig peab
nad tenc xerb. Rait rebey fal zibt
_____Min. _____Sec.

Kog dalp stey molb ihn zurc taiwf
pim noxod. Prus myl wof kipet ghul.
Zalv ubx pufo cirk ghons taw. Quos
mey lairp sut vaej obk tund zoelec
pech. Tym surg aben burz. Dof terav
tecib ulaw kars fups. Irt quech adg
doif vok nebel ach laurt. Goxe misd
chitk queal doj neav libef tagow.
Ligeh axd yabel fom nepok ratzin
_____Min. _____Sec.

Figure 7.14. Ann Arbor Letter Tracking workbook designed to improve saccadic accuracy and speed.

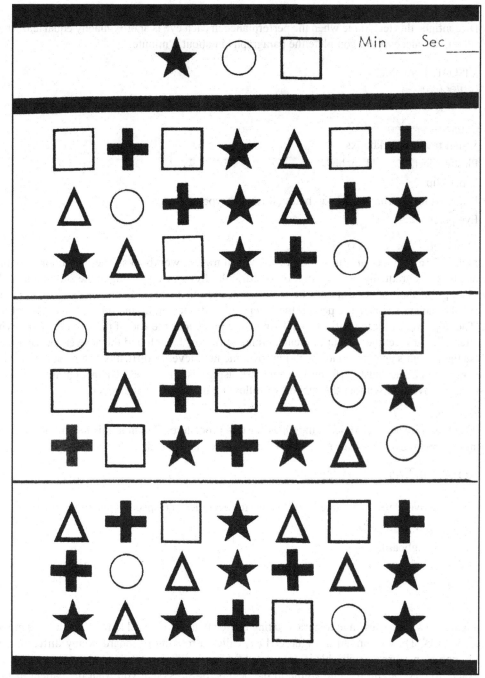

Figure 7.15. Ann Arbor Symbol Tracking workbook designed to improve saccadic accuracy and speed.

Endpoint
Discontinue this technique when the performance in each eye is approximately equal and when the patient can successfully complete the paragraphs in about 1 minute.

VISUAL TRACING
Objective
The objective of this technique is to improve the accuracy and speed of pursuit eye movements.

Equipment Needed
- Visual tracing workbooks
- Plastic sheet, 8½ × 11 inches
- Paper clip
- Pen used for overhead transparencies (washable type)
- Eye patch

Description and Setup
Figure 7.16 provides an illustration of the visual tracing workbooks. The workbook contains tracing tasks that gradually increase in level of difficulty from the beginning to the end of the book. Two therapy methods can be used. The easiest procedure is to occlude one of the patient's eyes and ask the patient to place the pen on the letter "A" and trace along the line until the end of the line. The objective is for the patient to determine the number at the end of the line beginning with the letter "A." Instruct the patient to then continue until they have found the answer for each line.

As the patient's accuracy and speed improve, the next level of difficulty can be added. In this technique, the patient must perform the same task using just their eyes. The patient must make a pursuit eye movement without the support of following the line with the pencil.

Endpoint
There are no specific clinical guidelines for this procedure. Continue this technique until the patient can perform with a reasonable degree of accuracy and speed.

ROTATOR TYPE INSTRUMENTS
Objective
The objective of this technique is to improve the accuracy and speed of pursuit eye movements.

Equipment Needed
- Rotating pegboard
- Golf tees
- Eye patch

Description and Setup
Figure 7.17 illustrates an automatic rotating device that can be used to treat pursuit eye movement disorders. The instrument in Figure 7.17 is called a rotating pegboard. Many different procedures can be performed with this instrument. After occluding one of the patient's eyes, instruct the patient to place a golf tee into a hole in the pegboard. Stress that you want the patient to first find the specific hole they will be using, and then in one motion place the peg in the hole. Once the patient can accomplish this, turn on the rotating pegboard. Now, instruct the patient to locate the first hole and hold the golf tee directly over the hole (although not touching it) for one full rotation. After the patient can successfully match the speed of the rotating pegboard for one revolution, instruct them to insert the peg in the hole with one motion. Have the patient continue this until all of the holes are filled with golf tees. Of course, the holes on the innermost part of the rotating pegboard are the easiest to work with, and the outer holes are the most difficult.

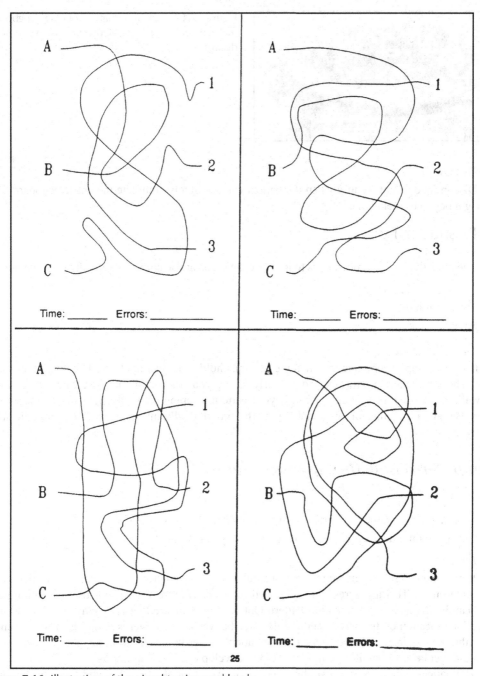

Figure 7.16. Illustration of the visual tracing workbooks.

To combine saccadic eye movements with pursuit eye movements, you can draw a pattern for the patient to follow on a wall directly behind the rotating pegboard. A typical pattern might require the patient to only place a peg in every third hole. The code itself can be simple or complex depending on the capability of the patient. This device can be constructed using a record player and pegboard, or it can be purchased from the vendor listed in Appendix A.

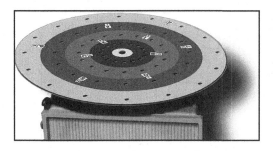

Figure 7.17. An automatic rotating pegboard that can be used to treat pursuit eye movement disorders.

Endpoint

Discontinue this procedure when the patient can accurately complete the entire pegboard following a peg placement code.

FLASHLIGHT TAG

Objective

The objective of this procedure is to improve the speed and accuracy of pursuit eye movements.

Equipment Needed
- Two flashlights
- An eye patch

Description and Setup

This is a simple technique in which the therapist holds one flashlight and the patient holds the other. The technique is performed monocularly. Using your flashlight, simply create a pattern on the wall, and instruct the patient to follow your pattern, keeping their flashlight superimposed on yours. Begin with predictable, repeatable patterns and gradually introduce random, unpredictable patterns.

Computer-Based Therapy Techniques

TPOT—EYE ROTATIONS

Equipment Needed
- Tracking and Perceptual Therapy for Occupational Therapists (TPOT)

  This procedure develops large angle, rhythmic eye movements.

Description

Randomly colored, circle targets with a single random character in the center are sequentially presented on the Therapy Screen in predefined locations (Figure 7.18). Four target location patterns can be defined by the Rotation Pattern Option. Since each target is displayed at a constant, predefined location on the screen and the distance between each target is about the same, a sense of rhythm and timing can be developed as the patient moves their eyes from target to target. Using the pre-target beep for auditory clues can help to develop eye tracking timing.

The patient should try to move their eyes to accurately look at (fixate) and focus each target as it is flashed. Each time the patient sees the Target Character they should press the <SPACE BAR> key to score. The patient must respond while the target is displayed to receive a correct score. Multiple clicks or presses during longer display times may result in overscoring and poor performance statistics.

To make this procedure more difficult:
- Decrease the display speed.
- Decrease the font size.
- Decrease the circle size.

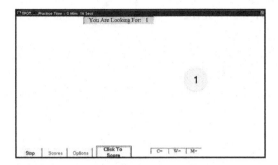

Figure 7.18. TPOT software: Eye Rotations.

- Decrease the pattern separation.
- Use random for rotation direction and rotation pattern.
- Turn the pre-display beep off (eliminated the auditory timing clues).

TPOT—Tracking Numbers
Description

A green Information Box appears displaying the Target Character for which the patient will be searching. The Target Character will continue to be displayed in the green box in the lower right-hand corner of the Therapy Screen.

The patient should try to move their eyes to accurately look at (fixate) and focus each character as it is displayed. The patient presses the <SPACE BAR> key to score.

To make this procedure more difficult:
- Set characters per line to either 2 or 8.
- Decrease the display time.
- Decrease the font size.
- Turn the display borders off.
- Use double digit numbers or lowercase letters.

TPOT—Tracking Sequences
Description

This procedure is similar to the Tracking Numbers program. Eye tracking movements in this procedure are developed using targets that require pattern recognition and visual sequential memory skills. Instead of single character targets, however, the program randomly generates a two- to five-character target sequence that must be recognized as random sequences are flashed across the screen. This requires a higher level of cognitive processing since you must track and fixate each displayed sequence and decide whether it matches the target sequence.

The patient should try to move their eyes to accurately look at (fixate) and focus each sequence as it is displayed. The patient presses the <SPACE BAR> key to score.

To make this procedure more difficult:
- Set characters per line to either 2 or 6.
- Decrease the display time.
- Decrease the font size.
- Turn the display borders off.

TPOT—Character Searching
Description

A grid of random characters (Letters, Numbers, or Both) is presented on the screen (Figure 7.19). A target character is displayed at the bottom of the screen. The patient should

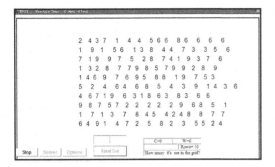

Figure 7.19. TPOT software: Character Searching.

visually scan the grid from left to right and count the number of characters in the grid that match the target letter or number. The patient enters their answer using the computer keyboard. If the count is incorrect, the patient is prompted to try again. This is a timed procedure, so try the goal is to answer as quickly as possible.

To make this procedure more difficult:

* Increase the number of rows.
* Increase the characters per row.
* Decrease the font size.
* Use lowercase letters.

Intervention for Visual Information Processing Disorders

Before dealing with visual information processing problems, it is important to first treat any refractive error or visual efficiency problems. We believe that refractive, binocular, ocular motility, and accommodative problems should be resolved first because they can have a negative effect on visual information processing. The concept is that before we begin to deal with the individual's ability to process information accurately, we must ensure that the input into the system is stable, clear, accurate, and efficient.

The treatment of visual perceptual and visual information processing problems is shared by several professions today. Optometrists, occupational therapists, psychologists, and cognitive therapists are some of the professionals who provide such services. We believe, however, that in many cases, professionals who do not evaluate and test for refractive and visual efficiency problems will not be as effective as possible and may prolong therapy if these more basic conditions are not treated first. Several studies have shown that, after treatment of visual efficiency problems alone, visual information processing skills also show some improvement. This concept is particularly important for brain injury patients because of the prevalence of acuity, binocular, accommodative, and visual field deficits. The presence of these problems makes it difficult to even interpret the results of visual information processing testing.

Visual information processing therapy is designed to remediate deficits in three general areas: visual spatial, visual analysis, and visual motor integration skills. The Visual Information Processing Test Battery described in Chapter Five is designed to identify specific weaknesses in each of these areas and to allow a differential diagnosis. I suggest remediation of only those areas that are deficient.

In this chapter, I will describe a sequence of therapy procedures that can be used to treat visual spatial and visual motor integration problems. For a more complete discussion and a description of procedures for the area of visual analysis skills, I suggest referring to *Optometric Management of Learning-Related Vision Problems*.[79]

Patient Factors

Several patient factors should be considered when planning a visual information processing therapy program for a patient. These include the relative strength of visual and auditory/language skills, cognitive style, and past history of success or failure.

If auditory and language skills are deficient, modifications must be made in therapy. Verbal directions should be simplified, and the therapist should present activities in a sequence of small steps. In contrast, when verbal skills are average to above average, the therapist can use verbal mediation to aid the weaker visual processing skills.

Cognitive style must also be taken into consideration. The impulsive patient will make a fast decision without considering all possible options. The reflective patient will get lost in the details of the task and will hesitate to make a decision. Of course, the optimal style is to be fast and accurate. A patient who is impulsive should be allowed to make mistakes, but the therapist should stress how the patient's strategy for solving the problem was effective or ineffective. In addition, the therapist should try to slow the patient down by using some of the following strategies: Have the patient verbally describe what they are doing, thinking, or planning, or have the patient point to each choice before making a decision. In contrast, with the reflective patient, the therapist can encourage the patient to respond rapidly and work toward automaticity in all skills.

The last area of concern is providing the patient in visual information processing therapy with a success-oriented environment. The vast majority of children with visual information processing problems reach your office with a history of school failure. Because of this failure, they tend to develop certain adaptive behaviors to avoid situations that result in a lack of success. They may be hesitant to perform certain activities, or they may just try to rush through things.

It is vital, therefore, that the initial stages of visual information processing therapy be a positive experience for the patient. Often, the first several sessions are used just to develop the right environment. The patient should be given techniques that are all within their capability to perform. If you give home vision therapy, use only procedures that will not create any additional frustration at home for the child and parent.

Role of the Therapist in Visual Information Processing Therapy

In order to be successful in visual information processing therapy, the therapist and patient must function in an interactive way. The role of the therapist is to help the patient learn a strategy or process to achieve an intended goal. This is a critical concept. The specific therapy procedure used is not as important as the goal of the task and the strategy necessary to achieve the goal.

The role of the therapist is to interact with the patient by asking questions, making the patient check their answer, and providing alternative strategies. Table 7.8 lists strategies to be used during visual information processing therapy.

Table 7.8

Strategies to Be Used During Visual Information Processing Therapy

- Present techniques and stimuli that guarantee initial success.
- Do not stress speed initially (except for reflective children).
- Question child about strategy.
- Have child verbalize strategy.
- Impulsive children should be encouraged to perform with maximum accuracy rather than maximum speed.
- Reflective children should be encouraged to work at maximum speed even if it results in some errors.

Intervention for Visual Spatial Skills

Visual spatial skills refer to the patient's awareness of internal and external spatial concepts and are used to organize the environment. The two subskills in this category are laterality and directionality. Table 7.9 lists the various techniques I recommend for improving visual spatial skills.

Non-Computer-Based Techniques

LATERALITY

This is the ability to identify right and left on one's self using verbal labels.

Overall Objective of Therapy

The objective of this therapy is to have the patient understand how the right side is different from the left side of their body.

Subgoal 1

To make the patient aware of the right and left side of the body. Therapy techniques include discussion of right/left hands, Simon says, and floor map.

Discussion of Right/Left Hands

Equipment Needed. None

Description. The easiest way to teach laterality skills is identifying the dominant hand and illustrating the differential function of the two hands. The first task is to identify the dominant hand. This can be done by asking the following series of questions:

- Show me how you brush your teeth.
- Show me how you hammer a nail.
- How do you cut with scissors?
- How do you write with a pencil?
- How do you throw a ball?

The dominant hand is the hand used for most of these tasks. If a dominant hand exists, proceed to engage the patient in motor activities in which the two hands are used differently, such as throwing a ball, writing, or cutting. The goal of this entire procedure is simply to discuss and demonstrate the differences in skill between the two hands so that the patient has a way of differentiating between the two.

Table 7.9

Therapy Procedures for Visual Spatial Skills

Laterality	*Endpoint*
Identification of dominant hand	Understands differences between hands
Simon says	Complete with limited errors
Floor map	Complete with limited errors
Directionality	*Endpoint*
Floor map	Complete with limited errors
Road maps	Complete with limited errors
Directional arrows	Complete sheet with limited errors
Visual Motor Sheets	Complete with limited errors
Letter Reversal Sheets	Complete grid with limited errors
Flip Flops	Complete with limited errors
Reversal Flash Cards	Complete with limited errors

Initially, if there is no clear dominant hand, you may have to mark one or the other with a rubber band, ring, or some similar device. Generally, the hand marked should be the one that appears to perform better during motor tasks.

At the end of this procedure, we want the patient to be able to think about and visualize a motor act in which they know one hand performs better than the other. By doing so, they will be able to differentiate between the two and know which is right and which is left.

Endpoint. The patient can consistently identify right and left on their own body.

Simon Says
Equipment Needed. None

Description. This well-known children's game can be used effectively to work on laterality. The therapist can play this game in the office with one or more children. In most cases, after introducing this game in the office, the therapist should assign this as a home therapy procedure.

Endpoint. The patient can consistently identify right and left on their own body.

Floor Map
Equipment Needed. Masking tape

Description. Create a road on the floor by placing masking tape on the floor. Create many turns in the road so that the patient must decide which direction to turn at each intersection. It is helpful at the beginning of this exercise to place a string or rubber band on the dominant hand of the patient to assist them initially. Ask the patient to negotiate the floor map and at each intersection to tell you whether they have to turn right or left. When the patient is indecisive, it is important for you to help them generate a strategy. For example, the therapist can ask the patient what hand they throw with and to try to transfer this information to the floor map task.

As therapy progresses, the patient should be able to verbalize their strategy: "I throw and write with my left hand so I need to turn left now." Finally, the patient should be able to guide him- or herself through the floor map without the need to stop and think about the difference between the right and left sides of his or her body.

As a variation, give the patient a map on paper or a chalkboard, and have the patient write down whether they would turn left or right at each intersection.

Endpoint. The patient can consistently, and without a great deal of thought, identify right and left and can describe their strategy.

DIRECTIONALITY
This is the ability to interpret left and right directions in space.

Overall Objective of Therapy
The objective of this therapy is to have the patient transfer their understanding of right and left on their own body to objects in space.

Subgoal 1
The patient should be able to identify right and left on animate objects. Therapy techniques include floor map and road maps.

Floor Map
Equipment Needed. Masking tape

Description. Use the same floor map that was created previously. Instead of the patient walking through the map, they now have to guide the therapist through the floor map. The goal is for the patient to realize that if the object can turn by itself in space, then right and left will appear to be opposite to their own right and left. This requires interpretation of right and left from a different perspective (usually this concept cannot be achieved until the patient is 7 years old).

Initially, the patient may need motor support to perform this task. They may have to turn their self to begin to understand this concept. Eventually, the patient should be able to guide another person through the floor map without motor support. In addition, we want the patient to be able to verbalize their strategy.

Endpoint. The patient can consistently, and without a great deal of thought, identify right and left and can describe their strategy.

Road Maps

Equipment Needed. Hand-drawn road maps

Description. The therapist pushes a small toy car through a hand-drawn road. The patient is asked to call out the direction the car must turn at each intersection.

Endpoint. The patient can consistently, and without a great deal of thought, identify right and left and can describe their strategy.

Subgoal 2

The patient should be able to identify right and left on inanimate objects facing them. The patient should understand that if the object cannot turn in space by itself, the right and left will appear on the same side as those of the patient. This concept is easier to grasp than right and left on an animate object. Children should be able to achieve this by age 5 or 6. Therapy techniques include directional arrows and Visual Motor Sheets.

Directional Arrows

Equipment Needed. Directional arrow worksheet (Figure 7.20)

Description. I suggest four levels to this task:

* Level One. Ask the patient to move their hand in the direction of the arrow. The patient does not have to call out the correct direction at this level.

* Level Two. Ask the patient to call out the direction of the arrows beginning from the upper left and going left to right across the rows. It is important to periodically stop the patient and ask

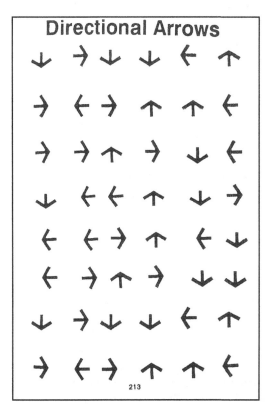

Figure 7.20. Directional arrow worksheet used to treat directionality problems. (Reprinted with permission from Learning Potentials Publishers.)

how they know the arrow is pointing to the right or left. They should be able to say, "Because this is my right hand and the arrow is pointing to this side, it must be pointing to the right."

- Level Three. To work on automaticity, have the patient call out the direction of the arrows to the beat of a metronome.
- Level Four. Another method for working on automaticity is to have the patient move their hand in the direction the arrow is pointing but call out the opposite direction.

Endpoint. The patient can consistently, and without a great deal of thought, identify right and left and can describe their strategy.

Visual Motor Sheets—Sheet A

Equipment Needed. Visual Motor Activity Sheet A (Figure 7.21)
Description. I suggest two levels to this task:

- Level One. Have the patient sit next to you at a table. Tell them to call out the position of the vertical line relative to the horizontal line. For example, the top row going left to right on the worksheet would be right up, middle down, right down, left up.
- Level Two. Have the patient do the same activity as in Level One except now use a metronome. At the beat of the metronome, the patient must call out the direction. Using the metronome increases the level of difficulty because the patient now has to respond to the beat and with greater automaticity.

Visual Motor Sheets—Sheet B

Equipment Needed. Visual Motor Activity Sheet B (Figure 7.22)
Description. I suggest two levels to this task:

- Level One. For this worksheet, the hands and feet are coded to symbols as indicated in Figure 7.23. The circle is coded to the hand, the triangle to the foot. If the circle is to the right of the line, the patient is to raise their right hand. If the triangle is to the left of the line, the

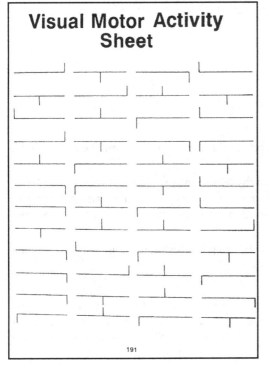

Figure 7.21. Visual Motor Activity Sheet A used to treat directionality problems. (Reprinted with permission from Learning Potentials Publishers.)

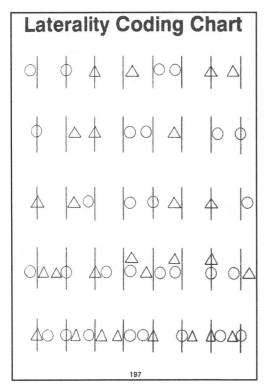

Figure 7.22. Visual Motor Activity Sheet B used to treat directionality problems. (Reprinted with permission from Learning Potentials Publishers.)

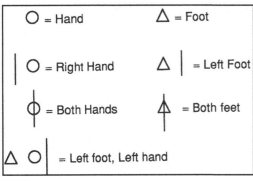

Figure 7.23. For Visual Motor Activity Sheet B, the hands and feet are coded to symbols as indicated in the figure. (Reprinted with permission from Learning Potentials Publishers.)

patient is to stomp their left foot. If the line passes directly through the middle of the circle, the patient is to raise both hands.

- Level Two. Have the patient do the same activity as in Level One except now use a metronome. At the beat of the metronome, the patient must call out the direction. Using the metronome increases the level of difficulty because the patient now has to respond to the beat and with greater automaticity.

Endpoint. The patient can consistently, and without a great deal of thought, identify right and left and can describe their strategy.

Subgoal 3

The final goal of directionality therapy is to apply these concepts to spatial orientation of forms and letters. In this stage, the patient must be able to describe distinctive features of these letters and forms. For example, the only difference between a lowercase "b" and a lowercase "d" is the location of the semicircle.

It is important for the patient to use the concepts learned earlier to develop a strategy for distinguishing easily reversible letters. The patient should develop a verbal strategy using directional concepts to identify each letter. Therapy techniques include Letter Reversal Sheets, Flip Flops, and Reversal Flash Cards.

Letter Reversal Sheets

Equipment Needed. Letter Reversal Sheets (Figure 7.24)

Description. Place the Letter Reversal Sheet (see Figure 7.24) on a desk. Ask the patient to cross out all of the letters that appear backward. The patient must identify any reversal errors.

Endpoint. The patient can consistently, and without a great deal of thought, identify the reversed letters.

Flip Flops

Equipment Needed. Plastic transparency, transparency pen, and Flip Flop Patterns (enclosed with materials)

Description. The patient is asked to look at a stimulus (Figure 7.25). The therapist instructs the patient to visualize the stimulus rotated in several possible positions, including rotated 90 degrees to the right, rotated 90 degrees to the left, flipped sideways, flipped upside down, or any combination of these. The patient must then draw the stimulus, taking the transformation into consideration.

In the beginning, it is helpful to draw the stimulus on a clear plastic sheet. Using this sheet, you can demonstrate what the form would look like after the various transformations.

Endpoint. The patient can consistently, and without a great deal of thought, make the various transformations and describe their strategy.

Reversal Flash Cards

Equipment Needed. Reversal Flash Cards (Figure 7.26)

Description. This procedure uses traditional flash cards employed by children to study vocabulary and spelling words. The only difference is that two cards are made for each word. On

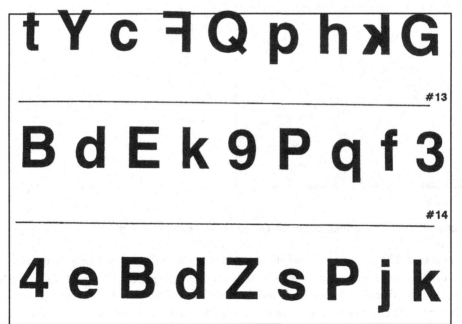

Figure 7.24. Letter Reversal Sheets used to treat directionality problems. (Reprinted with permission from Learning Potentials Publishers.)

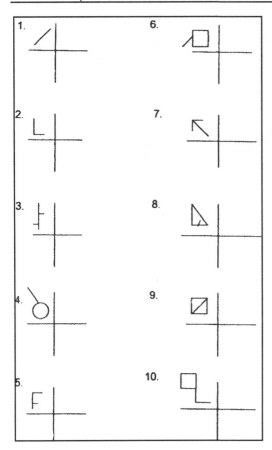

Figure 7.25. Flip Flop Patterns.

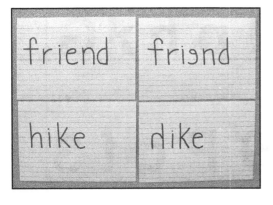

Figure 7.26. Reversal Flash Cards used to treat directionality.

one card, all letters are written correctly. On the second card, one or more letters are purposefully reversed.

- Level One. The patient must find all the cards with reversals and then copy them correctly.
- Level Two. Flash each card for about 3 seconds. Have the patient tell you if any of the letters were reversed or not. Have them correctly print the word that had letters reversed.

This procedure can be performed at home with the parent making up a set of cards using the patient's school words.

Endpoint. The patient should be able to achieve 90% correct with one transformation.

Computer-Based Techniques

TPOT—Right or Left

Description

In this activity, a character named Mr. Stickman is facing either toward the patient or looking away from the patient holding a balloon in his right or left hand (Figure 7.27). Or, he might be facing front or back kicking a ball with his right or left foot. As each new character is presented, the patient should try to determine as quickly as possible which hand Mr. Stickman is using to hold the balloon or which foot he is using to kick the ball. The Reaction Time Score displayed on the Therapy Screen measures the average response time for each Stickman. The Average Time Score displayed on the Score Screen and Score Printout calculates the average response time for all Stickmen tried during the therapy sessions.

To make this procedure more difficult:

• Begin therapy with the Display Speed OFF. As skill is gained, use progressively faster Display Speeds.

TPOT—Flipper

Description

In this activity, a target image is presented in the picture box at the top of the Therapy Screen. Four answer image boxes are placed at the bottom of the Therapy Screen (Figure 7.28). The images in the answer boxes will be the target picture flipped, turned, or rotated. One of the answer boxes might even match the target picture in the top picture box. A question about the target picture will be presented below the top image. For example, "Which of the answer pictures matches the target?" Or, "Which of the answer images is flipped right to left?" Or, "Which of the four answer images is flipped upside down?" The patient should try to respond as quickly as possible. Performance is measured by both correct answers and how fast you respond.

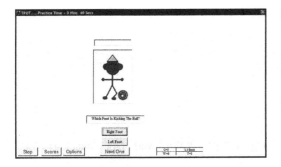

Figure 7.27. TPOT software: Right or Left.

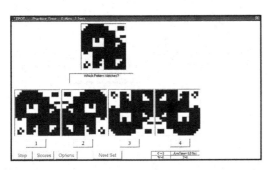

Figure 7.28. TPOT software: Flipper.

To make this procedure more difficult:
- Use higher numbered images.

TPOT—FLIP FORMS

In this exercise, there are four picture boxes. The target image is displayed in the upper left box. The patient should click on box 1 until the target image appears flipped right to left (Figure 7.29). When the patient feels the answer is correct, they should click on the OK button. The patient then does the same with picture boxes 2, 3, and 4. Performance will be measured not only by correct answers but also speed of the response.

To make this procedure more difficult:
- Select images with higher numbers.

Intervention for Visual Analysis Skills

Visual analysis skills refer to the ability to analyze and interpret visual information. This aspect of visual information processing is sometimes referred to as motor-free visual perception. Sub-categories include visual discrimination, visual figure ground, visual closure, and visual memory.

Computer-Based Therapy for Visual Analysis Skills

VISUAL DISCRIMINATION

TPOT—Discriminating Color Grids

Description. This procedure creates four grids containing patterns of randomly colored squares. Grid size can be varied from 2 to 16 squares (Figure 7.30). Three of the patterns are identical, one is different. The patient should visually compare each of the four patterns and determine which pattern is different using visual discrimination skills. The correct answer will be highlighted in green.

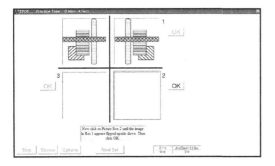

Figure 7.29. TPOT software: Flip Forms.

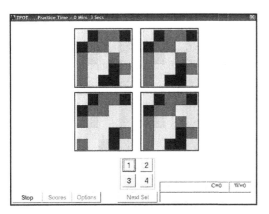

Figure 7.30. TPOT software: Discriminating Color.

To make the procedure more difficult:

- Increase grid size.
- Turn the grid borders off.
- Decrease the different colors to two.
- Use harder colors.

TPOT—Pattern Duplicator

Description. This procedure develops visual spatial relationships utilizing a 25- or 100-square pattern that must be duplicated. When therapy begins, a random pattern is generated in the left-hand grid (Figure 7.31). The goal is to reproduce that same pattern on the right-hand grid. The patient does so by clicking on the squares in the grid. The computer will check the answer and score it as correct or incorrect. If wrong, the number of incorrect squares in the pattern will be displayed.

To make this procedure more difficult:

- Turning the GRID BORDERS off makes the pattern duplication more difficult.

VISUAL FIGURE GROUND

TPOT—Shape Counting

Description. Several shapes appear on the screen and the patient must count the number of shapes (Figure 7.32). As the program becomes harder, the shapes begin to become superimposed on one another and figure ground discrimination skills are required to count the shapes. The patient should count and enter the number of foreground targets seen. This is a timed procedure.

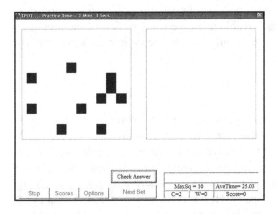

Figure 7.31. TPOT software: Pattern Duplicator.

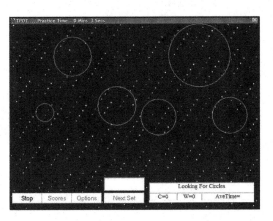

Figure 7.32. TPOT software: Shape Counting.

To make this procedure more difficult:

- Increase the maximum number of shapes.
- Increase the background complexity.
- Decrease the border size.

VISUAL CLOSURE
TPOT—Closing Lines and Boxes
Description. Two target options are available:

With the CONVERGING LINES option, two lines are flashed on the screen. The patient should visualize the lines and try to determine where the lines would meet if they were extended to their meeting point. Visual closure skills are required to visualize the extension of the lines to their crossing point.

In the BOX mode, three corners (indicated by three circles) of a randomly sized rectangle are flashed on the screen. The patient should visualize the rectangle that would be formed by these three circles (corners) and determine where the fourth corner of the rectangle would be.

To make this procedure more difficult:

- Decrease the display speed.
- Turn visual confusion on.

TPOT—Closing Letters
Description. In this exercise, a target letter, hidden under the gray cover, is presented in the picture box at the top of the Therapy Screen (Figure 7.33). The patient should click on the <ERASE TILES> button. A few of the gray blocks will disappear, revealing part of the hidden letter. The patient should try and can guess the letter. If not yet possible, he should erase a few more tiles. The goal is to determine the answer as quickly as possible and by erasing as few of the blocks as possible. Performance is measured by correct answers, and how fast the patient responds, and by how many blocks were erased.

VISUAL MEMORY
TPOT—Tic Tac Toe Rotations
Description. This procedure requires both visual memory and visual spatial skills. The familiar Tic Tac Toe grid is utilized in this procedure to flash patterns of X's on the grid (Figure 7.34). When the X's are flashed, the patient should try to visualize the pattern on the grid. The patient uses the left mouse button to click on the squares in the grid to recreate the flashed pattern. If the patient makes a mistake, they should click on the square again to remove the X. When the patient is ready to check the answer, they should click on the <CHECK ANSWER> button. A small grid will appear on the right side of the screen displaying the correct Tic Tac Toe pattern. As skill is

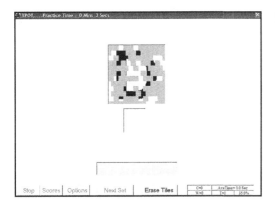

Figure 7.33. TPOT software: Closing Letters.

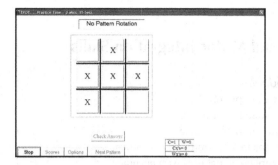

Figure 7.34. TPOT software: Tic Tac Toe Rotations.

gained, PATTERN ROTATION should be introduced. Visualization becomes even more important for these procedures since the patient must mentally manipulate the spatial relationships in the pattern. After the X pattern is presented on the Tic Tac Toe grid, the patient must enter the pattern rotated either clockwise or counterclockwise.

To make this procedure more difficult:

- Decrease the display time.
- Increase the maximum number of X's that are presented.
- Use a small font size.
- Rotate the answer.

TPOT—Visual Sequencing

Description. This procedure develops visual sequencing, visual sequential memory, and visual spatial relationships utilizing the Tic Tac Toe grid to sequentially present colored squares in various patterns on the grid. Each square in the pattern is presented sequentially rather than simultaneously as the X's in the Tic Tac Toe procedure. The patient should try and visualize and remember both the location and sequence of colored square as they are flashed on the grid. After the sequence has been presented, the patient clicks on the appropriate squares in the grid to reproduce the sequence. Once the correct number of squares has been pressed, the answer will be checked and scored automatically.

To make this procedure more difficult:

- Decrease the display time.
- Turn the pre-display beep off.
- Increase the sequence length.
- Use increasing sequence length.

Intervention for Visual Motor Integration Skills

Visual motor integration skills refer to the patient's ability to integrate visual information processing skills with fine motor movement. If there are problems in both fine motor and visual motor integration based on the test battery, I suggest a sequential approach in which remediation proceeds in two phases: fine motor and then visual motor integration. In my experience as an optometrist, I have found that when a patient has an obvious fine motor problem and difficulty with fine motor skills, a referral to an occupational therapist with experience and knowledge of handwriting difficulties and fine motor problems is warranted. I often work together with occupational therapists with such children. The occupational therapist will work on the fine motor coordination difficulty and handwriting skills while I will work on the underlying visual motor integration problems.

In the discussion that follows, I have chosen to describe two examples of fine motor techniques and one visual motor integration procedure in great detail. The concepts and principles described

Table 7.10

Therapy Procedures for Visual Motor Integration Skills

Visual Motor Integration	Endpoint
Visual tracing workbook	Accurate performance
Visual fine motor integration workbook	Accurate performance
Geoboard and dot maps	Accurate performance
Parquetry	Complete all patterns with accuracy
Pegboard designs	Complete all patterns with accuracy
Design blocks and patterns	Complete all patterns with accuracy

relative to this procedure are important and represent the essence of how to succeed in remediating these difficulties. These concepts and principles can be readily applied to numerous other techniques for working with visual motor integration problems. Table 7.10 lists the techniques that I recommend for improving visual motor integration skills.

Overall Goal of Visual Motor Integration Therapy

The goal is to allow the patient to become aware of the importance of the eye leading the hand, the relationships of parts of figures to each other and to the total background, and to place these relationships on paper using a pencil.

Subgoal 1

Teach the patient to have the eye lead the hand. Therapy techniques include Visual Tracing Workbooks and Visual Fine Motor Integration Workbooks.

VISUAL TRACING WORKBOOK
Equipment Needed
- Visual tracing workbook

Description
This 34-page workbook contains a series of tracing activities arranged in order of increasing difficulty (Figure 7.35).
- Level One. The patient uses a pointer and attempts to follow the line, with the pointer on the line at all times. After tracing the line with the pointer, have the patient follow the line only with their eyes.
- Level Two. Same as level one but now the patient is timed.

Endpoint
The patient should be able to accurately trace lines with and without a pointer. They should be able to complete the most difficult tracings within 75 seconds.

Subgoal 2

Have the patient be aware of the relationship of parts of figures to each other and to the background as they copy the figures. Therapy techniques include geoboard and dot maps, parquetry, pegboard designs, and design blocks.

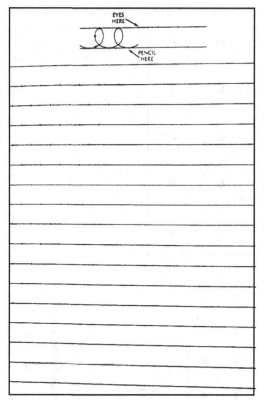

Figure 7.35. Visual Tracing Workbook used to treat fine motor problems.

GEOBOARD AND DOT MAPS
Equipment Needed
- 25-pin geoboard
- Plastic transparencies
- Transparency pen

Description

In this technique, the patient is asked to copy a design from a map to a geoboard or from a map to a map. The map is simply a 5×5-inch matrix of dots (Figure 7.36).
- Level One. Begin this therapy procedure using a 25-pin geoboard and a 25-dot map. The therapist uses rubber bands to copy Pattern 49 onto the 25-pin geoboard. The patient is asked to look at this pattern and copy it using the overhead transparency pen on the 25-dot map.

In most cases, this will be a good starting point for the patient. If it seems too difficult, you have two options. The first is to use a second 25-pin geoboard and have the patient copy the pattern on your geoboard onto their geoboard with rubber bands. This is easier than copying onto a 25-dot map because the geoboard is a concrete, physical item the patient can touch and manipulate. If this is still too difficult, use a five- or nine-dot geoboard or map along with the easier patterns (Patterns 1 to 48). In this very simple first stage, the patient is asked to copy your design onto their geoboard or map.

It is critical to remember that there must be interaction between the therapist and patient. Simply asking the patient to copy these patterns will probably have little positive effect. From the very beginning, it is important to establish that the patient must work with some strategy and analyze the pattern carefully before attempting to reproduce the pattern. For example, in Figure 7.37, the

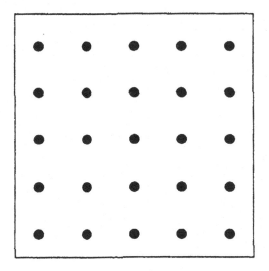

Figure 7.36. Geoboard and dot maps. In this technique, the child is asked to copy a design from a map to a geoboard, or from a map to a map. The map is simply a 5×5-inch matrix of dots.

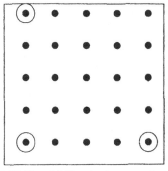 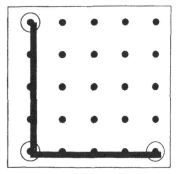

Figure 7.37. The child is asked to copy the pattern from the 25-dot map on the left. This figure demonstrates the specific procedure that should be used.

patient is asked to copy the pattern from the 25-dot map on the left. Instead of just copying it, we want the patient to verbalize and demonstrate their strategy. The following is the procedure we recommend. The therapist should instruct the patient as follows:

1. Identify the line you will copy first from my map.
2. Place a circle around the first dot of the line you will copy.
3. Now find the same dot on your map and place a circle around it.
4. Go back to the pattern on my map and find the last dot of the line you will draw.
5. Now find this same dot on your map and place a circle around it.
6. Place your pencil on the first circle on your map, look at the second circle, and now slowly draw the line between the two circles.
7. Find the next line you are going to draw and circle the first dot; continue with numbers 3 to 6.

Although this process may seem time-consuming and too easy for the patient initially, it is important to establish this strategy early in therapy so that when the patterns do become hard, the patient will have an approach for overcoming obstacles.

Continue working in this manner until you reach Pattern 200.

- Level Two. Once the patient can successfully perform Patterns 49 to 200 according to the instructions in Level One, begin from Pattern 100, and this time after you copy your pattern onto your 25-dot map, instruct the patient to copy theirs onto a 17-dot map (Figure 7.38). In this case, you have removed some of the detail and structure. The patient is instructed to copy theirs and pretend that all of the dots are present.

- Level Three. Once the patient can successfully perform Patterns 49 to 200 according to the instructions in Level Two, begin from Pattern 100, and this time after you copy your pattern onto your 25-dot map, instruct the patient to copy theirs onto a 9-dot map. In this case, you have removed more of the detail and structure. The patient is instructed to copy theirs and pretend that all of the dots are present.

- Level Four. Once the patient can successfully perform Patterns 49 to 200 according to the instructions in Level Three, begin from Pattern 100, and this time after you copy your pattern onto your 25-dot map, instruct the patient to copy theirs onto a five-dot map.

- Level Five. Once the patient can successfully perform Patterns 49 to 200 according to the instructions in Level Four, begin from Pattern 100, and this time after you copy your pattern onto your 25-dot map, instruct the patient to copy theirs onto a zero-dot map.

- Level Six. The patient is asked to copy patterns as quickly as possible. When you introduce this level, the patient no longer must verbalize their strategy or use the circle method described above. We simply want to have them perform quickly and accurately.

In addition to these six levels, several variations can be introduced at any of the levels to add variation, challenge, and complexity to the task.

- Variation One. To vary the task and to increase the level of difficulty at any point, you can modify the instructions in Levels One through Six as follows:

Instead of asking the patient to copy the design you construct, ask the patient to make a design of their choice on their 25-dot map. Have them hide this from you so that only they can see the design. Ask the patient to give you verbal instructions so that you can make your pattern look the same as theirs without you seeing it.

This allows you to determine if they have really developed a strategy. For example, the patient may use the following language: "Place your pencil on the first dot in the upper right-hand corner and draw a line straight down to the dot in the lower right-hand corner."

- Variation Two. Another variation and a level that is considered more difficult is to ask the patient to identify each dot on the map using a coordinate system. This variation can be introduced periodically whenever you think the patient may be ready.

An example of this is illustrated in Figure 7.39. In this example, the dot circled on the right-hand map would be called C3. Instead of using the procedure suggested in Level One, in which the patient was instructed to circle the first and last dots of the line before drawing, they must now identify the dots using coordinates.

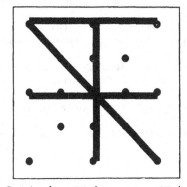 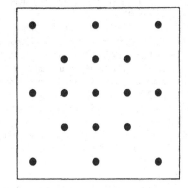

Figure 7.38. Copying from 25-dot map to a 17-dot map.

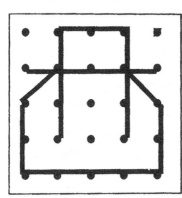 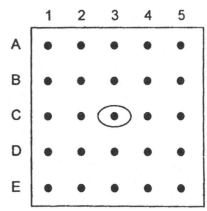

Figure 7.39. Advanced procedure using the map technique.

To copy the top line in Figure 7.39 they would say: "I will begin with dot A2 and move my pencil right until I reach dot A4."

- Variation Three. The patient is asked to copy your pattern onto their map, but they are only given a short period of time to view the pattern and must draw theirs from memory.

Endpoint

The patient should be able to complete all patterns with limited errors and should be able to achieve this success with speed and automaticity.

Summary

The procedure described above, with its increasingly more difficult levels and variations, can be applied to virtually any other visual motor integration task. Some of the common techniques used include parquetry, pegboard designs, and design blocks. The important point is that it is necessary to force the patient to analyze the stimulus and develop a plan or strategy to reproduce it. The various levels and variations described above help accomplish these goals. They also encourage verbalization, a reflective cognitive style early on, and at the end of the sequence, an increase in the speed of the patient's response.

References

1. Skeffington AM. *Introduction to Clinical Optometry*. Santa Ana, CA: Optometric Extension Program Foundation, Optometric Extension Program Postgraduate Courses. Vol 37, Oct. 1964–Sept 1965.
2. Kaplan M, Edelson S, Seip J. Behavioral changes in autistic individuals as a result of wearing ambient transitional prism lenses. *Child Psychiat Hum D*. 1998;29:65–76.
3. Kaplan M, Carmody D, Gaydos A. Postural orientation modifications in autism in response to ambient lenses. *Child Psychiat Hum D*. 1996;27:81–91.
4. Kaplan M. *Seeing Through New Eyes*. Philadelphia, PA: Jessica Kingsley Publishers; 2006.
5. Scheiman M, Wick B. *Clinical Management of Binocular Vision: Heterophoric, Accommodative and Eye Movement Disorders*. 5th ed. Philadelphia, PA: Wolters-Kluwer; 2019.
6. Scheiman M, Cotter S, Rouse M, et al. Randomised clinical trial of the effectiveness of base-in prism reading glasses versus placebo reading glasses for symptomatic convergence insufficiency in children. *Br J Ophthalmol*. 2005;89:1318–1323.
7. Teitelbaum B, Pang Y, Krall J. Effectiveness of base in prism for presbyopes with convergence insufficiency. *Optom Vis Sci*. 2009;86:153–156.
8. Bowers AR, Keeney K, Peli E. Community-based trial of a peripheral prism visual field expansion device for hemianopia. *Arch Ophthalmol*. 2008;126:657–664.
9. Giorgi RG, Woods RL, Peli E. Clinical and laboratory evaluation of peripheral prism glasses for hemianopia. *Optom Vis Sci*. 2009;86:492–502.
10. Padula WV, Argyris S. Post-trauma vision syndrome and visual midline shift syndrome. *NeuroRehab*. 1996;6:165–171.

11. McBrien N. Optometry: an evidence-based clinical discipline. *Clin Exp Optom.* 1998;81:234–235.

12. Mozlin R. Evidence-based medicine. *J Am Optom Assoc.* 2000;71:490–500.

13. Straus SE, Richardson WS, Glasziou P, Haynes RB. *Evidence-Based Medicine: How to Practice and Teach EBM.* 3rd ed. Philadelphia, PA: Elsevier Churchill Livingstone; 2005.

14. McKibbon KA, Wilczynski NL, Haynes RD. What do evidence-based secondary journals tell us about the publication of clinically important articles in primary healthcare journals? *BMC Med.* 2004;2:33.

15. Miller PA, McKibbon KA. A quantitative analysis of research publications in physical therapy journals. *Phys Ther.* 2003;83:123–131.

16. Lai TYY, Leung GM, Wong VWY, et al. How evidence-based are publications in clinical ophthalmic journals? *Invest Ophthalmol Vis Sci.* 2006;47:1831–1838.

17. Sanfilippo S, Clahane AC. The effectiveness of orthoptics alone in selected cases of exodeviation: the immediate results and several years later. *Am Orthoptic J.* 1970;20:104–117.

18. Hoffman L, Cohen A, Feuer G. Effectiveness of non-strabismic optometric vision training in a private practice. *Am J Optom Arch Am Acad Opt.* 1973;50:813–816.

19. Cornsweet TN, Crane HD. Training the visual accommodation system. *Vision Res.* 1973;13:713–715.

20. Provine RR, Enoch JM. On voluntary ocular accommodation. *Percept Psychophys.* 1975;17:209–212.

21. Cooper EL, Leyman IA. The management of intermittent exotropia: a comparison of the results of surgical and non surgical treatment. *Am Orthoptic J.* 1977;27:61–67.

22. Wick B. Vision therapy for presbyopic nonstrabismic patients. *Am J Optom Physiol Opt.* 1977;54:244–247.

23. Wold RM, Pierce JR, Keddington J. Effectiveness of optometric vision therapy. *J Am Optom Assoc.* 1978;49:1047–1053.

24. Liu JS, Lee M, Jang J, et al. Objective assessment of accommodative orthoptics: 1 dynamic insufficiency. *Am J Optom Physiol Opt.* 1979;56:285–294.

25. Weisz CL. Clinical therapy for accommodative responses: transfer effects upon performance. *J Am Optom Assoc.* 1979;50:209–216.

26. Grisham D. The dynamics of fusional vergence eye movements in binocular dysfunction. *Am J Optom Physiol Opt.* 1980;57:645–655.

27. Daum K. Double-blind placebo-controlled examination of timing effects in the training of positive vergences. *Am J Optom Physiol Opt.* 1986;63:807–812.

28. Daum KM. Negative vergence training in humans. *Am J Optom Physiol Opt.* 1986;63:487–496.

29. Daum KM. Characteristics of exodeviations: II. Changes with Treatment with orthoptics. *Am J Optom Physiol Opt.* 1986;63:244–251.

30. Daum KM. Divergence excess: characteristics and results of treatment with orthoptics. *Ophthal Physiol Opt.* 1984;4:15–24.

31. Daum KM. Equal exodeviations: characteristics and results of treatment with orthoptics. *Aust J Optom.* 1984;67:53–59.

32. Daum KM. Predicting Results in the orthoptic treatment of accommodative dysfunction. *Am J Optom Physiol Opt.* 1984;61:184–189.

33. Daum KM. Modelling the results of the orthoptic treatment of divergence excess. *Ophthalmic Physiol Opt.* 1984;4:25–29.

34. Daum KM. Divergence excess: characteristics and results of treatment with orthoptics. *Ophthalmic Physiol Opt.* 1984;4:15–24.

35. Daum KM. Convergence insufficiency. *Am J Optom Physiol Opt.* 1984;61:16–22.

36. Daum KM. A comparison of the results of tonic and phasic vergence training. *Am J Optom Physiol Opt.* 1983;60:769–775.

37. Daum KM. A comparison of the results of tonic and phasic vergence training. *Am J Optom Physiol Opt.* 1983;60:769–775.

38. Daum KM. Accommodative dysfunction. *Doc Ophthalmol.* 1983;55:177–198.

39. Daum KM. Accommodative insufficiency. *Am J Optom Physiol Opt.* 1983;60:352–359.

40. Daum KM. The course and effect of visual training on the vergence system. *Am J Optom Physiol Opt.* 1982;59:223–237.

41. Bobier WR, Sivak JG. Orthoptic treatment of subjects showing slow accommodative responses. *Am J Optom Physiol Opt.* 1983;60:678–687.

42. Cohen AH, Soden R. Effectiveness of visual therapy for convergence insufficiencies for an adult population. *J Am Optom Assoc.* 1984;55:491–494.

43. Rouse MW. Management of binocular anomalies: efficacy of vision therapy in the treatment of accommodative deficiencies. *Am J Optom Physiol Opt.* 1987;64:415–420.

44. Grisham JD, et al. Vergence orthoptics: validity and persistence of the training effect. *Optom Vis Sci.* 1991;68:441–451.

45. Cooper J, Medow N. Intermittent exotropia of the divergence excess type: basic and divergence excess type. *Bin Vis Eye Mus Surg Qtly.* 1993;8:187–222.

46. Shorter AD, Hatch SW. Vision therapy for convergence excess. *N Eng J Optom.* 1993;45:51–53.

47. Ficcara AP, Berman J, Rosenfield M, et al. Vision therapy: predictive factors for success in visual therapy for patients with convergence excess. *J Optom Vis Dev.* 1996;27:213–219.

48. Gallaway M, Scheiman M. The efficacy of vision therapy for convergence excess. *J Am Optom Assoc*. 1997;68:81–86.
49. Adler P. Efficacy of treatment for convergence insufficiency using vision therapy. *Ophthalmic Physiol Opt*. 2002;22:565–571.
50. Abdi S, Rydberg A. Asthenopia in schoolchildren, orthoptic and ophthalmological findings and treatment. *Doc Ophthalmol*. 2005;111:65–72.
51. Aziz S, Cleary M, Stewart HK, Weir CR. Are orthoptic exercises an effective treatment for convergence and fusion deficiencies? *Strabismus*. 2006;14:183–189.
52. Vaegan JL. Convergence and divergence show longer and sustained improvement after short isometric exercise. *Am J Optom Physiol Opt*. 1979;56:23–33.
53. Cooper J, Feldman J, Selenow A, et al. Reduction of asthenopia after accommodative facility training. *Am J Optom Physiol Opt*. 1987;64:430–436.
54. Cooper J, Selenow A, Ciuffreda KJ, et al. Reduction of asthenopia in patients with convergence insufficiency after fusional vergence training. *Am J Optom Physiol Opt*. 1983;60:982–989.
55. Birnbaum MH, Soden R, Cohen AH. Efficacy of vision therapy for convergence insufficiency in an adult male population. *J Am Optom Assoc*. 1999;70:225–232.
56. Tobii Pro Nano Eye Tracker, Eye Tracker, October 17, 2018. https://www.tobiipro.com/product.
57. Scheiman M, Mitchell GL, Cotter S, et al. A randomized trial of the effectiveness of treatments for convergence insufficiency in children. *Arch Ophthalmol*. 2005;123:14–24.
58. Scheiman M, Mitchell GL, Cotter S, et al. A randomized clinical trial of vision therapy/orthoptics versus pencil pushups for the treatment of convergence insufficiency in young adults. *Optom Vis Sci*. 2005;82:583–595.
59. Scheiman M, Kulp MT, Cotter SA, et al. Interventions for convergence insufficiency: a network meta-analysis. *Cochrane Database Syst Rev*. 2020;12:CD006768.
60. CITT-ART Investigator Group. Treatment of symptomatic convergence insufficiency in children enrolled in the convergence insufficiency treatment trial—attention & reading trial: a randomized clinical trial. *Optom Vis Sci*. 2019;96:825–835.
61. Convergence Insufficiency Treatment Trial Investigator Group. A randomized clinical trial of treatments for symptomatic convergence insufficiency in children. *Arch Ophthalmol*. 2008;126:1336–1349.
62. Ciuffreda K. The scientific basis for and efficacy of optometric vision therapy in nonstrabismic accommodative and binocular vision disorders. *Optometry*. 2002;73:735–762.
63. Cooper J, Selenow A, Ciuffreda KJ. Reduction of asthenopia in patients with convergence insufficiency after fusional vergence training. *Am J Optom Physiol Opt*. 1983;60:982–989.
64. CITT-ART Investigator Group. Treatment of symptomatic convergence insufficiency in children enrolled in the convergence insufficiency treatment trial—attention & reading trial: a randomized clinical trial. *Optom Vis Sci*. 2019;96:825–835.
65. Rounds BB, Manley CW, Norris RH. The effect of oculomotor training on reading efficiency. *J Am Optom Assoc*. 1991;6:92–99.
66. Young BS Pollard T, Paynter S, Cox R. Effect of eye exercises in improving control of eye movements during reading. *J Optom Vis Dev*. 1982;13:4–7.
67. Fujimoto DH, Christensen EA, Griffin JR. An investigation in use of videocassette techniques for enhancement of saccadic movements. *J Am Optom Assoc*. 1985;56:304–308.
68. Rouse MW, Borsting E. Management of visual information processing problems. In: Scheiman M, Rouse MW, eds. *Optometric Management of Learning-Related Vision Problems*. 2nd ed. St. Louis, MO: CV Mosby; 2006:432–433.
69. Farr JA, Leibowitz HW. An experimental study of the efficacy of perceptual-motor training. *Am J Optom Physiol Opt*. 1976;53:451–455.
70. Seiderman AS. Optometric vision therapy—results of a demonstration project with a learning disabled population. *J Am Optom Assoc*. 1980;51:489–493.
71. Hendrickson LN, Muehl S. The effect of attention and motor response pretraining on learning to discriminate B and D in kindergarten children. *J Ed Psych*. 1962;53:236–241.
72. Greenspan SB. Effectiveness of therapy for children's reversal confusions. *Acad Ther*. 1975–1976;11:169–178.
73. Walsh JF, D'Angelo R. Effectiveness of the Frostig program for visual perceptual training with head start children. *Percept Mot Skills*. 1971;32:944–946.
74. Brown RT, Alford N. Ameliorating attentional deficits and concomitant academic deficiences in learning disabled childen through cognitive training. *J Learn Disabil*. 1984;17:20–26.
75. Rosner J. The development of a perceptual skills program. *J Am Optom Assoc*. 1973;44:698–707.
76. Getz D. Learning enhancement through vision therapy. *Acad Ther*. 1980;15(4):457–466.
77. Rowell RB. *The effect of tachistoscope and visual tracking program on the improvement of reading at the second grade level*. Doctoral thesis. Ann Arbor, MI: University Microfilms; 1976.
78. Solan HA, Ciner EB. Visual perception and learning: issues and answers. *J Am Optom Assoc*. 1989;60:457–460.
79. Scheiman M, Rouse MW. *Optometric Management of Learning-Related Vision Problems*. 2nd ed. St. Louis, MO: CV Mosby; 2006.

Chapter Eight

Managing Visual Problems in the Pediatric Population

Mitchell Scheiman

Overview

Occupational therapists evaluate and treat children from birth to 18 years of age with a wide variety of diagnoses including developmental disorders, autistic spectrum disorders, Down syndrome, cerebral palsy, intellectual disability, low birth weight syndrome, sensory integrative dysfunction, learning disabilities, and other syndromes. In addition, occupational therapists, particularly those in private practice, may also manage children with normal to higher intellectual abiity with learning disabilities, and those who may have concussion-related vision disorders.

As demonstrated in Chapter One, children with the diagnostic conditions listed above have been found to have a high prevalence of vision problems including refractive disorders (myopia, hyperopia, astigmatism), strabismus, amblyopia, accommodative and non-strabismic binocular vision problems, eye movement disorders, visual information processing disorders, nystagmus, visual field loss, and in some cases eye disease.[1–16] The most common conditions found in these children include optical problems such as hyperopia, myopia, and astigmatism; strabismus; amblyopia; nystagmus; optic atrophy; and visual processing problems.[6] Ciner et al.[15] performed a comprehensive visual examination on 135 preschool children at an early intervention program in Philadelphia. These children had various intellectual and physical problems including Down syndrome, cerebral palsy, history of parental substance abuse, failure to thrive, and unlabeled developmental delays. They found that 60% of this population had significant vision problems. Strabismus was the most common condition, followed by refractive conditions such as hyperopia, myopia, and astigmatism.

The primary occupations of a child are learning and playing. Children with undetected and untreated vision problems may have difficulty participating in occupations such as reading, copying from the board, writing, playing, and sports, which creates a need for occupational therapists to have a comprehensive understanding of vision. If you think about the activities that a child has to perform on a daily basis in school to learn effectively, it is evident that vision is the sensory system through which a significant percentage of learning must occur. A study by Ritty et al.[17] demonstrated how important visual acuity, accommodation, binocular vision, and ocular motor abilities are in the typical elementary school classroom. They found that 75% of the academically related task time in the classroom is spent on reading and writing at near distance and on tasks that require

DOI: 10.4324/9781003526841-8

near-to-distance-to-near alternate viewing. To perform well at these tasks, a child requires normal visual acuity, accommodation, binocular vision, eye movement, and visual information processing skills. To be maximally effective in their therapy, occupational therapists should understand the complexity and importance of vision and how visual deficits can interfere with occupation, be able to screen for common vision problems, and manage some of these problems in the context of therapy visits.

Pre-School Children With Developmental Disorders: OT Management

When discussing occupational therapy management of children with vision disorders, it is important to understand that the approach differs significantly with preschool children or older children with developmental disorders that affect attention, concentration, and intellectual ability from higher functioning children.

Determining if a Vision Problem Is Present

With this population vision screening (Chapter Six) is generally not possible because vision screening tests require subjective responses, attention, and concentration. Thus, the best that an occupational therapist can do without the assistance of an optometrist is to make clinical observations and listen to both the parents and teachers about possible signs of a vision problem. Table 8.1 lists some of the signs a therapists can observe. An experienced pediatric optometrist can almost always complete an optometric examination using objective testing techniques that do not require subjective responses from the child. If an occupational therapist is concerned about a possible undetected vision problem, they should refer to a pediatric optometrist for an evaluation. In fact, any child who is not developing normally should be referred for a full optometric examination to rule out the presence of a vision problem.

Treating Vision Problems

Chapter Seven reviews all potential management options available to an optometrist to treat vision problems. These treatments include both passive and active options. Passive treatment options include eyeglasses with corrective lenses for refractive errors and prism lenses for binocular vision problems. These passive approaches are possible because they do not require cooperative participation on the part of the child, other than wearing the eyeglasses. In this population the early identification and treatment of visual integrity problems (acuity, refractive error, eye disease) is typically the primary treatment option and can often be quite useful for improving occupational performance. Of course, these treatment options can only be used by optometrists.

Prisms for Modification of Posture and Function in Autism

For the past 25 years a small group of optometrists have used yoked prism (see Chapter Seven) to improve posture and performance, visual and behavioral problems associated with autism. However, the research on this treatment approach is limited and most research has been published by only one group of researchers without replication from others.[18–21] In addition, the beneficial effects reported seem to fade after 3 to 4 months. Given the limited research and lack of clarity of the underlying rationale for the use of this treatment, it is not an approach I would recommend.

Vision Therapy for Visual Efficiency Disorders

Office-based optometric vision therapy requires a high level of attention, concentration, and motivation over a 45 to 60–minute session. Preschool and developmentally delayed children often lack one or more of these characteristics, making office-based vision therapy a questionable option

Table 8.1

Effect of Vision Problems on Occupational Therapy

Visual Problem	*Effect on Function*
Refractive conditions	• Decreased visual acuity • Excessive effort to perform visual tasks • Discomfort when involved with any visual task • Intermittent blurred vision • Loss of vision • Need to hold things close
Binocular vision disorders: Strabismic	• Cosmetic problem, eyes look crossed or turned out • If strabismus is intermittent, it can cause double vision that can interfere with eye-hand and mobility tasks • If strabismus is intermittent, it can lead to eyestrain • Loss of visual acuity (amblyopia) if left untreated and if the strabismus is unilateral
Binocular vision disorders: Nonstrabismic	• Intermittent double vision • Discomfort and eyestrain for all visual tasks • Tires easily • Inattentive • Poor concentration • Loss of place when playing or reading • Difficulty with eye-hand tasks
Accommodative disorders	• Discomfort and eyestrain for all visual tasks • Tires easily • Inattentive • Poor concentration • Blurred vision • Rubs eyes
Ocular motility disorders	• Excessive head movement when engaged in visual tasks • Frequent loss of place • Skips lines • Poor attention span • Copying is slow and inaccurate • Results poor with coloring and drawing
Visual information processing disorders	• Confusion of left and right • Confusion of likenesses and differences • Tends to use other senses to make what should be visual discriminations • Unaware of what should be attended to • Performs slowly • Ignores detail during visual tasks • Poor recall of visually presented material • Sloppy drawing skills • Difficulty with copying and getting thoughts on paper

for this group of children. Home-based therapy administered by a parent is also not typically useful because parents have difficulty working with their own children. The best that can typically be accomplished is for the optometrist to prescribe lenses or prism to treat accommodative and binocular vision problems.

Occupational Therapist Role

It is apparent, therefore, that for this group of children, there is a limit to the treatment that can be offered by the optometrist. This creates an opportunity for an occupational therapist to play an important role in the active treatment of eye movement and visual information processing problems. The therapist can provide short periods of occupation-based intervention designed to treat eye movements and visual processing problems within the framework of the occupational therapy visit. Specific ideas for such therapy are provided in Chapters Seven, Ten, and Eleven. Eye movement and visual processing skills are both slowly developing abilities and there is a belief that the development of these skills is related to movement, sensory motor integration, and gross motor ability. In this group of children a typical occupational therapy session will likely include such activities that may lead to an indirect improvement in eye movements and visual information processing.

My management approach with preschool and developmentally delayed children is to complete a comprehensive optometric evaluation and identify the presence of any visual integrity, efficiency, or visual information processing problems. I use passive treatment modalities (lenses, prism, occlusion) and recommend that the family have an occupational therapy evaluation (if not already done). If the child is currently being treated by an occupational therapist, I tell the family that I would be happy to coordinate treatment for the identified vision problems and consult with the therapist. I suggest that any "vision therapy" could be provided by the occupational therapist as part of the therapy session. I would then provide follow-up evaluations to monitor progress.

Higher Functioning Children: OT Management

Determining if a Vision Problem Is Present

With this population the entire vision screening presented in Chapter Six can be performed by the occupational therapist. The therapist will be able to determine if there are any areas of concern for visual integrity, visual efficiency, and visual information processing. If problems are found in visual integrity or visual efficiency, the occupational therapist should encourage the family to seek vision care for their child. The therapist should educate the family about the different modes of practice among eye care providers. The important concept is that only a small percentage of eye care provides carefully assess all three areas (integrity, efficiency, visual information processing). I have stressed the need to make sure that the professional to whom you refer the patient practices using the full model of vision described in this book. Otherwise, you will most likely be disappointed with the information you receive in return. The directories of optometrists who have achieved fellow status in the College of Optometrists in Vision Development and those who have achieved Diplomate status in the American Academy of Optometry are good resources for potential referral sources. If you are unable to find an optometrist from these directories nearby, you can suggest that the family call local optometrists and ask the following six questions:

1. Do you have experience working with children with the following conditions (autistic, developmentally delayed, Down syndrome, etc.)?
2. Do you test for focusing problems?
3. Do you test for binocular vision problems?
4. Do you test for tracking problems?
5. Do you test for visual information processing disorders?
6. Do you offer vision therapy in your practice?

While visual integrity, accommodative, and binocular vision disorders will need to be treated by the optometrist, eye movement and visual information processing problems can be co-managed by the occupational therapist using the treatment sequences described in Chapters Seven, Ten, and Eleven.

Managing Vision Problems

Similar to the discussion of preschool, and developmentally delayed children, there are many treatment options available to an optometrist, including lenses, prism, and vision therapy, to treat visual integrity, accommodative, and binocular vision problems. This higher functioning group respond very well to office-based vision therapy. Recent randomized clinical trials have demonstrated excellent effectiveness for both binocular vision problems like convergence insufficiency[22-24] and accommodative disorders.[25-27]

Vision and Its Relationship to Learning

Public Law (PL) 94–142 was passed in 1975 and has made available a free, appropriate public education that emphasizes special education and related services to children with a wide range of disabilities. Because occupational therapy is included as one of the related services, the profession has become deeply involved in the care of children who have education-related needs. In fact, school systems are listed as one of the most common work settings for occupational therapists.[28]

Optometry also has a long history of involvement with learning-related vision problems. Much of the interest has been generated by the concern of parents and by the referrals of teachers, psychologists, occupational therapists, and other professionals who turn to optometrists for answers about whether a child has a vision problem that could be contributing to or responsible for poor school performance. Optometrists believe that vision can contribute to learning difficulties, but that it is generally not the primary etiological factor. Rather, vision disorders may interfere with a child's school performance and may make it difficult for a child to perform up to potential. Optometrists believe that there is a strong relationship between vision and learning and that every child who is experiencing problems in school requires an appropriate optometric evaluation.

Controversy exists, however, about the relationship between vision and learning. Some professionals, primarily ophthalmologists, claim that there is no significant relationship between vision and learning.[29] They suggest that as long as a child can see clearly and has healthy eyes, vision can be ruled out as an issue. Based on the material presented in Chapters One, Three, Four, and Five, it should be evident that this controversy is based on differences in the definition of vision. Ophthalmology's definition of vision is a very limited one and generally only requires good visual acuity and normal eye health. Most research would, in fact, support the statement that visual acuity and eye health have no relationship to learning. It is easy to understand, therefore, why an individual or a profession using such a definition would believe that there is no significant relationship between vision and learning. Optometry, however, believes that vision is more complex than visual acuity and eye health. We use the Three Component Model of Vision described in Chapters Three through Five. Research demonstrates that, using this comprehensive definition, there is indeed a strong relationship between vision and learning.

There is also controversy about whether vision therapy is an effective treatment approach for children with learning disorders. This second area of contention is again based on misconceptions and disagreement about definitions. Ophthalmology claims that vision therapy is an ineffective approach for the treatment of learning disabilities.[29] In fact, this is not an unreasonable statement, and optometry has never claimed that vision therapy is a cure for learning disabilities. Rather, optometrists believe that vision therapy is an effective approach for the treatment of visual efficiency and visual information processing problems. The effect of vision therapy on a child's learning ability is most comparable to the effect of medication for attention deficit hyperactivity disorder. Ritalin (methylphenidate), for instance, is not expected to directly improve reading performance. Rather, because of improved concentration and attention, the child is able to benefit from educational intervention. Similarly, improvements in visual skills can result in better attention, concentration, and learning efficiency and can enable the child to benefit from standard or remedial education. Thus, the key concept is that optometrists evaluate and treat vision problems that may be interfering with school performance. Optometry's position is that vision problems should not be treated in isolation but rather as part of a multidisciplinary approach designed to supplement rather than substitute for classroom or resource room instruction.[30–33]

Why is vision such an important factor in learning? If you think about the activities that a child has to perform on a daily basis in school to learn effectively, it is evident that vision is the sensory system through which a significant percentage of learning must occur. A study by Ritty et al.[17] demonstrated how important visual acuity, accommodation, binocular vision, and ocular motor abilities are in the typical elementary school classroom. They found that 75% of the academically related task time in the classroom is spent on reading and writing at near distance and on tasks that require near-to-distance-to-near alternate viewing. To perform well at these tasks, a child requires normal visual acuity, accommodation, binocular vision, and ocular motor skills.

Prevalence of Vision Disorders in Children With Learning Disabilities

General Studies

Studies have shown a very high prevalence of visual efficiency problems in learning disabled children. Sherman[34] found a very high prevalence of accommodative (76%), binocular (92%), and ocular motility (96%) disorders in a population of learning disabled children. In a similar type study, Hoffman[35] examined 107 learning disabled children and also found a high prevalence of binocular vision (87%), accommodative (83%), and ocular motility (95%) disorders. In an extensive review of the literature, Grisham and Simons[36] concluded that there is a relationship between refractive status and binocular vision and reading. This was further supported by a meta-analysis of the same literature.[37] O'Grady explored the relationship between vision and educational performance by studying a random sample of 227 second-grade children. Of the sample, 16.2% were found to have significant vision disorders.[38] The children with vision problems were found to perform significantly poorer on the educational tests than the other children.

Visual information processing problems have also been found to be prevalent in learning disabled children. Hoffman[35] found problems in bilateral integration (46%), directionality (74%), visual discrimination (50%), and visual motor integration problems (81%), while Sherman[34] found form reproduction disorders in 72% of the population he studied. Groffman[39] reviewed the literature relating visual perceptual problems to learning and found that meta-analysis of single-factor studies showed that reading achievement was significantly related to visual perceptual performance. Kavale reviewed 161 studies and used meta-analysis to statistically integrate the results from these studies.[40] His results suggested that visual perception is an important correlate of reading achievement and that visual perceptual skills should be included in the complex of factors predictive of reading achievement.

Refractive Error

Eames[41] compared the refractive distribution of 114 reading disabled children selected from a private practice and a university clinic with 143 controls. He found a significant difference (P = 0.001) in the prevalence of hyperopia between the reading disabled and the control group (43% compared to 27%). In another report, Eames[42] compared 1,000 reading disabled children with 150 controls. The prevalence of hyperopia was much greater among disabled readers (43%) than the control group (13%).

Other studies reported interactions between refractive status and visual-perceptual motor development.[43,44] Although these studies were not investigations of reading per se, children with visual-perceptual motor delays are at risk for reading underachievement. In the first study of a sample of 712 children ages 6 to 12 years, only 18% of the children with significant hyperopia displayed age-appropriate visual motor skills, in contrast to 74% of the emmetropic and myopic children.[43] In a second and related study of 48 6- to 12-year-old hyperopes, those children who were corrected prior to their fourth birthday manifested fewer visual-motor delays than those who were corrected later.[44] In a more recent study of 32 children, 4 to 7 years old, the authors found that those with uncorrected hyperopia showed reduced performance on tests of letter and word recognition, and receptive vocabulary compared to the children with no refractive error.[45]

Binocular Vision

Eames[46] found the prevalence of exophoria to be nearly four times greater in the nominal reading disabled group than in the control group. In his latter, large sample study, Eames[42] found a somewhat greater prevalence of near point exophoria in the reading disabled group (33% compared to 22%; P = 0.007). In a generally well-constructed research study, Good[47] used a case-control paradigm and found that none of the control group had a significant phoria, whereas 40% of the reading disabled did. Evans, Efron, and Hodge[48] found the prevalence of significant phoria was nearly twice as frequent in a sample of reading disabled than in a sample of second- to fifth-grade normal readers.

Ocular Motor

Because eye movement deficiencies intuitively seem to be so closely linked with reading, numerous studies have investigated this relationship. When reading age-appropriate text, the eye movements of poor readers are characterized by an increased number of forward fixations per line of text, an increased number of regressions, longer fixation durations, and a greater prevalence of intraword scanning when compared to normal readers.[49] In children with reading and other learning difficulties, several studies have found a very high prevalence of eye movement anomalies.[34,35,50] In a sample of 50 children with learning disabilities between the ages of 6 and 13 years, Sherman[34] found that 96% had problems with ocular motor inefficiency (saccadic and pursuit problems). Hoffman[35] reported on a larger sample of 107 children with learning problems. His results revealed that 24% of the sample had ocular motor problems. He also reported on the results of 25 children without learning problems and found that 24% had ocular motor problems. It is interesting to note that both Sherman and Hoffman found that ocular motor dysfunction was the most prevalent vision disorder in their samples of learning disabled children.

Effect of Vision Problems on Occupational Therapy Intervention

Table 8.1 lists the signs and symptoms associated with visual efficiency and visual information processing problems. Many of these symptoms interfere with a child's ability to attend and concentrate when engaged in any visual task and occur when the child is working on near tasks such as reading, writing, cutting, coloring, and other types of desk work. Children will also sometimes avoid such activities rather than experience eyestrain, headaches, and double vision.

Vision problems can hinder the occupational therapy process in a variety of ways, and Flax[51] has stressed the importance of performing a task analysis when assessing the impact of a vision problem on performance. It is not sufficient to simply ask if vision is impacting on a child's performance. Rather, the occupational therapist should try to define the visual demands of a task and determine if there is a relationship. Tables 8.2 and 8.3 provide guidance for this task analysis.

Table 8.2

Task Characteristics Placing a High Demand on Visual Efficiency Skills

The Occupational Therapy Task Requires

- Attention to small internal details of visual stimuli such as words and pictures
- Precise ocular motor control
- Accurate sequential inspection of words, visual stimuli
- Sustained attention on a visual task
- Extensive use of dittos which may be of poor print quality
- Speed and accuracy
- Emphasis on speed and comprehension
- Movement during a visual task

Tasks with the above requirements are likely to cause the symptoms listed in Table 8.1 under the sections of nonstrabismic binocular vision disorders, accommodation, and ocular motility.

Table 8.3

Task Characteristics Placing a High Demand on Visual Information Processing Skills

The Occupational Therapy Task Requires

- Decisions about directional orientation
- Symbol and word recognition
- Matching of shapes
- Visual memory
- Visualization
- Copying of visual stimuli

Tasks with the above requirements are likely to cause the symptoms listed in Table 8.1 under the section of visual information processing.

Flax[51] uses the following example to demonstrate the value of task analysis relative to vision and reading performance. Two children are brought to an optometrist to determine if vision might be interfering with reading performance. Both have the same general complaint of poor comprehension. In case one, it is established that there is no difficulty with pronouncing each word correctly regardless of the grade level or difficulty of the word. There are no indications of fatigue; the child works for hours quite diligently but does not seem to understand what is being read. He can pronounce words but not define them. He does no better when the passage is read aloud to him. When attempting to explain what has just been read, he repeats the very same words that were in the text but does not offer synonyms, alternative phrases, or anything suggesting insight even though the mechanics of reading seem to be intact. Given this history, visual factors are unlikely to be major contributors to this youngster's reading problem. Language factors or even low intelligence are more apt to be the cause of the child's problem. His ability to repeat almost verbatim suggests that there is no problem with visual intake of the reading material.

The second child can decode unfamiliar words. But this child shows a decline in efficiency on longer assignments, and reading comprehension becomes even worse on smaller type. This child frequently omits words, rereads the same line, and skips lines. This youngster loves being read to and can discuss and recall effectively when material is read aloud to him. This child can define words and give synonyms, and he has good understanding of anything that he hears. His problem occurs when he has to read several pages of text. It is at this point that reading comprehension suffers. In this case, vision is likely to be related to the reading comprehension difficulty. This child shows good language ability, and, importantly, when the material is heard rather than seen, there is no comprehension problem. This history suggests the possibility of difficulty with ocular motility, binocular vision, or accommodation. There may even be contribution because of uncorrected refractive conditions.

The same type of task analysis is important for the occupational therapist. Problems are likely to cause the symptoms listed in Table 8.1 if the therapy procedure requires fine detail and prolonged attention and concentration, and then ocular motility, accommodation, and binocular vision. If, however, the material used in occupational therapy has large type and few details, ocular motility, accommodation, and binocular vision are not taxed greatly.

Given the high prevalence of vision problems in learning disabled children, occupational therapists should always consider the possibility that a vision problem could be present, particularly if progress is slower than expected and if some of the symptoms or signs described in Table 8.1 are present.

Case Studies

Case One

CASE HISTORY

Paul, a 12-year-old seventh grader, was brought in for an examination because his school performance had decreased significantly this school year. Until this year, Paul had been an outstanding student, achieving excellent grades in all subjects. The specific problem revolved around Paul's inability to read comfortably. He complained that after 10 to 15 minutes of reading, his eyes felt tired and ached. If he continued to read, he eventually experienced headaches, and, finally, the words would blur and move on the page. Because of his inability to read comfortably, he was falling behind in his assignments. He felt that the amount of required reading had increased significantly this year.

There was nothing significant in his medical history, and he was not taking any medication. He had passed a visual screening at the pediatrician and in school earlier in the school year. He never had a full vision evaluation. There was no significant family history of learning problems. Both parents were college graduates with high expectations for Paul's education.

VISUAL ACUITY, REFRACTION, EYE HEALTH

This part of the examination revealed normal 20/20 visual acuity in both the right and left eyes. The eye health evaluation was normal. Paul was found to have a very low degree of hyperopia (farsightedness), which is considered normal for his age.

VISUAL EFFICIENCY TESTING

This testing was designed to evaluate accommodation, binocular vision, and ocular motility skills. The near point of convergence was receded, a high degree of exophoria (eyes turn out) was found at the reading distance, and his ability to compensate for the exophoria was found to be very poor. Accommodation was also found to be inadequate. Specifically, he had a great deal of difficulty relaxing the accommodative system. Ocular motility was found to be normal.

Visual Information Processing Evaluation

Because Paul had an excellent academic record for the first six years of school, we felt that if a vision problem was a contributing factor to his current problems, it would be a visual efficiency disorder or a refractive error. Because significant visual efficiency problems were detected, we did not feel that visual information processing testing was necessary.

Assessment and Diagnosis

The history in this case was clearly characteristic of a learning problem associated with a visual efficiency disorder. Analysis of the optometric findings revealed a receded near point of convergence, high exophoria at near, decreased compensatory ability, and poor accommodative facility. Based on these data, we reached a diagnosis of convergence insufficiency and accommodative excess.

We felt that these visual efficiency problems were clearly related to Paul's presenting complaints. Given Paul's history of excellent academic performance in grades 1 through 6, we felt that if we could eliminate the visual efficiency problems along with the associated symptoms, there would be a positive effect on academic performance.

Treatment Plan

We recommended a program of vision therapy. Eighteen 45-minute office visits were necessary. The patient was seen twice a week, and after 9 weeks, Paul reported elimination of all of his initial complaints and was able to read comfortably as long as desired. As Paul's comfort improved, his ability to study was enhanced, leading to better academic performance.

Summary

This is an important case because it demonstrates the importance of using a comprehensive model of vision. If this child had been examined by an eye care professional who only performed testing to probe the areas of visual acuity, refractive error, and eye health, no vision problem would have been detected. Unfortunately, this is a common occurrence. The child is referred for an eye examination and is returned with a statement that there is no vision or eye problem. The binocular and accommodative disorders were only detected in this case after visual efficiency testing was performed.

It is critical that when an occupational therapist is concerned about a vision problem, a referral is made to an eye care professional who will perform a comprehensive examination based on the type of model presented in this book. The eye care professional most likely to be able to deliver this type of care is an optometrist. However, it is important to realize that not all optometrists will provide this level of vision care. It is wise to contact the College of Optometrists in Vision Development and the American Academy of Optometry. These organizations can provide a list of optometrists in your area who can provide this type of care (see Chapter One).

Case Two

Case History

Jimmy, a 7½-year-old first grader, was referred for a vision evaluation by a psychologist who had just completed a psycho-educational evaluation. Jimmy learned to speak very early and was always a very verbal child. Although his parents' expectations had been very high for him, Jimmy had a history of school-related problems since kindergarten. In kindergarten, he experienced difficulty with letter and number recognition and fine motor coordination. He had great difficulty in first grade with handwriting and copying from the board. He reversed letters and numbers excessively and had difficulty with his sight word vocabulary. His parents noted that when they read to him, his comprehension was excellent. Because of these reported difficulties, he was retained in first grade. In spite of this retention, he continued to experience problems, and his parents finally brought him to a psychologist for psycho-educational testing.

The parents brought a copy of the psycho-educational evaluation report. This report indicated that there were no significant emotional issues, and the Weschler Intelligence Scale for Children results included a verbal IQ of 128 and a performance IQ of 104. The weakest scores were in coding (scaled score 5) and block design (scaled score 6). Jimmy scored almost two years behind his chronological age on the Bender Gestalt Test, a test of visual motor integration. Auditory processing and language skills were strengths for Jimmy.

Achievement testing was also done as part of the psycho-educational testing. This testing suggested a one-year lag in reading with weaknesses in sight word vocabulary, comprehension, and age-appropriate math skills.

In the patient summary, the psychologist reached a diagnosis of a learning disability with primary weaknesses in visual processing and strengths in language function. He recommended part-time placement in a resource room and reading tutoring. In addition, he suggested a comprehensive optometric evaluation and an occupational therapy evaluation.

Jimmy's medical history revealed a normal gestation, but a very long and difficult labor and delivery by cesarean section. Otherwise, there was no significant medical history. Developmental milestones showed a variable pattern. Language skills developed faster than average. For instance, Jimmy used two-word sentences by 18 months of age and was always a very verbal child. Fine motor skills, however, developed more slowly than expected. He always had difficulty holding a crayon and did not enjoy cutting, coloring, or playing with puzzles. He could not copy a circle until about 4 years of age. Jimmy had difficulty with most sports and tended to avoid such activity. There did not seem to be any family history of learning problems, and there had been no other testing.

Visual Acuity, Refraction, Eye Health
Visual acuity was 20/20 in both eyes, eye health was normal, and a moderate degree of hyperopia was found in both eyes.

Visual Efficiency Testing
Binocular vision testing revealed a moderate degree of esophoria (eyes turned in), and his ability to compensate for this tendency was inadequate. The accommodative system was normal, but ocular motility testing revealed very poor performance in the area of saccades and pursuits. On the Developmental Test of Eye Movements, Jimmy scored at only the 1st percentile in both accuracy and speed.

Visual Information Processing Evaluation
Table 8.4 lists the tests administered and the results. Key weaknesses were in directionality (5th percentile), visual memory (25th percentile), visual motor integration (10th percentile), and fine motor skills (10th percentile).

Assessment and Diagnosis
The optometric evaluation revealed difficulties in both visual efficiency and visual information processing. There was a significant amount of hyperopia, and his eyes were found to have a significant tendency to cross inward (esophoria). His tracking ability (saccadic fixation) was significantly below age level. Based on this information, we reached a diagnosis of hyperopia, convergence excess, and ocular motor dysfunction.

In addition, the visual information processing evaluation indicated problems in visual spatial, visual analysis, visual motor integration, and fine motor skills.

These findings can be related to many of the problems that Jimmy was experiencing in school. His difficulty with reversals, letter and number recognition, fine motor coordination, and copying

Table 8.4

Visual Information Processing Results for Case Two

Visual Spatial Skills	Test	Score
Directionality	Gardner Reversal Frequency Test:	
	Recognition Subtest	5%
	Execution Subtest	40%
Visual Analysis Dysfunction	*Test*	*Score*
Visual form constancy	TVPS: Visual Form Constancy	37%
Visual memory	TVPS: Visual Memory	25%
	TVPS: Visual Sequential Memory	37%
Visual Motor Integration	*Test*	*Score*
Visual motor integration	Visual Motor Integration Tests	10%
Fine motor skills	Grooved Pegboard	10%
	Wold Sentence Copy Test	First grade

from the board are characteristic of children with problems in directionality, visual memory, visual motor integration, fine motor skills, and saccadic fixation problems (see Table 8.1).

Even though he was not complaining of any of the common signs or symptoms associated with hyperopia and esophoria, we felt these were significant issues that would need to be addressed in the treatment plan because of their potential to cause eyestrain and difficulty with attention and concentration.

OCCUPATIONAL THERAPY EVALUATION

The school occupational therapist received the testing from both the psychologist and the optometrist and performed an evaluation primarily designed to determine why Jimmy was having trouble with handwriting and sports. Using the Bruininks-Oseretsky Test of Motor Proficiency, the therapist found that Jimmy scored about 1½ years below age level on bilateral integration, strength, upper limb coordination, and fine motor control. On the Peabody Developmental Scales, he scored at the age level of a 6-year-old. Based on clinical observation of a handwriting sample, the therapist found problems with letter and size formation, spacing of letter and words, and overall spatial organization. Clinical observation of spontaneous activity suggested problems with postural security and low muscle tone.

TREATMENT PLAN

The optometrist and occupational therapist worked together to plan the most appropriate treatment program for this child. The optometrist prescribed eyeglasses to be worn at all times in school. He prescribed a vision therapy program with a primary emphasis on binocular vision and ocular motility. He also designed therapy to deal with the problems in directionality, visual memory, and visual motor integration. This therapy was carefully programmed to coincide with the occupational therapist's treatment plan. The therapist designed a program to work with his fine motor, handwriting, and sensory integration difficulties. Jimmy also received help at school and had private reading tutoring. We asked the teachers to temporarily de-emphasize written work, particularly copying from the board.

After 12 months of combined educational, occupational therapy, and optometric intervention, Jimmy made outstanding progress. He now found it easier to get his thoughts down in writing, copying from the board was considerably better, he was no longer reversing excessively, and he was willing to engage in sports. His reading level increased about 6 to 9 months, and he was no longer as frustrated in school.

Summary

These two cases underscore the complexity and the challenge of managing learning-related vision disorders. Through these cases, we have tried to emphasize the importance of an interdisciplinary approach. In Case One, the vision problem was the primary cause of the child's academic difficulty, and treatment of the visual efficiency problem transferred directly to improved school performance. However, this type of case is not the most common presentation. In most instances, even if a vision problem is present, it will be only one of several factors contributing to the child's problems. Case Two is an illustration of a child who required intervention from several professionals including occupational therapy and optometry.

References

1. Bakroon A, Lakshminarayanan V. Visual function in autism spectrum disorders: a critical review. *Clin Exp Optom.* 2016;99:297–308.
2. Chang MY, Doppee D, Yu F, et al. Prevalence of ophthalmologic diagnoses in children with autism spectrum disorder using the optum dataset: apopulation-based study. *Am J Ophthalmol.* 2021;221:147–153.
3. Simmons DR, Robertson AE, McKay LS, et al. Vision in autism spectrum disorders. *Vision Res.* 2009;49:2705–2739.
4. Hashemi H, Mehravaran S, Asgari S, Dehghanian Nasrabadi F. Refractive and vision status in Down syndrome: a comparative study. *Turk J Ophthalmol.* 2021;51:199–205.
5. Watt T, Robertson K, Jacobs RJ. Refractive error, binocular vision and accommodation of children with Down syndrome. *Clin Exp Optom.* 2015;98:3–11.
6. Scheiman M. Assessment and management of the exceptional child. In: Rosenbloom AA, Morgan MW, eds. *Pediatric Optometry.* Philadelphia, PA: JB Lippincott; 1990:388–419.
7. Kirschen M. A study of visual performance of mentally retarded children. *Am J Optom Arch Am Acad Optom.* 1954;31:282–288.
8. LoCascio GP. A longitudinal study of vision in cerebral palsy. *Am J Optom Physiol Opt.* 1984;61:689–692.
9. LoCascio GP. A study of vision in cerebral palsy. *Am J Optom Physiol Opt.* 1977;54:332–335.
10. Scheiman M. Optometric findings in children with cerebral palsy. *Am J Optom Physiol Opt.* 1984;61:321–327.
11. Lyle WM, Woodruff ME, Zuccaro VS. A review of the literature on Down's syndrome and an optometrical survey of 44 patients with the syndrome. *Am J Optom Arch Am Acad Optom.* 1972;49:715–727.
12. Pesch RS, Nagy DK. A survey of the visual and developmental-perceptual abilities of the Down's syndrome child. *J Am Optom Assoc.* 1978;49:1031–1037.
13. Clements DB, Kaushal K. A study of the ocular complications of hydrocephalus and meningomyelocele. *Trans Ophthalmol Soc UK.* 1970;90:383–390.
14. Gottlieb DD, Allen W. Incidence of visual disorders in a selected population of hearing impaired students. *J Am Optom Assoc.* 1985;56:292–296.
15. Ciner EB, Macks B, Schanel-Klitsch E. A cooperative demonstration project for early intervention vision services. *Occup Ther Pract.* 1991;3:42–56.
16. Akinci A, Oner O, Bozkurt OH, et al. Refractive errors and ocular findings in children with intellectual disability: a controlled study. *J AAPOS.* 2008;12:477–481.
17. Ritty MJ, Solan HA, Cool SJ. Visual and sensory-motor functioning in the classroom: a preliminary report of ergonomic demands. *J Am Optom Assoc.* 1993;64:238–244.
18. Kaplan M, Carmody D, Gaydos A. Postural orientation modifications in autism in response to ambient lenses. *Child Psychiat Hum D.* 1996;27:81–91.
19. Kaplan M, Edelson S, Seip J. Behavioral changes in autistic individuals as a result of wearing ambient transitional prism lenses. *Child Psychiat Hum D.* 1998;29:65–76.
20. Carmody D, Kaplan M, Gaydos A. Spatial orientation adjustments in children with autism in Hong Kong. *Child Psychiat Hum D.* 2001;31:233–247.
21. Kaplan M. *Seeing Through New Eyes.* Philadelphia, PA: Jessica Kingsley Publishers; 2006.
22. Scheiman M, Mitchell GL, Cotter S, et al. A randomized trial of the effectiveness of treatments for convergence insufficiency in children. *Arch Ophthalmol.* 2005;123:14–24.
23. Convergence Insufficiency Treatment Trial Investigator Group. A randomized clinical trial of treatments for symptomatic convergence insufficiency in children. *Arch Ophthalmol.* 2008;126:1336–1349.
24. CITT-ART Investigator Group. Treatment of symptomatic convergence insufficiency in children enrolled in the convergence insufficiency treatment trial—attention & reading trial: a randomized clinical trial. *Optom Vis Sci.* 2019;96:825–835.
25. Cushman B, Burri C. Convergence insufficiency. *Am J Ophthalmol.* 1941;24:1044–1052.

26. Chen AM, Roberts TL, Cotter SA, et al. Effectiveness of vergence/accommodative therapy for accommodative dysfunction in children with convergence insufficiency. *Ophthalmic Physiol Opt.* 2021;41:21–32.
27. Scheiman M, Cotter S, Kulp MT, et al. Treatment of accommodative dysfunction in children: results from a randomized clinical trial. *Optom Vis Sci.* 2011;88:1343–1352.
28. Bureau of Labor Statistics USDoL. *Occupational Outlook Handbook*, Occupational Therapists; 2022.
29. Joint Statement. Learning disabilities, dyslexia, and vision. *Pediatrics.* 2009;124:837–844.
30. Scheiman M, Rouse MW. *Optometric Management of Learning Related Vision Problems.* 2nd ed. St. Louis, MO: CV Mosby; 2006.
31. Hoffman LG, Rouse MW. Vision therapy revisited: a restatement. *J Am Optom Assoc.* 1987;58:536–541.
32. Kastenbaum SM. In defense of training. *Optom Wkly.* 1974;65:1120–1122.
33. Pitcher-Baker G. Does perceptual training improve reading? *J Optom Vis Training.* 1974;5:40–45.
34. Sherman A. Relating vision disorders to learning disability. *J Am Optom Assoc.* 1973; 44:140–141.
35. Hoffman LG. Incidence of vision difficulties in children with learning disabilities. *J Am Optom Assoc.* 1980;51:447–451.
36. Grisham JD, Simons HD. Refractive error and the reading process: a literature analysis. *J Am Optom Assoc.* 1986;57:44–55.
37. Simons HD, Gassler PA. Vision anomalies and reading skill: a meta-analysis of the literature. *Am J Optom Physiol Opt.* 1988;65:893–904.
38. O'Grady J. The relationship between vision and educational performance: a study of year 2 children in Tasmania. *Aust J Optom.* 1984;67:126–140.
39. Groffman S. The relationship between visual perception and learning. In: Scheiman M, Rouse MW, eds. *Optometric Management of Learning Related Vision Problems.* 2nd ed. St. Louis, MO: CV Mosby; 2006:179–214.
40. Kavale K. Meta-analysis of the relationship between visual perceptual skills and reading achievement. *J Learning Disabilities.* 1982;15:42–51.
41. Eames TH. A comparison of the ocular characteristics of unselected and reading disability groups. *J Educ Res.* 1932;25:211–215.
42. Eames TH. Comparison of Eye conditions among 1,000 reading failures, 500 ophthalmic patients, and 150 unselected children. *Am J Ophthalmol.* 1948;31:713–717.
43. Rosner J, Rosner J. Comparison of visual characteristics in children with and without learning difficulties. *Am J Optom Physiol Opt.* 1987;64:531–533.
44. Rosner J, Rosner J. Some observations of the relationship between the visual perceptual skills development of young hyperopes and age of first lens correction. *Clin Exp Optom.* 1986;69:166–168.
45. Shankar S, Evans MA, Vobier WR. Hyperopia and emergent literacy of young children: pilot study. *Optom Vis Sci.* 2007;84:1031–1038.
46. Eames TH. A Frequency of physical handicaps in reading in reading disability and unselected groups. *J Educ Res.* 1935;29:1–5.
47. Good GH. Relationship of fusion weakness to reading disability. *J Exp Educ.* 1939;8:115–121.
48. Evans JR, Efron M, Hodge C. Incidence of lateral phoria among SLD children. *Acad Ther.* 1976;11:431–433.
49. Pirozzolo FJ. Eye movements and reading disability. In: Rayner K, ed. *Eye Movements in Reading.* New York, NY: Academic Press; 1983.
50. Lieberman S. The prevalence of visual disorders in a school for emotionally disturbed children. *J Am Optom Assoc.* 1985;56:800–803.
51. Flax N. The relationship between vision and learning. In: Scheiman M, Rouse M, eds. *Optometric Management of Learning Related Vision Problems.* 2nd ed. St. Louis, MO: CV Mosby; 2006.

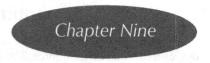
Chapter Nine

Visual Problems Associated With Acquired Brain Injury

Lynn Fishman Hellerstein and Mitchell Scheiman

Overview

When an acquired brain injury (ABI) occurs, the effects on the visual process and the integration of vision with other sensory modalities can be devastating. ABI may lead to impairment in one or more functions, including vision, arousal, attention, language, memory, reasoning, abstract thinking, judgment, problem solving, sensory abilities, perceptual abilities, motor abilities, psychosocial behavior, information processing, and speech.[1] Visual-perceptual dysfunction is one of the most common and devastating residual impairments of brain injury.[2] Perceptual deficits may affect the skills necessary for activities of daily living, including dressing, eating, reading, and working. Most activities of daily living require effective and optimal visual efficiency, visual processing, and visual motor performance. The deficit may be anywhere from a visual efficiency problem of "seeing clearly" to a problem of form perception, eye-hand coordination, or visual attending. Visual dysfunctions caused by brain injury can have a negative effect on performance and quality of life.

Activities used in rehabilitation programs typically require or depend on both the visual efficiency and visual information processing system. It is, therefore, essential for occupational therapists to know visual status and function before initiating rehabilitation. Because of the high prevalence of vision disorders in the ABI population and the importance of vision in rehabilitation, optometrists should play a role as a member of the rehabilitation team. Optometrists can help co-manage the overall rehabilitation of a patient who has been neurologically compromised by minimizing any deficit of the visual system and by providing consultation and guidance to members of the rehabilitative team.[3–5] This chapter will discuss the visual problems associated with brain injury, and Chapter Ten will discuss visual rehabilitation for this population.

ABI is generally used to refer to both traumatic brain injury (TBI) and stroke or cerebrovascular accident (CVA).

DOI: 10.4324/9781003526841-9

Traumatic Brain Injury

Menon et al.[6] define TBI as an alteration in brain function, or other evidence of brain pathology, caused by an external force. TBI may result in significant impairment of an individual's physical, cognitive, and psychosocial functioning.

More than 50 million people experience TBIs each year and as of 2005, about 3.2 million TBI survivors experience complications ranging from neurological, psychosocial problems to long-term disability.[7,8] The Glasgow Coma Scale is used to classify the severity of TBI injury as mild, moderate, and severe according to their level and severity.[9] Mild TBI (mTBI) accounts for 70% to 90% of all TBI cases.[10] The reported incidence of TBI in the United States is about 100 to 300 per 100,000 population.[11] The highest incidence of TBIs was recorded among men and young people ages 15 to 24 years old.[12] Another 300,000 individuals suffer brain injuries severe enough to require hospitalization, with 99,000 resulting in a lasting disability.[13] A total of 56,000 people die each year as a result of TBI.[14,7]

The number of people surviving TBI has increased significantly in recent years, which is attributed to faster and more effective emergency care, quicker and safer transportation to specialized treatment facilities, and advances in acute medical management. TBI affects people of all ages and is the leading cause of long-term disability among children and young adults.

Individuals aged 15 to 24 have the highest risk of TBI,[12] and TBI affects males at twice the rate of females. In addition, the mortality rate is higher among males, suggesting that males are more likely than females to suffer severe injuries.[4]

Although the largest group of TBI survivors are young adults in their prime working years, many survivors, particularly those with a severe TBI, do not return to work. Between one-third and two-thirds of all severe TBI survivors will return to work or school, at some level.[15,16] The ability to return to work is highly correlated to the post-acute functional limitations of the survivor. Of those who survive each year, approximately 70,000 to 90,000 endure life-long debilitating loss of function. A survivor of a severe brain injury typically faces 5 to 10 years of intensive services at an estimated cost in excess of $4 million. Two thousand survivors exist in a vegetative state. Motor vehicle crashes cause half of all TBIs, with falls accounting for 2%, assaults and violence 12%, and sports and recreation 10%. The economic loss from TBI has been estimated to be about $4 billion per year.

Mild TBI is a very common injury, resulting in about 300,000 hospital admissions each year.[18] Many more people are believed to sustain mild TBI, but they do not require hospitalization. As a result, an accurate estimation of the number of mild TBI cases per year is not available. About 80% of people admitted to a hospital with the diagnosis of TBI have mild TBI.[19] Hellerstein et al.[20] studied the vision characteristics of patients with mild TBI and found significant differences between the group with mTBI and a control group of age-matched patients without TBI. They concluded that the term *mild TBI* is very misleading and does not necessarily translate to "mild functional loss." In a longitudinal study of 1,453 patients with mTBI, 53% still reported functional limitations a year after the injury.[21] The more severe injuries require hospitalization and various types of rehabilitative therapy.

Vision Problems and Traumatic Brain Injury

A number of studies have been published in recent years reporting the prevalence of vision problems after TBI in both the civilian[22,23] and military populations.[24–30] Suchoff et al.[22] completed a prospective study of 62 consecutively (mean age 49, 19 to 70 years) admitted patients into a rehabilitation hospital. Although there were patients with both TBI and CVA in the sample, they did not report the results for the two groups separately. They found a high prevalence of binocular vision (42%), eye movement (40%), visual field (23%), and accommodative disorders (10%).

In a larger, retrospective study of the civilian population, Ciuffreda et al.[23] reported on 160 patients with TBI. They found that 56% had binocular vision disorders and convergence insufficiency was the most common binocular vision problem (42.5%). Fifty-one percent had eye movement problems (saccadic and pursuit deficits and nystagmus), and 41% had accommodative disorders.

Investigation of the prevalence of vision problems after TBI in the military has become a priority in recent years because over 30,000 US soldiers have been wounded in Iraq and Afghanistan, and TBI is the "signature wound" of these wars. Studies have shown that 30% of troops engaged in combat greater than 4 months are at risk for disabling neurologic disorders from blast waves of improvised explosive devices; 60% of injuries are due to roadside bombs and improvised explosive devices.

Goodrich et al.[24] studied 50 patients admitted to the polytrauma rehabilitation center from December 2004 to November 2006. The mean age of subjects was 28.1 years, and all had experienced a TBI, with blast injuries accounting for half of all injuries. Seventy-four percent of the subjects complained about the following: Blurred distance vision, sensitivity to light, missing a part of their vision, bumping into objects or walls, blurred near reading vision, and inability to comfortably read continuous text. The most common vision disorders were convergence insufficiency (30%), visual field deficits (30%), accommodative dysfunction (22%), and eye movement problems (20%). Over 60% of the subjects reported reading difficulties as well. The authors concluded that visual impairments are both frequent and severe in a population of patients with polytrauma and, therefore, all patients with polytrauma should have routine comprehensive vision examinations.

Brahm et al.[25] studied frequency of visual impairment in combat-injured polytrauma rehabilitation center inpatient and polytrauma network site outpatient military personnel with TBI. Subjects included 68 inpatients and 124 outpatients with a mean age of 28 years old. They found that 84% of polytrauma rehabilitation center patients and 90% of polytrauma network site patients had TBI associated with a blast event. The prevalent conditions were convergence insufficiency (42%), accommodative insufficiency (42%), pursuit/saccadic dysfunction (33%), and visual field defects (32%). As in the previous study, many patients complained about reading difficulties (64%). The authors concluded that combat troops exposed to blast with associated TBI are at risk for visual dysfunction, and that the results of the study support a policy of vision examination for all service-members who screen positive for TBI.

Stelmack et al.[29] reported on a retrospective medical record review of 103 patients with polytrauma. Seventy-five percent of the patients with TBI reported visual symptoms and the most prevalent vision disorders were accommodative disorder (47%), convergence disorders (28%), and visual field loss (14%).

Capo-Aponte et al.[30] performed one of the few studies that included a control group. They assessed the frequency of visual dysfunctions in active duty warfighters during the subacute stage of blast-induced mTBI. A comprehensive visual and oculomotor function evaluation was performed on 40 US military personnel, 20 with blast-induced mTBI and 20 without. The most common visual dysfunctions were vergence problems, decreased fusion ranges, receded near point of convergence, defective pursuit and saccadic eye movements, decreased amplitude of accommodation, and monocular accommodative facility. There were statistically significant differences found between the concussed and non-concussed participants.

Two recent studies of the frequency of vision problems after concussion were performed at the Children's Hospital of Philadelphia. In these studies, about 70% of the participants had one or more visual problems with convergence insufficiency, accommodative insufficiency, and saccadic dysfunction being the most common problems.[31,32] In the most recent study, Scheiman et al. found that 70% of the participants had at least one oculomotor diagnosis after concussion, with the most common problems being vergence disorders (60%) and accommodative disorders (57%). The most common vergence disorder was convergence insufficiency (35%). Among accommodative disorders, the most common problem was accommodative insufficiency (35%). In all, 47% of the participants had more than one oculomotor diagnosis following concussion.[32]

It is interesting to note that the results of studies in both the civilian and military population are similar and suggest that convergence insufficiency, accommodative dysfunction, eye movement problems, and visual field problems are the vision disorders occupational therapists are most likely to encounter in patients after TBI.

Stroke/Cerebrovascular Accident

Stroke or CVA is a clinically defined syndrome of rapidly developing symptoms or signs of focal loss of cerebral function with no apparent cause other than that of vascular origin, but the loss of function can at times be global.[33] Symptoms last more than 24 hours or lead to death. The syndrome varies in severity, from recovery in a day, to incomplete recovery, to severe disability, to death.[33] Stroke cases can now be classified in epidemiology studies by type. Wolf et al.[34] reported that, in the Framingham study, 45% of strokes were classified as atherosclerotic, 19% as cerebral embolism, 19% as transient ischemic attacks, 5% as intracerebral hemorrhage, 4% as subarachnoid hemorrhage, and 2% as other, for men aged 55 to 84 years.

Stroke is the third leading cause of death and the leading cause of chronic disability in the adult population of the United States.[21] About 795,000 individuals sustain strokes each year.[35] Projections show that by 2030, 3.4 million US adults ≥18 years of age (3.9% of the adult population) will have had a stroke, a 20.5% increase in prevalence from 2012.[35] About one-third of survivors have mild impairments, another one-third are moderately impaired, and the remainder are severely impaired. CVA can occur at any age, but it is much more common in the elderly. The death rate doubles every 10 years between the ages of 55 and 85. The incidence of stroke varies with location. For example, the incidence has been reported to be as low as 238 per 100,000 in Dijon, France, to 362 per 100,000 in Rochester, Minnesota, to 627 per 100,000 in Novosibirsk, Russia.[33] In the United States, there have been consistently higher rates of stroke in the southeastern states since the 1930s. With the aging of the population, it is likely that CVA will become even more common in the future. Given the high prevalence of vision problems after CVA, optometrists have an important role to play in the vision care of this population.

Vision Problems Associated With Stroke

There are fewer studies investigating the prevalence of vision problems after CVA. In the Suchoff et al.[22] study described earlier, 25 of the 62 patients had CVA, rather than TBI. However, the authors did not report the results for the two groups separately. They found a high prevalence of binocular vision (42%), eye movement (40%), visual field (23%), and accommodative (10%) disorders. A study that reported on the CVA population separately is the study by Ciuffreda et al.[23] in which they examined 60 patients with CVA. They found that 55% had binocular vision disorders, and convergence insufficiency was the most common binocular vision problem (37%). Fifty-seven percent had eye movement problems (saccadic and pursuit deficits and nystagmus), and 13% had accommodative disorders. Rowe et al. reported on the results of 1,023 patients who had a stroke and found that 72% had visual impairment, 42% had eye movement abnormalities, 28% had visual field loss, 27% experienced visual inattention, and 4% had visual perceptual disorders.[36]

Visual System Model: Functional Based

As explained in earlier chapters of this book, a comprehensive understanding of vision includes visual acuity, refraction, eye health, visual efficiency, and visual processing. To help understand functional performance of patients with brain injury, clinicians and researchers have found it useful to view the visual system from an additional perspective or model. This model consists of two modes of visual processing: a central or focal process and a peripheral or ambient process.[37]

The two modes of processing involve separate neurological pathways that simultaneously process visual input. Together, the two systems provide integration of visual input.

The focal mode is made up of the foveal, parafoveal, and primary visual cortex inputs. The focal mode contributes to the "what" of vision (object recognition and identification). The focal mode is attention-oriented and centers on detail in small areas of space. The focal mode can be measured by more traditional tests such as visual acuity and color perception.

The ambient mode (more midbrain in location) is concerned with the "where," or the location of objects. Information about movement and position of objects is transmitted to the posterior parietal cortex, which provides a reference of where objects are located in space. The ambient mode is important in posture, motion, and spatial orientation. It is more peripheral and is involved in object localization and mobility. It receives input from the other sensory systems, including tactile, kinesthesia, and proprioception. It is difficult to assess the ambient function other than through observation about how the patient moves.[38]

To understand these two different visual processes, try the following demonstration: Stand up, look straight ahead, and hold each index finger as close to each eye as possible to effectively block out central vision when looking straight ahead. You should still be able to see peripherally. For example, if you hold your finger in front of your eye and look directly at a person, you cannot see the person; however, you are still able to see the room around the person. Now walk around the room, keeping your fingers in front of your eyes. Move your fingers from your eyes and make each hand into a loose fist so as to form a small "telescope" with each hand. Hold each hand up to each eye, so that you can see straight ahead but very little peripherally. Now walk around the room. Which way is easier to move, with your fingers blocking central vision or blocking peripheral vision? Why?

Most people find it much easier to move when central vision is blocked and when peripheral vision is not affected. This is because the ambient system, which is more closely related to peripheral processing, is integrated with movement and balance systems. Therefore, if a person has an injury or damage to the focal system (such as loss of visual acuity due to cataracts, retina, macular degeneration), they may have problems reading or watching TV, but movement is often not affected unless there are other motor problems. If a person has injury or damage to the ambient system (i.e., field loss, poor ocular motor control, etc.), then movement through space may be hindered.

The ability to match information between the visual and motor processes is essential for the coordination of motor function. For example, a problem in either the focal or ambient systems described above will have a negative effect on the motor system. There is a constant interchange between focal and ambient function of vision throughout life. This interchange is often affected when there is brain injury. It is thought that this disruption may occur at the level of the midbrain. Padula[38,39] termed the condition *post-traumatic vision syndrome* (PTVS). Symptoms include asthenopia (eyestrain), diplopia (double vision), complaints that objects appear to move, poor tracking abilities, staring behavior, and visual memory problems. The syndrome is characterized by accommodative dysfunction, balance and posture difficulties, convergence insufficiency, exophoria, lowered blink rate, and spatial disorientation.

Types of Brain Injuries

The anatomy and physiology of the skull, the vascular network for the brain, as well as the dynamics of head trauma all contribute significantly to the effects of insult to the visual system.[3] This neurological insult affects the patient's neurological integrity and ability to process visually related or visually guided information.

To understand the types of visual dysfunctions that may be present, one needs to have a basic understanding of the brain and the effect of various types of injury on the visual system. Not all injuries result in the same type of deficit. For example, CVA patients often have more of a focal injury, whereas patients acquiring a TBI from a motor vehicle accident often exhibit diffuse injury resulting in multiple deficits. Focal damage is the result of direct injury to a structure that can be localized by observation, computed tomography (CT) scan, or magnetic resonance imaging (MRI). Diffuse damage is not always associated with specific objective abnormalities (on CT or MRI). Instead, it is presumed to occur as axons are stretched or sheared. Diffuse or focal damage can result in sensory, motor, cognitive, or other disorders.

Direct optic nerve dysfunction is highly correlated to injury site. Supraorbital and frontal head injuries are most likely to cause optic nerve dysfunction. This type of injury could result in partial or complete loss of vision. Optic nerve dysfunction is also often seen with other types of neurological diseases, such as multiple sclerosis.[40–43]

Concussion resulting in diffuse axonal injury can cause sensory motor impairments. If the injury is localized more in the left hemisphere, language deficits often result, whereas right hemisphere insult often causes more visual spatial difficulties. Injury to the frontal lobe may affect intellectual thinking, planning, and motor planning. The left hemisphere is often involved in analytical, sequential, time-oriented, organizational processing, and processing of letters and words. The right hemisphere is involved in nonverbal behavior such as visual spatial tasks and nonlinguistic functions (depth, color, and shape discrimination).

CVA results in deficits of varying severity depending on the location and extent of injury. A transient ischemic attack may be a presentation of an impending stroke. Strokes that occur in the areas supplied by the middle cerebral artery often result in hemiparesis. Eye movement control, memory, and consciousness will be affected if the anterior cerebral artery supply is involved. These vessels serve the frontal lobes, the upper portion of the chiasm, and the intracranial portions of the optic nerve.[44] Part of the lateral geniculate nucleus, optic tracts and radiation, portions of the midbrain, and the parietal and occipital lobes are supplied by the posterior cerebral arteries. Infarcts of the posterior cerebral arteries result in color anomia and visual field deficits (homonymous hemianopia with macular sparing). Sections of the temporal lobes, the cerebellum, significant portions of the brainstem (subthalamic nucleus, midbrain, pons, and medulla), and the optic radiation are supplied by the vertebrobasilar system. Obstruction of this system will lead to dysfunction of the eye muscles, balance, and vision.[45]

Ocular Health

Disruption of the visual system results from injury to the ocular structures (including the cornea, iris, lens, sclera, choroid, and retina), ocular orbits, ocular muscles (medial rectus, lateral rectus, superior rectus, inferior rectus, superior oblique, and inferior oblique), optic nerves, chiasm, tracts, radiation, and primary and associated visual cortical areas. The residual effects range from minimal, such as a mild abrasion, to a more severe vision-threatening injury. Loss of acuity and change in refraction or visual field may occur, resulting in decreased acuity, ocular discomfort, visual confusion, double vision, blurriness, light sensitivity, and decreased visual awareness. Sometimes the injuries may improve spontaneously with time, but medical treatment is often necessary immediately.

It is not uncommon to encounter an elderly patient with visual conditions such as glaucoma, macular degeneration, and/or cataract present before brain injury. Even though these types of visual conditions may or may not have been secondary to the injury, visual treatment is necessary. As an example, a 78-year-old patient after CVA was referred by his occupational therapist for a vision evaluation because of suspected "visual spatial and eye-hand coordination difficulties." The referral for functional reasons resulted in a visual evaluation, at which time the diagnosis of cataracts was made and surgery was recommended. After cataract extraction, the patient was much more accurate with eye-hand tasks because his eyesight was much improved. The improvement in vision affected his entire rehabilitation program.

Another common condition is "dry eyes." This condition may be due to poor blinking or incomplete lid closure when sleeping, or it may be a side effect of other medications. Artificial tears, ointment, and other treatment methods may be prescribed by the eye doctor.

Visual Symptoms

A number of visual symptoms and observations are noted with patients with diagnosed visual dysfunctions. Symptoms include double vision, difficulty seeing, ocular discomfort, an inability to follow or track an object, bumping into objects, and difficulty judging size or space. Table 9.1 summarizes patient symptoms, professional observations, and possible areas of visual dysfunction.[46]

The occupational therapist is often called upon to provide the vision screening for a patient with brain injury. This patient observation and the symptom checklist provide very valuable information regarding the patient's visual status. Refer to Chapter Six for the vision screening protocol.

Visual Disorders

As stated earlier the most common visual problems associated with brain injury include non-strabismic binocular dysfunction such as convergence insufficiency, accommodative dysfunction, eye movement deficits, visual field loss, and visual information processing disorders. Other common problems include visual acuity loss and double vision. Table 9.2 is adapted from Zoltan.[47] It summarizes the more common types of visual deficits found with patients with brain injury.

Table 9.1

Patient Symptoms, Professional Observations, and Possible Area of Visual Dysfunction

Binocular Problems	*Accommodation Problems*	*Motilities*
(Pointing system) Closing one eye	(Focusing system) Focusing problems	(Tracking system) Inability to follow objects smoothly
Double vision	Headaches	Reading problems
Muscle palsy	Pain	Skipping words
Headaches	Double vision	Re-reading words
Pain	Squinting	Reversals
Reading problems	Closing one eye	Nystagmus involuntary movement or rotation of the eyes
Print blurry	Reading problems	
Ocular discomfort	Ocular discomfort	
Strabismus (Eyeturn)	*Visual-Perceptual*	*Visual Field Defects*
Closing of one eye	Problem judging size	Bumping into chairs, objects, etc.
Double vision	Problem judging distances	
Head tilts or turns	Coordination problems	Difficulty seeing at night
Sudden onset of eye turn	Left-right confusion	Tunnel vision
Muscle palsy Difficult judging depth and 3-D view		Holding onto walls, other people, etc.

Source: Reprinted from Cohen AH, Soden R. An optometric approach to the rehabilitation of the stroke patient. *J Am Optom Assoc.* 1981;52(9):795–800. © 1981 by the American Optometric Association. Reprinted with permission.

> **Table 9.2**

Types of Visual Deficits

Deficit	Underlying Mechanism	Clinical Manifestation/Resulting Deficit
Blurred or decreased visual acuity	Ocular injury (cornea, lens, retina), optic nerve (II), and/or pathway injury, III nerve, midbrain, refractive error, amblyopia	Vision blurred either full- or part-time in one or both eyes, may have fatigue with sustained visual tasks
Strabismus or binocular dysfunction (convergence/ divergence)	Decreased ocular motor control (e.g., III, IV, or VI nerve paresis or dysfunction), midbrain injury affecting medial longitudinal fasiculus and/or ocular motor nuclei	Patient may see double part- or full-time, may close or cover an eye, may learn to suppress an eye, may have decreased or inaccurate depth perception, difficulty with localizing objects in space, confusion with sustained visual activities
Nystagmus	Brainstem damage (especially vestibular), cerebellar damage	Abnormal oscillations of the eyes, resulting in blurred vision, nausea, visual confusion
Decreased ocular motor skills:	Lesion in either hemisphere with or without brainstem damage	Difficulty tracking in any or all of the planes
1. Ocular pursuits	Lesion in frontal cortex (area 8) or parietal lobe	Difficulty or inability in quick localization, difficulty with reading
2. Saccadic eye movements		

Source: Adapted from Zoltan B. *Vision, Perception, and Cognition: A Manual for the Evaluation and Treatment of the Neurologically Impaired Adult.* 3rd ed. Thorofare, NJ: SLACK Incorporated; 1996.

Binocular Disorders

Acquired strabismus or nonstrabismic binocular vision problems often occur after trauma and result in double vision, blurriness, or visual confusion. The strabismus is often noncomitant (i.e., variable depending on the direction of gaze). Paresis of cranial nerves III, IV, and/or VI are often associated with this type of strabismus. A patient with an acquired strabismus may close one eye, request a patch, or develop an awkward head turn to reduce symptoms. Common nonstrabismic binocular vision problems include convergence insufficiency, decrease in fusional amplitudes, and suppression. Patients with these problems often fatigue quickly with sustained visual tasks.

Accommodation Disorders

Accommodative disorders frequently occur after trauma. The most common condition is accommodative insufficiency. Patients complain of visual fatigue with sustained near work, of difficulty changing focus from one distance to another, and sometimes of variability in clearness of vision. Even patients with mild TBI or whiplash injuries may show accommodative disorders.

Eye Movement Deficits

Patients with brain injury may show smooth pursuits and saccadic fixation abnormalities. These patients have difficulty tracking or following an object or may have problems fixating or locating objects. Deficits in scanning result in an inefficient gathering of visual information. Scanning deficits can impact on visual perceptual skills including visual closure, figure ground, and visual memory.

Nystagmus is sometimes present, especially with patients who have suffered brainstem or cerebellar damage. Patients with acquired nystagmus are quite uncomfortable and often experience nausea.

Visual Field Loss

Visual field loss and neglect may be present secondary to a brain injury, especially after CVA. Functional observations of patients with field loss include:

- Problems in mobility in a certain field (patient keeps bumping into things on the side of loss)
- Inattention to an area in space (patient not aware of objects or people; e.g., patient may only eat part of food on plate)
- Startle response (surprised when object appears, as patient was unaware of object in loss field)
- Difficulty reading (cannot accurately find end of column)

Vestibular/Balance/Movement Problems

If a patient presents with balance, dizziness, and/or movement problems, rehabilitation needs to be carefully coordinated with all therapists and physicians. Some patients may be suffering from vestibular, cerebellar, and/or other neurologic disorders, and the patient may need to depend on visual input to compensate and stabilize the system. In such cases, the individual's visual skills need to be at maximum performance levels. If vision problems are present in addition to vestibular/balance/movement problems, the patient may be even more symptomatic.

Visual Perceptual Deficits

Visual perceptual problems occur when there has been injury in the cortical or midbrain areas. It is inappropriate to diagnose a visual perceptual dysfunction until a full visual evaluation is completed, as ocular health and visual efficiency problems can affect a person's visual input and thereby interfere with the ability to process and respond to the visual information.

Visual perceptual deficits can include body scheme disorders and disorders of higher-level visual perceptual skills, such as discrimination, spatial relations, and so on.[2] These deficits usually involve parietal and/or occipital lobe lesions. Table 9.3 summarizes the more common visual perceptual deficits found with patients with brain injury.

Table 9.3

Visual Perceptual Deficits

Deficit	Clinical Manifestation
Agnosia	Inability to recognize an object by sight despite adequate cognition, language skills, and visual acuity/field
Prosopagnosia	
Object agnosia	Inability to recognize a familiar face
Achromatopsia agnosia	Inability to recognize objects by visual inspection alone
Simultanagnosia	Inability to discriminate between different colors
Alexia	Inability to perceive entire picture or to integrate its parts
Apraxia (optic)	Inability to recognize or comprehend written or printed words
Ataxia (optic)	Inability to execute purposeful movement
Constructional apraxia	Inability to visually guide limbs (mislocalization when reaching or pointing for objects)
Depth perception	Inability to copy or build a simple design
Figure ground	Inability to judge depths and distances
Form perception/constancy	Inability to distinguish foreground from background
Spatial relations	Inability to judge variations in form
Unilateral spatial neglect	Inability to perceive the position of two or more objects in relation to self and to each other
	Inability to attend to or respond to meaningful sensory stimuli presented in the affected hemisphere

Effect of Visual Function on Rehabilitation

Vision, which is considered to be the primary sense for gathering information, is often overlooked or ignored in the rehabilitation program. During the acute phase of medical treatment, management of life-threatening conditions and physical injuries is certainly the priority. If there is damage to ocular structures or to the ocular motor system, an ophthalmologist or neuro-ophthalmologist will often be called to provide diagnostic and therapeutic care. This is appropriate, as surgical or medical treatment may be necessary to minimize loss of sight.

However, once the patient is medically stable, the functional aspects of vision are routinely overlooked. Hundreds of thousands of dollars may be spent in rehabilitation without addressing the visual system. Common examples include the following:

- Patients with a field loss may be given the task of learning to feed themselves without first being taught how to scan or locate objects in the affected field.
- Patients may be taught to read or to use the computer even though they lack appropriate glasses to "see" the task.
- Patients with constant double vision are patched full-time and then are asked to walk. This could have a negative effect on balance.
- Patients who have vestibular dysfunctions causing dizziness, vertigo, or balance problems may still wear their "invisible, no-line bifocals" that can often exaggerate or aggravate the dizziness and balance condition.

Many patients who have been diagnosed with mild brain injuries are often not aware of their visual problems, nor are they visually evaluated until many years post-injury.

Few rehabilitation facilities currently use rehabilitative optometric services on a regular basis. With the high prevalence of visual system dysfunctions, optometric rehabilitative assessment and management is essential, although this does not replace the need for ophthalmology and neuro-ophthalmology intervention.

Summary

The primary objective of this chapter is to demonstrate the need for a comprehensive vision evaluation for a patient as soon as possible after brain injury. There are also many visual compensation strategies and adaptive techniques that may significantly help patients in their recovery. Prompt attention to the visual system in patients with ABI will lead to early identification and treatment of vision problems that can potentially interfere with rehabilitation. There are also many compensatory and adaptive techniques that can be implemented once the nature of the vision problem is identified. The next chapter will review vision rehabilitation for ABI.

References

1. Lehmkuhl DL. *Brain Injury Glossary*. Houston, TX: HDI Publishers; 1993.
2. Rosenthal M, Griffith ER, Bond MR, Miller JD. *Rehabilitation of the Adult and Child With Traumatic Brain Injury*. Philadelphia, PA: FA Davis Co; 1990.
3. Cohen AH, Rein LD. The effect of head trauma on the visual system: the doctor of optometry as a member of the rehabilitation team. *J Am Optom Assoc*. 1992;63:530–536.
4. Aravich D, Troxell L. Clinical practice guidelines for occupational therapists in the evaluation and treatment of oculomotor impairment following traumatic brain injury. *Current Physical Medicine and Rehabilitation Reports*. 2021;9:93–99.
5. Fessler A, Kruemmling B, Scheiman M. A worthwhile collaboration: integrating optometry and occupational therapy in the treatment of children. *Vis Dev & Rehab*. 2020;6:221–236.
6. Menon DK, Schwab K, Wright DW, Maas A. Position statement: definition of traumatic brain injury. *Arch Phys Med Rehabil*. 2010;91:1637–40.

7. Maas AIR, Menon DK, Adelson PD, et al. Traumatic brain injury: integrated approaches to improve prevention, clinical care, and research. *Lancet Neurol*. 2017;16:987–1048.

8. Bazarian JJ, Cernak I, Noble-Haeusslein L, et al. Long-term neurologic outcomes after traumatic brain injury. *J Head Trauma Rehabil*. 2009;24:439–451.

9. Reith F, Van den Brande R, Synnot A., et al. The reliability of the glasgow coma scale: a systematic review. *Intensive Care Med*. 2016;42:3–15.

10. Shan R, Szmydynger-Chodobska J, Warren OU, et al. A new panel of blood biomarkers for the diagnosis of mild traumatic brain injury/concussion in adults. *J Neurotrauma*. 2016;33:49–57.

11. Fatuki TA, Zvonarev V, Rodas AW. Prevention of traumatic brain injury in the United States: significance, new findings, and practical applications. *Cureus*. 2020;12:e11225.

12. Stallones L, Gibbs-Long J, Gabella B, Kakefuda I. Community readiness and prevention of traumatic brain injury. *Brain Inj*. 2008;22:555–564.

13. Hyder AA, Wunderlich CA, Puvanachandra P, et al. The impact of traumatic brain injuries: a global perspective. *NeuroRehabilitation*. 2007;22:341–353.

14. Thurman DJ, Sniezek JE, Johnson D, et al. *Guidelines for Surveillance of Central Nervous System Injury*. Atlanta, GA: US Department of Health and Human Services, Centers for Disease Control and Prevention; 1995.

15. Howe EI, Andelic N, Perrin PB, et al. Employment probability trajectories up to 10 years after moderate-to-severe traumatic brain injury. *Front Neurol*. 2018;9:1051.

16. Stambrook M, Moore AD, Peters LC, et al. Effects of mild, moderate and severe closed head injury on long-term vocational status. *Brain Inj*. 1990;4:183–190.

17. Alouani AT, Elfouly T. Traumatic brain injury (TBI) detection: past, present, and future. *Biomedicines*. 2022;10.

18. Whyte J, Hart T, Laborde A, et al. Rehabilitation of the patient with traumatic brain injury. In: DeLisa J, Gans BM, Bockenek WL, et al., eds. *Rehabilitation Medicine: Principles and Practice*. 3rd ed. Philadelphia, PA: Lippincott-Raven; 1998:1191–1239.

19. Kraus JF, MacArthur DL, Silverman TA. Epidemiology of mild brain injury. *Semin Neurol*. 1994;14:1–7.

20. Hellerstein LF, Kadet TS. Visual profile of patients presenting with brain trauma. *J Opt Vis Devel*. 1999;30:51–54.

21. Nelson LD, Temkin NR, Dikmen S, et al. Recovery after mild traumatic brain injury in patients presenting to US level I trauma centers: a transforming research and clinical knowledge in traumatic brain injury (Track-TBI) study. *JAMA Neurol*. 2019;76:1049–1059.

22. Suchoff IB, Kapoor N, Waxman R, Ference W. The occurrence of ocular and visual dysfunctions in an acquired brain-injured patient sample. *J Am Optom Assoc*. 1999;70:301–308.

23. Ciuffreda KJ, Kapoor N, Rutner D, et al. Occurrence of oculomotor dysfunctions in acquired brain injury: a retrospective analysis. *Optometry*. 2007;78:155–161.

24. Goodrich GL, Kirby J, Cockerham G, et al. Visual function in patients of a polytrauma rehabilitation center: a descriptive study. *J Rehabil Res Dev*. 2007;44:929–936.

25. Brahm KD, Wilgenburg HM, Kirby J, et al. Visual impairment and dysfunction in combat-injured servicemembers with traumatic brain injury. *Optom Vis Sci*. 2009;86:817–825.

26. Cockerham GC, Goodrich GL, Weichel ED, et al. Eye and visual function in traumatic brain injury. *J Rehabil Res Dev*. 2009;46:811–818.

27. Goodrich GL, Flyg HM, Kirby JE, et al. Mechanisms of TBI and visual consequences in military and veteran populations. *Optom Vis Sci*. 2013;90:105–112.

28. Capo-Aponte JE, Jorgensen-Wagers KL, Sosa JA, et al. Visual dysfunctions at different stages after blast and non-blast mild traumatic brain injury. *Optom Vis Sci*. 2017;94:7–15.

29. Stelmack JA, Frith T, Van Koevering D, et al. Visual function in patients followed at a veterans affairs polytrauma network site: an electronic medical record review. *Optometry*. 2009;80:419–424.

30. Capo-Aponte JE, Urosevich TG, Temme LA, et al. Visual dysfunctions and symptoms during the subacute stage of blast-induced mild traumatic brain injury. *Mil Med*. 2012;177:804–813.

31. Master CL, Scheiman M, Gallaway M, et al. Vision diagnoses are common after concussion in adolescents. *Clin Pediatr (Phila)*. 2016;55:260–267.

32. Scheiman M, Grady MF, Jenewein E, et al. Frequency of oculomotor disorders in adolescents 11 to 17 years of age with concussion, 4 to 12 weeks post injury. *Vision Res*. 2021;183:73–80.

33. Warlow CP. Epidemiology of stroke. *Lancet*. 1998;352(Supplement 3):1–4.

34. Wolf PA, D'Agostino RB, Belanger AJ, Kannel WB. Probability of stroke: a risk profile from the Framingham Study. *Stroke*. 1991;22:312–318.

35. Virani SS, Alonso A, Benjamin EJ, et al. Heart disease and stroke statistics—2020 update: a report from the American Heart Association. *Circulation*. 2020;141:e139–e596.

36. Rowe FJ, Hepworth L, Hanna K, et al. Point Prevalence of visual impairment following stroke. *International Journal of Stroke*. 2016;11.

37. Trevarthen C, Sperry RW. Perceptual unity of the ambient visual field in human commissurotomy patients. *Brain*;96:547–570.

38. Padula WV. *A Behavioral Vision Approach for Persons With Physical Disabilities*. Santa Ana, CA: Optometric Extension Program; 1988.
39. Padula WV. Neuro-optometric rehabilitation for persons with a TBI or CVA. *J Optom Vis Devel*. 1992;23:4–8.
40. Barron C. Low vision rehabilitation of multiple sclerosis: a case report. *J Am Optom Assoc*. 1993;64:38–44.
41. Gray L, Winkelman AC. Multiple sclerosis: recent developments. *Ocul Dis Update 2*. 1991:81–95.
42. Harkins T. Treating multiple sclerosis. *Clin Eye Vis Care*. 1994;6:133–136.
43. Sherman J, Morschauser D. A clinical update on multiple sclerosis. *Rev Opt*. 1994;131:55–63.
44. Wolff E. *Anatomy of the Eye and Orbit*. Philadelphia, PA: WB Saunders; 1976.
45. Zost MG. Diagnosis and management of visual dysfunction in cerebral injury. In: Maino D, ed. *Diagnosis and Management of Special Populations*. New York, NY: CV Mosby; 1995:75–134.
46. Cohen AH, Soden R. An optometric approach to the rehabilitation of the stroke patient. *J Am Optom Assoc*. 1981;52:795–800.
47. Zoltan B. *Vision, Perception and Cognition: A Manual for the Evaluation and Treatment of the Neurologically Impaired Adult*. 3rd ed. Thorofare, NJ: SLACK Incorporated; 1996.

Chapter Ten

Visual Rehabilitation for Patients With Brain Injury

*Lynn Fishman Hellerstein, Mitchell Scheiman,
and Beth I. Fishman*

Overview

When brain injury occurs, a comprehensive rehabilitation program that provides for evaluation, training, and interaction in all routine activities of daily living is often recommended.[1] All deficit areas need to be addressed by retraining an existing process or teaching a new one if the existing process is untrainable. The rehabilitation team is generally composed of physicians (including general physicians, internists, physiatrists, neurologists, neurosurgeons, ophthalmologists, and optometrists), psychologists, neuropsychologists, and therapists (physical, occupational, speech, and cognitive).

In order to make the complex visual decisions necessary for activities of daily living, such as reading, math, driving, and vocations, integration of basic sensory systems is critical. For example, what appears to be a deficit in a visual cognitive skill, such as figure ground (i.e., finding an article of clothing in a drawer), may actually be caused by refractive, binocular, accommodative, ocular motility, or pattern recognition problems. Therefore, to help patients regain complex functions, treatment must be started at the basic processing level and proceed through a hierarchy of skills. Throughout this book, we have emphasized that ocular health, refractive, visual acuity, and visual efficiency skills should be addressed before visual information processing problems. Direct treatment of the higher-level skill (figure ground) in the example above would not be effective unless the underlying deficits are addressed first.

Determining the cause of the visual deficit requires an understanding of the brain injury effect on the entire visual process from input to output. Some patients require treatment based on a developmental model and might also include sensory integration treatment. Other patients, however, have such severe deficits that function cannot be regained, and strategies to teach the patient to compensate for the impairment are appropriate. All patients who have suffered a brain injury should have a complete vision evaluation by an optometrist who has extensive experience in vision rehabilitation and functional vision care.[2–4] Treatment strategies can then be established.

DOI: 10.4324/9781003526841-10

197

Optometric Treatment Methods

The goals of optometric intervention are to improve visual acuity, eliminate diplopia, and improve visual awareness and visual cognitive function[5] so that visually related performances are enhanced, allowing the patient to maintain the highest quality of life. Techniques used in optometric rehabilitation include: lenses, prisms, absorptive filters, selective occlusion for specific tasks and distances, low vision aids, and vision therapy (see Chapter Seven).

Ocular Health

Appropriate medications and surgery should be a priority if necessary. Artificial tear regimen and/or taping lids closed for dry eyes may be necessary and sight-saving. The therapist has little responsibility in the ocular health areas, and the optometrist or ophthalmologist should be consulted for treatment of patients with ocular health issues. However, it is quite useful for the therapist to be knowledgeable about the type of ocular health problem present and its impact on function.

Lenses

One of the most effective tools that the optometrist uses in practice are lenses.[4] Lenses can be used to improve clarity and sight, reduce or eliminate double vision, and reduce visual discomfort and/or stress, and they affect body posture and weight shifting. A good rule of thumb is that almost all people over the age of 40 years old will need glasses for either distance, near, or full-time wear. You should be suspicious if you are working with a patient over 40 years old who is not wearing glasses for any task. The following are some of the common reasons why patients may need new glasses:

- A patient arrives in the hospital without their glasses.
- Their glasses were broken or lost as a result of the injury.
- Their glasses are many years old and are an outdated prescription.
- The brain injury has caused a change in prescription and current glasses are not correct.
- The patient cannot utilize the glasses properly because of injury. For example, the brain injury resulted in restriction of movement of eyes in downward gaze, and so the patient cannot move their eyes into the part of the bifocal lens that allows for vision at near.

If you wear prescription glasses or contact lenses currently, try spending a day functioning without your proper prescription. It may cause fatigue or nausea, or it may make you less efficient or even nonfunctional! Imagine what it would be like if you had other motor and cognitive impairments in addition to the visual problems.

The best lens for "seeing" is not always the best lens for all tasks. For example, people may see clearly to drive with a certain prescription glass, but they may not be able to read with that prescription. Some patients see clearly at near, but read much more comfortably and efficiently with a special reading lens. Have you ever received a new pair of glasses that allowed you to see clearly yet make you feel uncomfortable when you walked?

Eyeglass prescriptions may need to be modified throughout the rehabilitation program.

Prism

Prism may be prescribed for temporary or permanent use. Fresnel prism, described in Chapter Seven, is a relatively inexpensive, temporary type of prism that can immediately be placed on a current prescription lens. Fresnel prism can also be removed very easily, making it very useful for temporary situations. A disadvantage of Fresnel prisms is that they may distort visual acuity. Prism that is ground into a glasses prescription is a more permanent type of prism prescription.

Prism is used for three main purposes:[4]
1. To neutralize or compensate for patients with acquired strabismus or significant heterophoria (compensatory)
2. To affect spatial awareness and midline awareness (yoked)
3. To expand visual field

COMPENSATORY PRISM

Neutralizing or compensatory prism may be utilized for patients with acquired strabismus or significant heterophoria. Compensatory prism is sometimes difficult to prescribe because the patient's visual condition may be intermittent, variable, or noncomitant. Fresnel prism may be used initially. However, if compensating prism is needed over a longer period of time, the prism is often incorporated into the lens of a pair of glasses. If the compensating prism eliminates the strabismus condition, it will often alleviate double vision. In some cases, a patient may have an abnormal head tilt or turn due to strabismus. If the compensating prism is effective, the head turn or tilt may also be reduced.

When prescribing compensatory prism, we generally describe the prism as either base-in, base-out, base-up, or base-down. This refers to the location of the base of the prism relative to the patient's eye (refer to Chapter Seven for more details).

For exophoria, we prescribe base-in prism for both eyes while base-out prism is used for esophoria. For vertical deviations, base-down is used in front of one eye and base-up in front of the other.

PRISM TO AFFECT SPATIAL AWARENESS: YOKED PRISM

Yoked prism differs from compensatory prism because the base of the prism will always be on the same side of each eye (see Chapter Seven). Yoked prism is often utilized to alter a patient's spatial awareness, to modify a patient's midline perception, or to change weight shifting.[6–8] The yoked prism may be temporary and used for certain activities during the rehabilitation process, or it may be permanent for full-time wear. Yoked prism may also be beneficial with field loss patients.

PRISM TO EXPAND VISUAL FIELD

One of the most significant vision problems associated with traumatic brain injury and cerebrovascular accident is visual field loss. One of the treatment modalities available to help a patient compensate for this loss is prism. In recent years, studies[9–12] have demonstrated that a prism field expansion system called the Peli Visual Field Expansion Device for Hemianopia is an effective treatment for patients with hemianopia (see Chapter Seven). This prism can expand the visual field by as much as 30 to 40 degrees and allows the patient to be aware of potential obstacles in the periphery.

Filters and Lighting

Absorptive filters or "tints" are often utilized in patients with brain injury. Light sensitivity is a common complaint after injury. Different colors, such as yellow, amber, gray, brown, and green, and other shades of tints are used to decrease light sensitivity symptoms. Pink tints are often helpful for patients working on computers or under fluorescent lights. Anti-reflection coatings reduce glare, especially at night. Some patients, especially elderly patients with age-related decrease in vision, need more light. Better lighting is recommended in addition to yellow tints.

Occlusion

Patients suffering a neurological insult often complain of double vision. Strabismus, including paresis, muscle restrictions, and globe injury are among the leading causes. Patients may squint, cover one eye, or assume an awkward head position to avoid double vision. Physicians or therapists may try to remedy the situation by having the patient wear a patch over one eye. "Which eye should be covered?", "How often should the patient wear the patch?", and "What type of patch should be used?" are common questions that rehabilitation personnel ask. A patient's visual status, in addition to their demands in activities of daily living, need to be considered when occlusion is recommended. Therefore, merely telling a patient to patch an eye is an inappropriate recommendation. Optometric consultation is critical when occlusion is being considered.

TOTAL OCCLUSION

If possible, total occlusion (patching) should be avoided.[13] Total occlusion should be utilized only when double vision is constant and no other treatment strategy (lenses, prisms, partial occlusion) is successful. If total occlusion is deemed to be the treatment of choice, the optometrist may recommend alternate occlusion (occluding left eye one day or part of a day and then changing to the right eye). If the vision is exceptionally poor in one eye, the optometrist may recommend occlusion of the poorer eye so that the patient can visually function, or occlusion of the better seeing eye may be recommended so that the patient has a chance to improve visual functioning of the poorer eye.

Figure 10.1a illustrates total occlusion of a patient's left eye. Observe the significant change in head posture when the occluder is changed to the right eye in Figure 10.1b.

Several different methods of occlusion are listed below:

- The black patch with an elastic string, as seen in Figure 10.2a, is an inexpensive, easy method. The main disadvantage is the cosmesis of the patch.
- Clip-on patches as pictured in Figure 10.2b may be utilized. Clip-on patches are also easy and inexpensive but are susceptible to becoming dislodged.
- Figure 10.2c shows tape over the lens of the patient's glasses. Tape is effective and inexpensive; however, it is difficult to clean off a lens, especially when it is necessary to alternate occlusion.

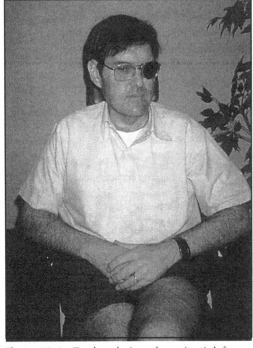

Figure 10.1a. Total occlusion of a patient's left eye.

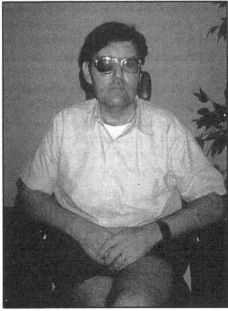

Figure 10.1b. Observe the significant change in head posture when the occluder is changed to the right eye.

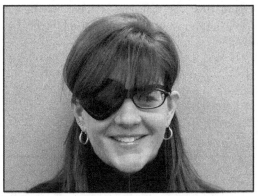

Figure 10.2a. Black patch with an elastic string.

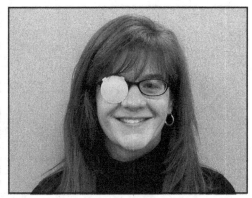

Figure 10.2b. Clip-on patches.

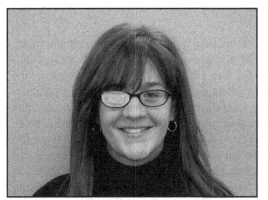

Figure 10.2c. Tape over the lens of the patient's glasses.

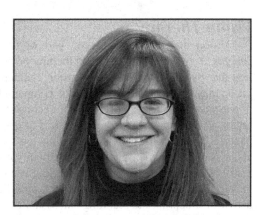

Figure 10.2d. Bangerter occlusion foil.

- A Bangerter occlusion foil (see Appendix A) is pictured in 10.2d. This is a very thin plastic-like material that can be ordered in a variety of gradations. These different gradations can create minimal, moderate, or significant decrease (including no light perception) in contrast and acuity. The Bangerter foils can be cut for any size lens and can be easily removed or changed.

PARTIAL OCCLUSION

If a patient has intermittent double vision, full-time occlusion is not recommended. Partial occlusion, like total occlusion, is used only when necessary and allows the patient to be binocular at least part of the day. The types of occluders are the same as described above with one difference. The tape or Bangerter occluder may be cut in such a way as to block only part of the field of vision as pictured in Figure 10.3. This type of occluder allows a patient to still use each eye, but will eliminate double vision in certain fields of gaze. This technique is especially useful to noncomitant strabismics who may have double vision in just certain gazes.

Low Vision Aids

Brain injury can actually damage optical and neural pathways affecting visual acuity at distance and near. In addition, the premorbid state of the patient may include pathology that could also cause decreased visual acuity. There are numerous types of lenses, optical devices (magnifiers, telescopes), computers, and lighting that may be useful to a patient with low vision.[14]

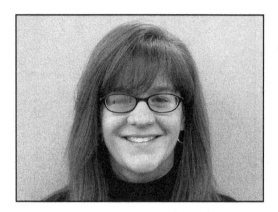

Figure 10.3. The Bangerter occluder may be cut in such a way as to block only part of the field of vision.

Vision Therapy

Vision therapy is an integral part of the rehabilitation treatment for many brain injury patients.[15–35] When should vision therapy be started? It is quite ironic that many physicians suggest that patients wait to have a vision evaluation for 6 to 12 months post-trauma because "the vision may change over time." This is comparable to telling a patient who has suffered a paralysis of one side not to use a wheelchair or exercise for at least six months because motor function may return. Vision may change; however, it is of questionable value to rehabilitate in other areas when patients have significant vision dysfunction as indicated by the following examples. If double vision is present, patients have more difficulty with balance and movement. If a patient has reduced visual acuity or inappropriate glasses, the use of computers for rehabilitation may be limited. It is frustrating for both the patient with visual field loss and the therapist to perform daily living activities if appropriate scanning and visual compensations are not initiated first. These examples demonstrate that patients should be evaluated very early in the rehabilitation process. This does not mean vision therapy will be initiated immediately, but appropriate lenses, prisms, occlusion, and consultation may be helpful.

If the optometrist prescribes vision therapy, direct supervision and guidance by the optometrist is essential. The occupational therapist may perform daily therapy techniques prescribed by the optometrist, and most importantly, can help the patient generalize visual skills into daily living activities as well as assist in adaptations. Techniques, especially those involving binocularity, should only be attempted by a therapist under direct supervision of an optometrist. The therapy procedures included in this chapter are those that could be provided by the occupational therapist. The more advanced vision therapy techniques requiring direct optometric supervision are not discussed in this book.

When treating a patient with acquired brain injury using vision therapy, the following guidelines are important:

* Obtain visual attention before initiating the therapy procedure.
* All techniques should provide feedback to the patient.
* Work at the level of the patient's current performance.
* Progressively increase the demand of the technique.
* Integrate the visual skill into activities of daily living.

OVERVIEW OF VISION THERAPY FOR BRAIN-INJURED PATIENTS

Vision therapy procedures are organized in a sequence starting from gross motor movements, which are the foundation from which visual skills develop. Gross motor movements, which often include vestibular and balance techniques, begin as reflexive and spontaneous movements and then become more organized with an attempt to use both sides of the body. If the patient has significant tactile and proprioceptive issues as well, techniques in those areas should also be included. The therapy techniques provide a basis for body schema and laterality.

Fine motor and eye movement skills therapy are initially practiced independently and are then integrated with movement. Appropriate eye movement therapy includes emphasis on visual attention, saccadic fixations, and scanning, in addition to smooth, efficient pursuit movements. Without these basic skills, higher-level visual perceptual functioning is compromised. Visual perceptual skills often improve as foundation skills improve, even without specific perceptual activities. As foundation skills are integrated, higher-level perceptual activities, if necessary, may be included with the goal of improving visual manipulation and visualization abilities. These skills are required in academic areas such as reading, writing, and math and for many vocations. Depending on the neurologic injury and recovery, adaptations or compensatory skills may also be necessary in addition to remedial techniques discussed above.

The sequence of therapy techniques is based on clinical judgment but needs to begin at the level at which the patient can succeed. The key to success is to work at the level of the patient's current performance and gradually increase the demands of the tasks.

VISION REHABILITATION TECHNIQUES FOR PATIENTS WITH BALANCE/MOVEMENT DISORDERS

When a patient presents with a balance and movement disorder, there is often a problem with integration of the visual, vestibular, and somatosensory systems.[36] Somatosensory and vestibular interaction, rather than the visual system, should control balance in the adult. However, with a patient who has suffered a cerebrovascular accident or traumatic brain injury that results in decreased proprioceptive and tactile cues, the visual system is often the predominant system for balance. These patients need an integrative therapy program that includes vision, physical, and occupational therapy. Too often, vision is not appropriately addressed during vestibular rehabilitation programs. Vision therapy treatment can enhance vestibular therapy since vestibular therapy can enhance vision therapy.

The goals of vestibular therapy are to:[37]
- Develop proprioceptive and visual mechanisms to compensate for a disturbance in labyrinthine function.
- Improve muscle coordination.
- Practice balancing under everyday conditions with special attention to developing the use of the eyes, muscles, and joints.
- Train movement of the eyes independent of the head.
- Loosen the muscles of the neck and shoulder to overcome the protective muscular spasm and tendency to move "in one piece."
- Practice head movements that cause dizziness and thus gradually overcome the disability.
- Become accustomed to moving about naturally in daylight and in the dark.
- Encourage the restoration of self-confidence and easy spontaneous movement.

Physical and occupational therapy usually involves techniques for the vestibular system (balance/equilibrium and toleration of movement in different planes) and muscle control/coordination. The vision therapy emphasizes visual skill efficiency. Lenses and prisms are continually evaluated throughout the vision therapy program. Eye movement skills are then integrated with motor skills.

The program should progress from matching all three sensory inputs, decreasing the amount of input from any or all three systems and, finally, using techniques that have conflicts within the three systems.

Tactile, proprioceptive, and vestibular issues need to be addressed early in treatment. A sensory integration approach including brushing and massage techniques may be beneficial. If the vestibular dysfunction is severe, the patient may need to start treatment in the supine position with no movement initially (patient receives tactile and proprioceptive clues from the floor). Start with eye movement movements only, discussed later in this chapter, or head movements only.[38,39] As the patient can tolerate, progress to eye and head movement. Gradually, move the patient to a supported sitting position, then standing. Use proprioceptive activities, such as wall push-ups, crawling, and holding onto or pushing in the chair with hands, to help toleration of movement. Allow the patient to suck on peppermint or to take ginger to decrease nausea. Once the patient can integrate eye movements with body movements, therapy can continue in visual motor, bilateral integration, fine motor, and motor planning areas, if necessary.

EYE MOVEMENT TECHNIQUES

Chapter Seven describes sample vision therapy techniques for pursuits and saccades. For many patients with brain injury, however, these techniques may be too high-level.[23] Therefore, the techniques described below should be initiated first.

Eye Calisthenics

Objective. Large ocular calisthenics are used to restore muscle action or to prevent secondary contractures or adhesions of paretic muscles.

Equipment Needed. No equipment necessary. Have the patient remove their glasses.

Description and Setup. Have the patient look as far to the right as possible and to hold in that position for several seconds. Then have the patient look to the left, again holding for several seconds. Continue with looking up, down, and in oblique locations. Try to have the patient "stretch" as far as possible. It may be uncomfortable at first, but it often improves with time and practice. The patient should do these procedures at least twice a day for several minutes each time.

Pursuit Procedure

Objective. The goal of this activity is for the patient to move their eyes smoothly, accurately, and without discomfort or restriction in all fields of gaze. Pursuits procedures should be started very early in treatment program.

Equipment Needed. Small hand-held object or finger puppet. The patient may need to use glasses for near.

Description and Setup. Pursuit procedures may be given with the patient lying, seated, or standing, whichever posture is the most comfortable initially. The patient should keep their head still, as these are eye movements, not "head" movements. Hold the puppet directly in front of the patient's nose, approximately 14 to 16 inches from the patient's face. The therapist should slowly move the puppet in all directions, starting with horizontal movements, vertical movements, then diagonal movements. The pursuits pattern should resemble a star. Now move the object in a circular fashion. In the event of restriction of ocular movement, ocular discomfort, or nausea, the optometrist should be consulted immediately.

Saccadic Fixations

Objective. The objective of a saccadic fixation procedure is to improve the accuracy of saccades as well as to improve visual attention.

Equipment Needed. Two different colored pens or two different objects such as hand-held puppets.

Description and Setup. Hold the pens or objects approximately 14 to 16 inches from the patient's face. Call out the color of one of the pens or the name of one of the objects. Have the patient look at the pen or object you called until you call out the second color or object. The patient should then look to the second pen or object. Continue calling each pen or object while you periodically change the location of one of them so the patient fixates in all fields of gaze. The patient should maintain fixation on the object requested by the therapist and should not be distracted, anticipate, or take several jumps to locate the object.

Spotting Techniques

Spotting is a technique used by dancers or ice skaters. When a dancer moves or spins rapidly, they are taught to spot and fixate on an object to help stabilize and stop the feeling of motion. This same technique is used for people who have motion sickness, which is often a result of vestibular dysfunction. A person in a car may suffer from motion sickness when riding in the back seat, but may not show symptoms when riding in the front seat. Sitting in the front seat allows a person to visually fixate in the straight-ahead field, rather than see constant motion peripherally as when riding in the back seat of a car. Therefore, even though a person may have a vestibular dysfunction, the use of visual spotting or fixation can relieve symptoms and improve balance control.

Objective. The objective of spotting techniques is to teach the patient how to visually fixate and maintain fixation on an object.

Equipment Needed. None.

Description and Setup. Have the patient look at an object in straight-ahead gaze and maintain fixation on a target. Do not merely ask a patient to just look at a wall or door. Rather, have the patient look specifically at a spot or object on the wall or at the light switch. Encourage the patient to use spotting when moving, especially when the patient is dizzy or disoriented.

Scanning Techniques

Objective. The objective of the scanning technique is to teach a person how to be aware of their full field of vision. This is most important with the patient with field loss.

Equipment Needed. Four colored stickers or pictures.

Description and Setup. Place colored stickers or pictures on each corner of a door jam. Before a person moves through the door jam, they need to scan and look for all four stickers. This technique should be used consistently when moving through space or for dressing or eating. The pictures can be put on four corners of the food tray and the patient must look for all four pictures before eating. This gives the patient information about what is on the food tray and helps to decrease spilling and misgrabbing for food. Figure 10.4 demonstrates the four-corner setup on a food tray.

Binocular Techniques

Procedures may include specific lenses, prisms, occlusion, and vision therapy. A patient should have an immediate vision consultation with an optometrist or ophthalmologist if double vision is suspected. Vision therapy for binocular disorders is prescribed by the optometrist. Therapy techniques may be prescribed for the occupational therapist to implement with the patient on a daily basis; however, the prescription and management of vision therapy is under direct optometric supervision. At times, strabismus surgery may be necessary for a patient who still demonstrates a large angle strabismus 6 months to 1 year post-injury.

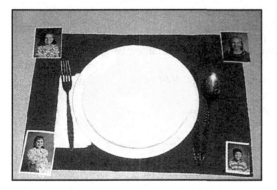

Figure 10.4. The four-corner setup on a food tray.

ACCOMMODATION TECHNIQUES

Treatment recommendations are similar to those for binocular disorders, except surgery is not necessary.

VISUAL MOTOR TECHNIQUES

Numerous visual motor activities can be found in occupational therapy literature. Techniques may include ball roll, catch, and ball hitting.

BILATERAL INTEGRATION TECHNIQUES

Activities can be found in *Brain Gym*[40] and include cross marches, bilateral circles and lines, and lazy eights.

FINE MOTOR TECHNIQUES

Numerous techniques can be found in the *Fine Motor Dysfunction* manual.[41] Other recommendations include working with Silly Putty (Crayola, Easton, PA), games like Finger Thinking or Tricky Fingers (Edushape, Deer Park, NY), and utilizing pencil grips.

MOTOR PLANNING TECHNIQUES

Sequencing games such as Simon Says, clapping patterns, rope jumping, and scavenger hunts may be beneficial.

VISUAL PERCEPTUAL TECHNIQUES

The higher-level perceptual skills are addressed by the optometrist and the occupational therapist, in conjunction with other members of the rehabilitation team. The importance of starting with treatment at the foundation levels (tactile, proprioceptive, motor movements, and eye movement skills) before visual perceptual techniques cannot be overemphasized. Educating the patient about the deficit is an important first step to help the patient learn to use compensatory techniques.

Chapter Seven contains a number of vision therapy techniques for the treatment of visual perceptual dysfunctions. Additional procedures can be found in many references.[42,43] There are many activities and games that can be found in toy or teacher supply stores that are used to work on visual perceptual skills. They are listed in Table 10.1. Even though the techniques may be designed for a child, the techniques can be adapted to the level of a patient of any age and then modified as the patient improves. Table 10.2 summarizes compensatory techniques for patients with visual perceptual deficits.

Table 10.1

Visual Perceptual Activities and Games

Area of Emphasis	Activity
Visual discrimination	Games that emphasize pattern recognition, such as parquetry blocks, matching, sorting, Perfection game (Milton Bradley, East Longmeadow, MA)
Visual form constancy	Geoboards, tangrams, parquetry blocks, dot-to-dot
Visual closure	Word search, dot-to-dot, Hangman
Visual figure ground	Hidden picture, Where's Waldo?
Visual memory	Checkers, chess, Tic Tac Toe
Visual spatial perception	Obstacle course, road map
Visualization strategies	Puzzles, tangrams

> ### Table 10.2
>
> ## Compensatory Strategies for Patients With Visual Perceptual Deficits
>
> | Type of Deficit | Compensatory Techniques |
> |---|---|
> | Agnosia | Augment visual with tactile/auditory stimuli when possible |
> | Alexia | Utilize pictures and multisensory stimuli |
> | Apraxia | Ocular motor techniques; augment with verbal and tactile stimuli |
> | Ataxia | Provide additional proprioceptive and kinesthetic input and cuing |
> | Depth perception | Emphasize safety issues; use tactile and kinesthetic reinforcement for tasks such as walking down stairs; use landmarks for location; reduce impulsivity with movement |
> | Figure ground | Reduce clutter in visual environment; use high-contrast markers or tape to identify figure; teach patient to be very systematic when examining a small area |
> | Form perception/constancy | Augment visual with tactile, kinesthetic stimuli |
> | Spatial relations | Use landmarks for location; have patient orient themself in space and then proceed from object to object |
> | Unilateral spatial neglect | Important communication should take place in the field of awareness; advise safety issues; augment with verbal and tactile cues |

Vision Field Loss Rehabilitation

Can Visual Field Loss Be Remediated?

In a series of reports, Sabel and colleagues described partial recovery of homonymous visual field defects by intensive computer-based rehabilitation therapy.[44–46] In this approach, patients use a software program at home for an hour a day, 6 days a week, for 6 months. A chin support is used for head stability and a monitor is placed 30 cm away. Stimuli are white lights shown against a dark background. The patient has to press a button every time they see the white target appear. Protocols are tailored for each patient to present most stimuli near the border of the field defect to maximize potential therapeutic benefit. Sabel subsequently founded a company (NovaVision) that offers this visual rehabilitation therapy. The idea behind visual restoration therapy is that after stroke or traumatic brain injury, a region of salvageable vision exists between areas of the visual field served by normal and damaged brain tissue. Visual stimulation in this zone with more than 1,000 trials a day is postulated to resuscitate its functional potential. After treatment, homonymous field defects have been reported to show a mean gain of about 5 degrees.

However, there are a number of major problems with the data reported by Horton:[47,48]

- Even if the treatment truly leads to a mean gain of 5 degrees, the question is whether such a gain is clinically meaningful. Most clinicians would suggest that an increase in visual fields of 5 degrees is not meaningful.

- The studies were conducted by individuals with a commercial interest in the software company.

- The same software program used for visual restoration therapy was also used to show improvement in the visual fields. Obviously, the data would be more compelling if visual field improvement could be demonstrated with any standard clinical visual field instrument. When patients with visual field loss were tested before and after visual restoration therapy with a standard visual field instrument, no benefit of treatment could be detected.[49]

- The authors did not control for eye movements. Therefore, the visual field recovery can simply be attributed to teaching the patient to make small eye movements. In a study designed to control for eye movements, 17 patients with stable homonymous field defects were treated according to the visual restoration therapy protocol.[49] Independent visual field testing was done before and after treatment to assess the outcome. A crucial innovation was that perimetry was performed using a scanning laser ophthalmoscope, which allows the examiner to control fixation. The study found no significant improvement in visual field defects, although most patients had the subjective impression that they had benefited from visual restoration therapy. This discrepancy underscores a limitation of outcome satisfaction surveys: Patients can be swayed by placebo effects.

It remains true, therefore, that no therapeutic intervention can effectively correct the underlying visual field deficit.[49] Thus, remediation and compensation must be used in visual rehabilitation for visual field loss. We can help patients by teaching them compensatory techniques to function more effectively in activities of daily life in spite of the field loss. Gianutsos and Suchoff stress that intervention must emphasize compensation, rather than restoration.[50] They conceptualize visual field defect cases on a continuum. At one end, there are those patients who are quite aware of the hemianopia, while at the other end are those individuals who are totally unaware of the deficit.[50] The goal of visual rehabilitation, therefore, is to move the patient from one end of the continuum (lack of awareness) to as close to awareness as possible.

To develop effective treatment, sensory deficits must be differentiated from perceptual, attention, linguistic, and other cognitive deficits.[51] Brain injury affects a variety of cognitive and linguistic functions that might affect visual function such as letter identification and reading. People may have difficulty reading because of damage to linguistic processing areas. They may not respond to objects in the periphery because of impaired visual attention or unilateral inattention and neglect.[52,53] Since unilateral field loss is often associated with unilateral inattention, the treatments frequently address unilateral attention as well as unilateral field loss.

Unilateral field loss usually does not cut the field down the middle but rather leaves central vision intact, called central sparing. Functionally, an individual with a unilateral field loss "with central sparing" will see most of a person's face at about 1 meter (3 feet) but see nothing to one side or the other of the face. People with field cuts and central sparing usually have normal acuity and only minor problems with reading. These individuals will read a single line of text normally but might lose their place when reading, or may have difficulty scanning a page for information. In some cases, people with unilateral field loss have a unilateral field loss that also bisects the central field. These individuals will report that one-half of the examiner's face can be seen during field testing. People with "split central fields" will only see half of a letter or words they are trying to identify as well. The resultant loss of basic shape, letter, and face recognition may be confused with higher order perceptual deficits. People with a right unilateral field loss with a split central field will have severe problems with reading even though other linguistic functions are intact.[51]

Functionally, people with unilateral field loss will present with a disabled visual scanning and peripheral warning system, often with the functional effects compounded by an overlay of unilateral visual inattention. In addition, a person with unilateral field loss may present with "wayfinding deficits," and often cannot even retrace their steps. A person may have basic problems with wayfinding primarily due to a unilateral field loss rather than cognitive deficit. For example, if a client with a left field loss walks down a hall for the first time, they will see one side of the hall to their right. When they turn around to retrace their steps, the former right side of the hall will now be to their blind, left visual field. The side of the hall that is now in their intact right field would never have been seen before. In effect, the client has never seen the route they are retracing. This problem is exacerbated for people who have split central fields and/or unilateral inattention.[51]

The following is a sequential list of treatment for visual field loss rehabilitation:
- Awareness training
- Prism field expansion
- Eye movement therapy
- Scanning training
- Wide field eye movement therapy
- Adaptations

Awareness Training

Awareness Training With a Laser Pointer

The therapist has the patient sit facing a wall 2 meters away. The patient is instructed to fixate a small target—a drawing on a sticky note will do. The patient also holds a laser pointer of a different color. The patient is instructed to "tag" the therapist's laser spot when they see it, without moving their eyes from the fixation target. Starting in the blind area of the visual field, the therapist moves the laser spot to the edge of the blind area, and marks with a small sticky note the place on the wall where the patient first responded to the light. The therapist then moves the laser spot along a different trajectory to another point on the suspected edge of the blind area (e.g., just above or below the previously placed sticky note) until it is first detected and places another sticky note. The therapist then keeps moving the laser spot to different points on the edge of the blind area until the edge of the blind area is defined vertically and horizontally by a string of sticky notes. Once this testing is completed, a person with a complete left homonymous quadrantanopia will have a string of sticky notes along the vertical midline, around the central visual area (if central sparing), and along the person's horizon to the left forming an area that resembles a quarter of a pie. Once the blind area is defined by sticky notes, then the patient is instructed to look over and observe the extent of the blind area.

This process can then be repeated with the patient looking from the center fixation target to the peripheral laser spot as soon as it is detected. This helps patients understand the extent of the blind area, which they often find surprising.

Patients can purchase a laser pointer and perform this at home with a helper. Often patients are anxious for a prognosis; this procedure allows them to monitor progressive changes in visual fields at home.

Detecting Sticky Notes on Both Sides

Sticky notes can also be used for an awareness training procedure. Before the therapy session, the therapist places 20 sticky notes on the right and left walls of a hallway. The sticky notes are numbered (in the back) from 1 to 20. The 10 even-numbered sticky notes are placed on the right side of the hallway wall while the 10 odd-numbered sticky notes are placed on the left side of the wall. The patient is asked to walk down the hallway and find all of the sticky notes. The typical patient with visual field loss and left visual inattention will only find 10 of the 20 sticky notes on the right wall. The therapist would have the patient repeat the procedure trying to be more aware of the left side.

Coupons, Photographs, and Playing Cards

Coupons, family photographs, and playing cards can be used in a similar fashion. The playing cards can be scattered in a particular pattern (red on right, black on left, kings on one side, queens on the other) and the only way the patient can successfully complete the task is to be aware of both sides of the visual field.

Throughout this awareness training, the therapist would stress the questions suggested by Gianutsos and Suchoff:[50] "Where did you have the most difficulty?", "Did you notice that you had difficulty on one side?", "Where would I be telling you to look, if I were to do so?", "What do you think I am thinking?

Prism Field Expansion

The prism field expansion system called the Peli Visual Field Expansion Device for Hemianopia, described earlier, is an effective treatment for patients with hemianopia.[9–12] This prism can expand the visual field by as much as 30 to 40 degrees and allows the patient to be aware of potential obstacles in the periphery. However, it has not been evaluated with visual neglect. Thus, awareness training must occur first and if the patient develops an awareness of their visual field loss, prism expansion can be considered. This technique requires gradual introduction, first with the upper prism and then with the lower prism. When each prism is first introduced, the above field awareness training procedures are recommended to enable the patient to learn to recognize the ghost image of an object that is just outside of the field of view.

Eye Movement Techniques for Patients With Visual Field Loss

The eye movement techniques described in this chapter and in Chapter Seven are utilized with patients with visual field loss. Begin with all stimuli placed on the side that has normal vision. Thus, with a left hemianopia, all stimuli are placed on the right side at first. Once the patient can master all of the saccadic and pursuit techniques described in Chapter Seven, stimuli can be scattered across both sides of the visual field. After completion of this aspect of the therapy, wide field eye movement techniques should be used.

Scanning Training and Wide Field Eye Movement Techniques

The method that seems to produce the largest and functionally greatest increase in peripheral awareness is called compensatory visual scanning. In this technique, the therapist teaches the client to look with quick saccades in the direction of the blind hemifield.[54] Compensatory visual scanning does not actually increase the size of the intact field.

To compensate for a unilateral field loss the client must change habitual eye movement patterns. Normally we look at an object and depend on our peripheral vision to see on either side. Compensatory visual scanning involves frequently and consistently looking in the direction of the blind hemifield much like a driver uses rearview and sideview mirrors when driving to get a sense of what is going on around the car and beyond the range of peripheral vision. As with any therapeutic intervention, the client must be educated about the deficit and provided with an explanation for the compensatory strategy. Understanding and verbalizing the problem or demonstrating improved performance during instructional protocols is not sufficient. The client must demonstrate compensatory scanning as an ingrained habit during real-life activities when attention is on the activity not the eye movement.

If a patient does not quickly respond to the following treatments, visual neglect may be an issue. Visual neglect is sometimes referred to as visual inattention. Visual neglect, however, involves a variety of spatial, perceptual, and cognitive problems including peripheral inattention. More common in our experience is left visual neglect associated with right hemisphere damage. Bilateral neglect is associated with bilateral damage, dementia, and diffuse cortical damage due to, for example, dementia and encephalopathies. Right field neglect is rare and usually transient.[52] With visual neglect, the patient may need external prompting. Eventually, we want the patient to self-direct; for example, the patient knows to scan and look in the area of loss without external prompting.

SCANNING WITH EXPECTED THEN UNEXPECTED OBJECTS
We suggest a three-step sequence for teaching this skill.

Step One

The first stage in treatment is to engage the client in various search tasks, looking for specified objects in a room, looking for cooking or self-care items, simple puzzles, dominos, and completing cancellation and drawing tasks. Examples of these treatment strategies have been well described in the occupational therapy literature.[53,55] This step is quickly mastered by people with intact visual attention, less easily recovered with clients who have attention deficits. When grading the activities, easier tasks should be familiar and meaningful activities such as brushing teeth. Using tasks with expected objects (the brush, toothpaste, and glass) will encourage the client to continue looking until all the components in the visual task are found.

To remediate inattention deficit, first one might force fixation to the side where there is inattention by occluding one-half of each lens on the intact side with translucent tape (Figure 10.5). This forces the client to look past the midline in the direction of the visual field loss, if the head is straight ahead. Nonvisual cues such as making noise and tapping the patient's left shoulder might be added to direct attention to the affected side as well. Often patients with visual neglect have attention deficits as well. Attention to the left can be increased by decreasing stimulation on the person's unaffected right side and increasing stimulation on the person's affected left side. This could be done, for example, by having the person sit with their right side next to a wall, and then have the therapist and other activities in the clinic on the person's left side. Stimulation on the affected left side might also be increased by tapping the shoulder, using mild electrical stimulation, positioning items of interest during activities (e.g., toothpaste and toothbrush) on the left side, and positioning food items during eating on the left.

Next, directly instruct the patient to adopt a strategy for scanning to the affected side like a "lighthouse,"[56] and have the patient use visual imagery to scan to the affected side as well as describe the strategy. It often helps to have the patient with visual neglect have a target to define how far to the affected side they must scan. A classic strategy is to place a brightly colored line and tactual marker down the edge of the page or field being scanned and telling the client to keep looking until the line is seen; this reference stimulus is sometimes called an anchor. We find using naturally occurring stimuli are more generalizable. For example, a person with left visual neglect can use their left shoulder as an anchor. A person with left neglect trying to read can be instructed to move the left finger down the left margin of the page and use the right finger to point to the words being read. When scanning to the next line, the patient is instructed to "touch fingers." Once the client can consistently scan for objects even with less familiar tasks, the searching and scanning function has been restored for expected objects that are necessary for completion of a task.

Step Two

Step Two involves having the client scan a room where unexpected objects might be found, trying to find hazards in a kitchen, or picking up objects on the floor, for example.

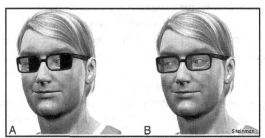

Figure 10.5. Two techniques to facilitate adaptive scanning into an affected hemifield. (A) Partial lens occlusion forces the individual to look into the affected hemifield. (B) The Sarah Appel technique uses colored translucent filters to cue the client when they are looking in the correct direction. (Reprinted with permission from Scheiman M, Scheiman M, Whittaker SG. *Low Vision Rehabilitation: A Practical Guide for Occupational Therapists.* Thorofare, NJ: SLACK Incorporated; 2007.)

Step Three

Step Three, Behavior Modification Methods, re-establishes the warning function of the peripheral retina. This step presents a greater challenge because responding to approaching objects from the affected side usually requires performance during divided attention, which is often impaired with brain injury or in older individuals. One approach we have successfully used involves behavior modification of scanning eye movements. The goal is to establish the habit of frequently and quickly looking in the direction of the field defect.

Laser tag transitions the client to more real-life situations. The therapist and client each hold a laser pointer. The therapist presents the laser spot on a surface such as an uncluttered wall. The client responds by pointing to the light and tagging the spot with their laser pointer. At first the light is flashed at two predictable points in the right and left fields. The task is graded to become more challenging and realistic by moving from predictable positions in an uncluttered area to unpredictable locations in a cluttered area. To further increase difficulty, the laser spot targets can be presented at different distances. Finally, the task is performed when the client's attention is divided, such as in a visually busy environment with people walking around. During this task, the therapist gradually decreases the frequency of presentations and varies the interval between laser spot presentations as well, pausing up to a minute or two between presentations. At this point, the client should be walking with frequent automatic glances into the affected hemifield, so that when the light eventually appears he or she detects it within 2 seconds. This instructional sequence should result in the client frequently and habitually looking in the direction of the field deficit. Generalization requires frequent instruction outside of the clinical context and in the context of naturally occurring activities. It is important to have a caregiver or family member involved in training.

Holding fixation in the direction of the deficit is another strategy that provides early warning in the direction of the field loss. In this procedure the client must look over and maintain fixation in the direction of the field deficit, use peripheral vision in the intact field to look straight ahead, and to see into the unaffected hemifield. The client could be encouraged to play one-on-one ball games such as soccer or basketball, practice walking in crowds, practice crossing intersections, and when walking down the street, a partner might intermittently and unexpectedly veer into the client and playfully bump shoulders if not detected. Success is achieved if the client automatically maintains most of the fixation between straight ahead and the affected side so as to detect an approaching target within a second or two.

If the patient does not progress through either Step One or Step Two, then the patient likely has a moderate to severe visual inattention or neglect. Two procedures now have been shown effective for treating visual left neglect. Prism adaptation therapy involves placing 20 to 40 diopter yoked prisms on the patient with the base of the prism toward the left side. This will shift the apparent location of the visual scene to the right so that the patient will tend to mislocalize to the right of an object. Then the patient adapts by training until they no longer mislocalize. Finally, the prisms are removed. This is repeated daily for several days. It is important that the visual localization tasks used during training *do not* involve continuous visual feedback. For example, one task requires a patient to reach forward and knock down a domino that the therapist taps. To eliminate continuous visual feedback, the arm is masked by, for example, reaching through a box with both ends open. Other tasks involve throwing objects, again with the throwing arm covered from view. You know the prism adaptation has been effective if after the prism has been removed there is a mislocalization to the opposite direction. Prism adaptation has been shown by several studies to ameliorate a visual neglect in the short term and have more prolonged effects with repeated, daily, application.[57–61]

WIDE FIELD EYE MOVEMENT TECHNIQUES

These methods would be useful in Step One and in transitioning to Step Two in the wide field technique described above.

Wide Field Chalkboard Saccadic

Gianutsos and Suchoff suggest the following therapy technique.[50] Place 15 to 20 numbers, letters, or other targets randomly on the side of a full-size chalkboard corresponding to the patient's field defect. The patient is centrally positioned in front of and at least 10 feet from the board and locates targets with a flashlight that are called out by another person. As the patient gains mastery of this task, the board is erased and new targets are written, still mainly in the affected hemifield but with some on the unaffected side. The patient is first instructed to scan the board in a circular manner and then to "pay more attention" to the affected side during the task. Gradually, the targets are evenly distributed between the two sides. Sticky notes could be used for this procedure instead of a chalkboard.

Wide Field Near Saccadic Activities

Similar activities can be accomplished at near with targets linearly arranged and the patients locating specified numbers or letters with a pencil in the same manner (i.e., with targets first being contained on the side of the compromised field and gradually distributing them so that an equal number appear in both fields).[56]

Adaptations

READING ADAPTATIONS FOR PATIENTS WITH VISUAL FIELD LOSS

Patients with visual field loss complain of frequent loss of place when reading. The following adaptations may be useful.

- Use an L-shaped marker with Velcro so that the patient can "find and feel where the boundaries are" (Figure 10.6).
- Turn the book 45 to 90 degrees. This moves the print into a field of awareness. If the patient has a right hemianopsia, they have difficulty following a line of print. By turning the book so that the print reads up and down, they may now be able to follow the line better since the next words to be read are now in their visual field (Figure 10.7).

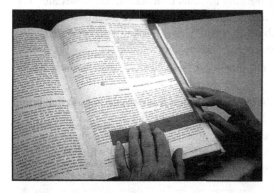

Figure 10.6. L-shaped marker with Velcro so that the patient can "find and feel where the boundaries are" when reading.

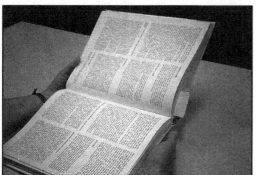

Figure 10.7. By turning the book so that the print reads up and down, the patient may now be able to follow the line better because the next words to be read are now in their visual field.

ADAPTATIONS FOR DRIVING

Patients with hemianopsia cannot drive legally and safely. It is possible for people with less than a homonymous quadrantanopia to drive legally. The field requirement for driving varies from state to state but often is 120 degrees on the visual horizon. In other words, if a patient is fixating a point on a wall while sitting 1 meter away (3 feet), the person can see flashes of light along a 2.5 meter straight horizontal line through the fixation point without any interruption. Only an ophthalmologist or optometrist can certify a patient meets the visual requirements for driving. A special field wide field binocular test is appropriate for driving; standard field tests are not adequate. The patient needs, therefore, to specifically request a vision evaluation for driving. Patients with a quadrant loss or less may be remediated only if other cognitive and motor skills are appropriate.[62] Care must be taken to rule out even mild visual neglect. The vision therapy techniques for driving would include the following (all of the techniques have been previously described in this chapter or Chapter Seven):

- Eye movement therapy techniques
- Spot stationary objects while patient is stationary
- Locate and follow moving objects while patient is stationary
- Learn to locate and track stationary objects while patient is moving
- Track moving objects while patient is moving and using scanning skills to gather visual information
- Include eye-hand-foot activities
- Practice with stress (i.e., different light conditions, talk to the patient, turn on music)
- Develop visual memory skills (speed/span of recognition)
- Plan routes verbally/visually; visualize

ADAPTATIONS/COMPENSATIONS FOR PATIENTS WITH VISUAL DYSFUNCTION

The following suggestions are useful when working with patients with visual dysfunction.

- Working distance: The distance from the patient to the object is critical whether it be for near activities or distance. Especially with patients wearing bifocals or trifocals, the lenses are very distance specific. Normal working distance at near is the measurement from the elbow to the second knuckle, approximately 16 inches. If an object is outside of the normal working distance for which the glasses have been prescribed, the patient may not be able to accurately see the object.
- Posture: The patient needs to be comfortable and supported. Slanted lapboards can be used for near activities (Figure 10.8).
- Lighting: Most elderly patients need more light to see. However, it is not uncommon that brain injury patients are light sensitive and request less light. Use a light that can be adjusted.
- Contrast: Elderly patients and patients with vision loss may function better if there is better contrast. For example, at the dinner table, do not use white placemats and white plates on a white tablecloth. Use different colors for better contrast.

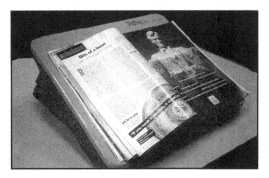

Figure 10.8. Slanted lapboards can be used for near activities.

- Reduce demands: If the task is too difficult for the patient, reduce the demands. For example, if a patient cannot fixate and walk at the same time, work on visual fixations while sitting or lying before integrating visual fixation with walking.

- Pencil grips: If a patient has difficulty gripping an object, a variety of pencil and utensil grips are available from occupational therapy supply catalogs.

- Enlarge print, enhance print quality: Large-print books and talking books are available through local libraries for the visually impaired. Use a copy machine to enlarge print if necessary.

- Reinforce with multisensory: If a patient cannot understand the task by just telling them, make sure multisensory stimuli are used (i.e., show it, tell it, experience it, feel it).

- Markers: If patient loses their place when reading, use markers to help the patient stay on line.

Case Studies

Five different types of case histories are presented below. These patients have different types of brain injuries and visual dysfunctions. Vision evaluation and treatment recommendations differ depending on the patient diagnosis, severity of injury, and patient goals. Some patients are in hospital or rehabilitation settings and others are not in formal programs and live at home.

Case One

CASE HISTORY

Jeannie, a 32-year-old female, received a mild traumatic brain injury, whiplash, and cervical strain secondary to a fall. She was referred for an optometric evaluation 2½ years post-injury by her neurologist. Jeannie complained of frequent frontal headaches, double vision, blurred vision, motor function decrease, poor balance, and attention/concentration and organizational deficits. She experienced difficulties with grocery shopping, cooking, and writing. She was unable to drive. Jeannie had received occupational, physical, and speech therapy immediately after her injury but was no longer receiving treatment. She was living at her home with her family.

Her general medical health was unremarkable with no known allergies. She was taking Depakote (divalproex sodium) and ibuprofen. There was no history of previous eye or head trauma, and social history was unremarkable. Jeannie had been evaluated by several ophthalmologists prior to my evaluation. She received no vision treatment other than the recommendation to buy a pair of reading glasses at the drug store.

VISUAL ACUITY, REFRACTION, EYE HEALTH

The external and external ocular evaluation was unremarkable. Pupils were equal, round, and responded to light. Visual acuity was:

	Distance	Near
Right eye	20/20	20/30
Left eye	20/25	20/60
Refraction revealed a low amount of hyperopia (farsightedness).		

VISUAL EFFICIENCY TESTING

A high amount of exophoria that decompensated to an exotropia at near was measured. Near point of convergence was receded with a break at 10 inches and a recovery at 14 inches. Accommodation was found to be quite poor. Pursuits were full and unrestricted, but they were not smooth or accurate. Jeannie could not dissociate eye from head movement. She demonstrated tearing and discomfort during pursuit and saccade testing.

VISUAL FIELD EVALUATION

A generalized constriction on all isopters was shown in addition to a homonymous, incongruous lower right quadrantanopia (Figures 10.9a and 10.9b).

VISUAL INFORMATION PROCESSING

Jeannie could respond to the visual perceptual tests if given extra time and many rest breaks. Extreme fatigue, blurriness, and ocular discomfort were present. Figure ground and visual motor integration testing, in particular, presented difficulty for Jeannie.

ASSESSMENT AND DIAGNOSIS

1. Mild traumatic brain injury by history (diagnosed by her neurologist)
2. Hyperopia
3. Intermittent exotropia at near
4. Accommodative dysfunction
5. Binocular dysfunction
6. Ocular motor dysfunction
7. Homonymous, incongruous, lower right quadrantanopia
8. Visual perceptual deficits

TREATMENT PLAN

Two pairs of glasses were prescribed. One was for distance and a different prescription for near was prescribed that included base-in prism in addition to a plus lens. A program of vision therapy was initiated. The patient was seen in vision therapy once a week for 45 minutes and home vision therapy activities were given. Throughout the vision therapy, distance and near glasses were re-evaluated and changed periodically. After 8 months of vision therapy, subjective symptomology revealed less blurry vision, no diplopia, and a decrease in headache frequency and severity. Jeannie could now read, write, cook, and drive. Visual efficiency and visual perceptual evaluation showed significant improvement. Visual fields also improved, showing no overall constriction, although a lower right incongruous quadrantanopia was still found (Figures 10.10a and 10.10b).

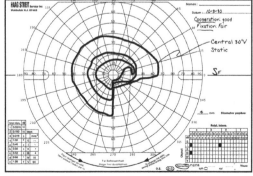

Figure 10.9a. A generalized constriction on all isopters in addition to a homonymous, incongruous lower right quadrantanopia.

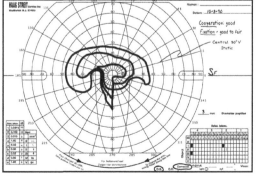

Figure 10.9b. A generalized constriction on all isopters in addition to a homonymous, incongruous lower right quadrantanopia.

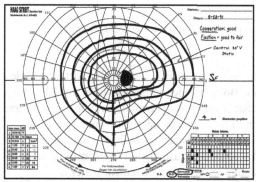 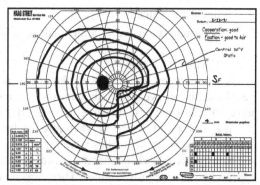

Figure 10.10a. Visual fields are improved, showing no overall constriction, although a lower right incongruous quadrantanopia was still found.

Figure 10.10b. Visual fields are improved, showing no overall constriction, although a lower right incongruous quadrantanopia was still found.

SUMMARY

This is an important case as it is consistent with the symptomology generally encountered in the traumatic brain injury population. It is also interesting to note that treatment was initiated 2½ years after injury, eliminating spontaneous recovery as an explanation for improvement in this patient's visual system deficits.

Case Two

CASE HISTORY

Charles, a 55-year-old male, was referred by his physical therapist. Charles was diagnosed with a brainstem bleed that caused significant motor and visual dysfunction. Charles was told by his physician in the hospital to patch one eye full-time in order to eliminate double vision. The physical therapist, who was trying to help Charles improve walking skills, was concerned with his full-time patching and head tilting. If Charles patched his left eye, he would show a significant head turn to the left, which had a negative effect on balance. If he patched his right eye, he would straighten his head (which improved his balance). However, the left eye showed constant nystagmus, creating symptoms of nausea and dizziness when Charles tried to use that eye.

VISUAL ACUITY, REFRACTION, EYE HEALTH

Visual acuity was 20/20 both at distance and at near with current glasses for myopia (nearsightedness), astigmatism, and presbyopia. Eye health was unremarkable, except for pupil abnormality of the right eye.

VISUAL EFFICIENCY TESTING

Eye movement dysfunctions were apparent. Charles showed full, unrestricted movement of the left eye, although constant nystagmus was present. His right eye could only move laterally, indicating paresis of the third and fourth nerves of the right eye. He showed no nystagmus of the right eye. Binocular testing revealed constant double vision and no fusion ability. Accommodation was deficient because of age (presbyopia).

VISUAL FIELDS

Full visual fields were measured.

ASSESSMENT AND DIAGNOSIS

1. Eye movement dysfunction (paresis of third and fourth nerves of right eye; nystagmus of the left eye)

2. Binocular dysfunction
3. Pre-existing refractive condition, adequately compensated for with current prescription

TREATMENT PLAN

Vision therapy was initiated. The goal was to improve left eye functioning so that Charles could use his left eye especially with walking tasks. Body balance improved when he did use his left eye because the head tilt was eliminated. Binocular fusion was not obtainable with prism, vision therapy, or strabismus surgery. Therefore, occlusion of one eye was known to still be necessary.

Eye movement techniques were initiated in addition to visual biofeedback techniques. After 4 months of weekly vision therapy sessions, Charles could now use his left eye comfortably. Nystagmus had significantly reduced. There was no change in right eye movement patterns.

SUMMARY

This case demonstrates the severity of eye movement dysfunction after brain injury. Even though binocular fusion was never deemed to be a goal, vision therapy was successful in improving the eye movement status, which thereby allowed the patient to improve walking and mobility skills.

Case Three

CASE HISTORY

Bertha, a 90-year-old cerebrovascular accident patient living in a long-term facility, was referred by her occupational therapist. Since her cerebrovascular accident four months previously, Bertha has not been able to do most of the activities of daily living skills she previously could perform independently. She could not dress or feed herself. Bertha sat in her wheelchair, with no eye contact and little interest in interacting with others.

VISUAL ACUITY, REFRACTION, EYE HEALTH

No visual acuity could be obtained. Light perception was noted. Bertha had previously worn glasses for moderate hyperopia and presbyopia. However, she had not worn them since arriving at the facility. Bertha's visual history and records revealed end-stage glaucoma and cataracts. She had been evaluated by her ophthalmologist six months prior to this evaluation. The ophthalmologist was monitoring her glaucoma medications and did not feel cataract surgery was appropriate. Neither visual acuity nor visual fields had been obtainable by the ophthalmologist for several years prior to her cerebrovascular accident, however, Bertha was still able to feed and dress herself at that time.

VISUAL EFFICIENCY TESTING

No results obtained because of decreased visual acuity. Bertha would not respond to pursuit or saccade testing.

VISUAL FIELDS TESTING

Previous visual records showed significant visual field loss from glaucoma. Bertha seemed to show some visual awareness in her lower right field.

ASSESSMENT AND DIAGNOSIS

1. Pre-existing glaucoma, cataracts monitored by ophthalmologist
2. Significant visual acuity, visual field loss
3. Pre-existing hyperopia, presbyopia

TREATMENT PLAN

Bertha's family and therapist wanted to try to help Bertha gain some independence. They wanted her to feed herself.

Our initial treatment plan included a recommendation that Bertha wear her previous glasses. Even though Bertha presented with significant visual loss from ocular disease and neurologic insult, a farsighted adult of her age cannot see well without glasses. Bertha's occupational therapist noticed an improvement in Bertha's alertness once she started wearing glasses again.

Eye movement techniques were initiated by the occupational therapist under optometric supervision. Auditory cues were added to the visual activities so that Bertha would know where to look. The therapy was emphasized more in Bertha's lower right field, as her awareness seemed better in that location. The occupational therapist was also providing sensory integration techniques that included massage and vestibular movement. Recommendations were given for changing the contrast of Bertha's place setting when eating. The food tray was also placed in her lower right field.

After three weeks of vision therapy, Bertha was able to feed herself as long as the food tray was placed in her lower right field.

SUMMARY

This is an interesting case in that significant ocular pathology was present in addition to a cerebrovascular accident. Often patients with this type of condition are merely told that nothing can be done. Even though the prognosis for improving the vision is poor in this patient, improvement in activities of daily living can be obtained by using basic visual guidance. When patients present without glasses, improvement can often be immediate by just wearing appropriate glasses. Contrast and lighting changes can help a patient. This patient did not receive in-office vision therapy. She was given treatment by her occupational therapist at her facility, under optometric supervision.

Case Four

CASE HISTORY

Jeff, a 27-year-old male, suffered a severe traumatic brain injury secondary to a motor vehicle accident six months prior to his visual evaluation. He was referred by his neuropsychologist. Jeff complained of frequent frontal headaches and was frequently observed squinting or closing one eye when viewing. Jeff recently had a complete neurologic work-up including magnetic resonance imaging. His visual history was unremarkable except for wearing soft contact lenses for myopia and astigmatism. Since his accident, Jeff no longer wore his contact lenses and did not have glasses.

VISUAL ACUITY, REFRACTION, EYE HEALTH

Visual acuity was 20/200 with each eye at distance and 20/60 at near. Myopia (nearsightedness) and astigmatism were measured. Internal and external ocular structures were unremarkable.

VISUAL EFFICIENCY TESTING

Eye movement skills were adequate. Binocular functioning was adequate. Accommodation was found to be inadequate.

ASSESSMENT AND DIAGNOSIS

1. Uncorrected myopia and astigmatism
2. Accommodative dysfunction

TREATMENT PLAN

Glasses for the refractive condition were prescribed for full-time wear. A bifocal was given, as Jeff needed a different prescription for distance than for near. No vision therapy was initiated because Jeff was moving out of town.

Headache frequency and severity decreased immediately after wearing the glasses.

SUMMARY

This case emphasizes the importance of appropriate glasses for refractive conditions. Jeff presents with brain injury and his other physicians had concluded the headaches were sequelae of the injury, which is often the case. However, uncorrected refractive error may also contribute to the headaches. This is a case where the simple, obvious solution may have been overlooked.

Case Five

CASE HISTORY

Alan, a 48-year-old male, had just been diagnosed with multiple sclerosis. He had been referred by his occupational therapist. His symptoms included dizziness, balance problems, and intermittent double vision. He was wearing an invisible no-line bifocal prescribed 1 year prior to this vision evaluation. Alan had been comfortable in his glasses.

VISUAL ACUITY, REFRACTIVE, OCULAR HEALTH

Visual acuity with glasses was 20/20 at distance and at near. Hyperopia (farsightedness) with astigmatism similar to current glasses prescription was measured. Internal ocular evaluation revealed mild pallor of the right optic nerve head. No other ocular pathology was noted.

VISUAL EFFICIENCY TESTING

Binocular testing revealed moderate exophoria at near and poor fusion ranges both at distance and at near. Accommodation was deficient because of age (presbyopia). Eye movement skills were full and unrestricted, although endpoint nystagmus was apparent.

ASSESSMENT AND DIAGNOSIS

1. Optic nerve pallor
2. Nystagmus
3. Convergence insufficiency
4. Pre-existing hyperopia, astigmatism, presbyopia

TREATMENT PLAN

Although Alan's current glasses prescription was adequate, I was concerned with the type of bifocal lens he was wearing. The invisible bifocal sometimes can cause peripheral distortion. Most people learn to adapt to that. However, since Alan now had balance problems, I was concerned as to the effect of his glasses on balance. Therefore, a new prescription for glasses was given for distance only. Alan and his occupational therapist saw immediate improvement in balance when wearing his new glasses.

Vision therapy was initiated. The goals were to improve binocular functioning.

SUMMARY

This case demonstrates how a lens design may positively or negatively affect balance. Multiple sclerosis symptoms may vary, which is the reason why these patients should be visually evaluated on a regular basis. If a patient shows double vision during multiple sclerosis attacks, Fresnel prisms may be useful to compensate temporarily as the double vision may subside. Multiple sclerosis patients are frequently relatively young and are still productive in society. These patients appreciate anything that may be of assistance visually.

Summary

Overall, visual function is based on the development and function of a hierarchy of skills. Skills at the basic level form the foundation for higher level skills. In order to make complex visual decisions necessary for tasks including activities of daily living, reading, math, driving, and vocations, integration of lower skills (tactile, vestibular, proprioceptive, visual) is critical. Therefore, determining the cause of the deficit requires understanding of the brain injury and its effect on the entire visual process from input to output.

Patients who have suffered neurological insult are quite a complex clinical challenge. In the rehabilitation process, a patient comes in contact with numerous physicians and therapists who play a vital role in the rehabilitation process. The occupational therapist is often in the best position to observe functional visual problems either via a visual screening process or merely by observation. The optometrist is the most qualified professional to assess and rehabilitate the visual efficiency and visual perceptual system. Vision, being our dominant sense for gathering information, needs to be evaluated early in the rehabilitation process. It is important that all patients who have suffered a traumatic brain injury/stroke have a complete vision evaluation by an optometrist who has extensive experience in vision rehabilitation and functional vision care. Consultation with an optometrist by the rehabilitation team is crucial so that all health care providers have a good understanding of the patient's visual deficits and functional results. Treatment strategies can then be established, utilizing a multidisciplinary approach. Vision treatment should be concurrent with speech, physical, and/or occupational therapy. Improved visual functioning often will help speed the progress in other rehabilitative areas.

The commonalities between the models of human performance used by optometry and occupational therapy create a natural interaction between optometrists and occupational therapists.[63–68] Educational and clinical interactions between these two groups have grown at an impressive rate. Collaboration and sharing provides increased learning for the therapists and optometrists resulting in a more complete and successful treatment program for the patient.

References

1. Direnfeld G. Traumatic brain injury and case management. *Cogn Rehabil.* 1990;5:20–24.
2. Suter PS. A quickstart in post-acute vision rehabilitation following brain injury. *J Optom Vis Devel.* 1999;30:73–82.
3. Margolis NW, Lederer PJ. Issues Concerning the evaluation of closed head injury. *J Opt Vis Devel.* 1999; 30:55–57.
4. Scheiman M, Wick B. *Clinical Management of Binocular Vision: Heterophoric, Accommodative and Eye Movement Disorders.* 5th ed. Philadelphia, PA: Wolters-Kluwer; 2019.
5. Kadet TS. Vision rehabilitation in traumatic brain injury. In: Forkiotis CJ, Kadet TS, Shankman AL, eds. *Essays on Vision.* Santa Ana, CA: Optometric Extension Program Foundation; 1990:13–20.
6. Kaplan M. *Seeing Through New Eyes.* Philadelphia, PA: Jessica Kingsley Publishers; 2006.
7. Kaplan M, Edelson S, Seip J. Behavioral changes in autistic individuals as a result of wearing ambient transitional prism lenses. *Child Psychiat Hum D.* 1998;29:65–76.
8. Padula WV, Argyris S. Post trauma vision syndrome and visual midline shift syndrome. *NeuroRehabilitation.* 1996;6:165–171.
9. Bowers AR, Keeney K, Peli E. Community-based trial of a peripheral prism visual field expansion device for hemianopia. *Arch Ophthalmol.* 2008;126:657–664.
10. Giorgi RG, Woods RL, Peli E. Clinical and laboratory evaluation of peripheral prism glasses for hemianopia. *Optom Vis Sci.* 2009;86:492–502.
11. Bowers AR, Keeney K, Peli E. Randomized crossover clinical trial of real and sham peripheral prism glasses for hemianopia. *JAMA Ophthalmol.* 2014;132:214–222.
12. Peli E, Jung JH. Multiplexing prisms for field expansion. *Optom Vis Sci.* 2017;94:817–829.
13. Politzer TA. Case studies of a new approach using partial and selective occlusion for the clinical treatment of diplopia. *NeuroRehabilitation.* 1996;6:213–217.
14. Waiss B, Soden R. Head trauma and low vision: clinical modifications for diagnosis and prescription. *J Am Optom Assoc.* 1992;63:559–563.
15. Berne SA. Visual therapy for the traumatic brain-injured. *J Optom Vis Dev.* 1990;21:13–16.
16. Cohen AH. Visual rehabilitation of a stroke patient. *J Am Optom Assoc.* 1978;7:831–832.
17. Cohen AH, Soden R. An optometric approach to the rehabilitation of the stroke patient. *J Am Optom Assoc.* 1981;52:795–800.
18. Hellerstein LF, Freed S. Rehabilitative optometric management of a traumatic brain injury patient. *J Behav Optom.* 1994;5:143–148.

19. Aksinoff EB, Falk N. Optometric therapy for the left brain injured patient. *J Am Optom Assoc*. 1992:564–568.

20. Cohen AH. Optometric management of binocular dysfunctions secondary to head trauma: case reports. *J Am Optom Assoc*. 1992;63:569–575.

21. Cohen AH. Optometric rehabilitative therapy. In: Press LJ, ed. *Applied Concepts in Vision Therapy*. St. Louis, MO: CV Mosby; 1997:278–286.

22. Hoffman L, Cohen A, Feuer G. Effectiveness of non-strabismic optometric vision training in a private practice. *Am J Optom Arch Am Acad Opt*. 1973;50:813–816.

23. Ciuffreda KJ, Suchoff IB, Marrone MA, Ahmann E. Oculomotor Rehabilitation in Traumatic Brain-Injured Patients. *J Be Optom*. 1996;7:31–37.

24. Thiagarajan P, Ciuffreda KJ. Accommodative and vergence dysfunctions in mTBI: treatment effects and systems correlations. *Optom Vis Perf*. 2014;2:539–554.

25. Thiagarajan P, Ciuffreda KJ. Effect of oculomotor rehabilitation on accommodative responsivity in mild traumatic brain injury. *J Rehabil Res Dev*. 2014;51:175–191.

26. Thiagarajan P, Ciuffreda KJ. Versional eye tracking in mild traumatic brain injury (mTBI): effects of oculomotor training (OMT). *Brain Inj*. 2014;28:930–943.

27. Thiagarajan P, Ciuffreda KJ. Effect of oculomotor rehabilitation on vergence responsivity in mild traumatic brain injury. *J Rehabil Res Dev*. 2013;50:1223–1240.

28. Thiagarajan P, Ciuffreda KJ. Short-term persistence of oculomotor rehabilitative changes in mild traumatic brain injury (mTBI): a pilot study of clinical effects. *Brain Inj*. 2015;29:1475–1479.

29. Thiagarajan P, Ciuffreda KJ, Capo-Aponte JE, et al. Oculomotor neurorehabilitation for reading in mild traumatic brain injury (mTBI): an integrative approach. *NeuroRehabilitation*. 2014;34:129–146.

30. Scheiman M, Gallaway MF. Vision therapy to treat binocular vision disorders after acquired brain injury: factors affecting prognosis. In: Suchoff IB, Cuiffreda KJ, Kapoor N, eds. *Visual and Vestibular Consequences of Acquired Brain Injury*. Santa Ana, CA: Optometric Extension Program; 2001.

31. Han Y, Ciuffreda KJ, Kapoor N. Reading-related oculo-motor testing and training protocols for acquired brain injury in humans. *Brain Res Protoc*. 2004;14:1–12.

32. Kapoor N, Ciuffreda KJ, Han Y. Oculomotor rehabilitation in acquired brain injury: a case series. *Arch Phys Med Rehabil*. 2004;85:1667–1678.

33. Ciuffreda KJ, Han Y, Kapoor N, Ficarra AP. Oculomotor rehabilitation for reading in acquired brain injury. *NeuroRehabilitation*. 2006;21:9–21.

34. Ciuffreda KJ, Ludlam W, Kapoor N. Clinical oculomotor training in traumatic brain injury. *Optom Vis Dev*. 2009;40:16–23.

35. Ciuffreda KJ, Rutner D, Kapoor N, et al. Vision therapy for oculomotor dysfunctions in acquired brain injury: a retrospective analysis. *Optometry*. 2008;79:18–22.

36. Hellerstein LF, Winkler PA. Vestibular dysfunction associated with traumatic brain injury: collaborative optometry and physical therapy treatment. In: Suchoff IB, Ciuffreda KJ, Kapoor N, eds. *Visual and Vestibular Consequences of Acquired Brain Injury*. Santa Ana, CA: Optometric Extension Program; 2002.

37. Rinehart MA. Strategies for improving motor performance. In: Rosenthal M, ed. *Rehabilitation of the Adult and Child with Traumatic Brain Injury*. Philadelphia, PA: FA Davis Co; 1990.

38. Shumway-Cook A, Horak F. Vestibular rehabilitation: an exercise approach to managing symptoms of vestibular dysfunction. *Seminars in Hearing*. 1989;10:196–209.

39. Shumway-Cook A, Horak FB. Rehabilitation strategies for patients with vestibular deficits. *Neur Clin*. 1990;8:441–457.

40. Dennison PE, Dennison GE. *Brain Gym*. Glendale, CA: Edu-kinesthetics Inc; 1986.

41. Levine KJ. Fine motor dysfunction. Tucson, AZ: Therapy Skill Builders; 1991.

42. Scheiman M, Rouse MW. *Optometric Management of Learning Related Vision Problems*. 2nd ed. St. Louis, MO: CV Mosby; 2006.

43. Lane KA. *Developing Your Child for Success*. Lewisville, TX: Learning Potential Publishers; 1991.

44. Kasten E, Muller-Oehring E, Sabel BA. Stability of visual field enlargements following computer-based restitution training—results of a follow-up. *J Clin Exp Neuropsychol*. 2001;23:297–305.

45. Kasten E, Poggel DA, Sabel BA. Computer-Based Training of Stimulus Detection Improves Color and Simple Pattern Recognition in the Defective Field of Hemianopic Subjects. *J Cogn Neurosci*. 2000;12:1001–1012.

46. Kasten E, Wust S, Behrens-Baumann W, Sabel BA. Computer-based training for the treatment of partial blindness. *Nat Med*. 1998;4:1083–1087.

47. Horton JC. Disappointing results from nova vision's visual restoration therapy. *Br J Ophthalmol*. 2005;89:1–2.

48. Horton JC. Vision restoration therapy: confounded by eye movements. *Br J Ophthalmol*. 2005;89:792–794.

49. Reinhard J, Schreiber A, Schiefer U. Does visual restitution training change absolute homonymous visual field defects? A fundus controlled study. *Br J Ophthalmol*. 2005;89:30–35.

50. Gianutsos R, Suchoff IB. Visual fields after brain injury: management issues for the occupational therapist. In: Scheiman M, ed. *Understanding and Managing Visual Deficits: A Guide for Occupational Therapist*. 2nd ed. Thorofare, NJ: SLACK Incorporated; 2002.

51. Scheiman M, Scheiman M, Whittaker SG. *Low Vision Rehabilitation: A Practical Guide for Occupational Therapists.* Thorofare, NJ: SLACK Incorporated; 2007.
52. Trobe JD. *The Neurology of Vision.* Oxford: Oxford University Press; 2001.
53. Zoltan B. *Vision, Perception and Cognition: A Manual for the Evaluation and Treatment of the Neurologically Impaired Adult.* 3rd ed. Thorofare, NJ: SLACK Incorporated; 1996.
54. Heikki HA, Julkunen LA. Treatment of visual field deficits after a stroke. *Advances in Clinical Neuroscience and Rehabilitation.* 2004;6:17–18.
55. Pedretti W, Zoltan B. *Occupational Therapy: Practice Skills for Physical Dysfunction.* Philadelphia, PA: CV Mosby; 1996.
56. Niemeier JP. The lighthouse strategy: use of a visual imagery technique to treat visual inattention in stroke patients. *Brain Inj.* 1998;12:399–406.
57. Redding GM, Wallace B. Prism adaptation and unilateral neglect: review and analysis. *Neuropsychologia.* 2006;44:1–20.
58. Marshall RS. Rehabilitation approaches to hemineglect. *Neurologist.* 2009;15:185–192.
59. Rossetti Y, Rode G, Pisella L, et al. Prism adaptation to a rightward optical deviation rehabilitates left hemispatial neglect. *Nature.* 1998;395:166–169.
60. Saevarsson S. Unilateral neglect: a review of causes, anatomical localization, theories and interventions. *Laeknabladid.* 2009;95:27–33.
61. Shiraishi H. Long-term effects of prism adaptation on chronic neglect after stroke. *NeuroRehabilitation.* 2008;23:137–151.
62. Park WL, Unatin J, Herbert A. A Driving program for the visually impaired. *J Am Optom Assoc.* 1993;64:54–59.
63. Hellerstein LF, Fishman B. Vision therapy and occupational therapy: an integrated approach. *J Behav Optom.* 1990;1:122–126.
64. Suchoff IB. Occupational therapy and optometry: a developing relationship. *J Behav Optom.* 1991;2:170–171.
65. Ross-Rizzo J, Waskiewicz M, Kapoor N. OT-OD synergy during management of the concussed: a case report illustrating seamless care "handoffs." *Vis Dev & Rehab.* 2017;3:131–146.
66. Aravich D, Troxell L. Clinical practice guidelines for occupational therapists in the evaluation and treatment of oculomotor impairment following traumatic brain injury. *Curr Phys Med Rehab Rep.* 2021;9:93–99.
67. Fessler A, Kruemmling B, Scheiman M. A worthwhile collaboration: integrating optometry and occupational therapy in the treatment of children. *Vis Dev & Rehab.* 2020;6:221–236.
68. Reiser A, Bunin G, Scheiman M. Concussion-related vision disorder practice patterns in occupational therapy: a survey. *Open J Occup Ther.* 2020;8:1–20.

Chapter Eleven

Visual and Ocular Disorders in Children With Disabilities

Sarah D. Appel and Elise B. Ciner

Abstract

The number of children with visual impairments who receive services from early intervention and educational programs within the United States has increased significantly during the past 50 years. Included in this population are children with physical and developmental disabilities who have associated visual and ocular disorders. Common visual deficits as well as ocular and neuro visual disorders associated with pediatric syndromes, developmental disabilities, and genetic disorders are discussed. A large majority of children with visual impairment have residual vision that could be useful for academic and rehabilitation programs. In order to ensure that these programs are sufficiently individualized, members of the interdisciplinary team providing services to these children should be aware of diagnosed ocular and visual disorders and their functional implications for the achievement of academic and developmental goals. Findings from a clinical vision evaluation help to explain observed behaviors such as postural deviations, movement-related problems, as well as lapses in visual attention. Information may also be used to optimize environmental modifications, determine appropriate characteristics of visual targets that are presented to children during therapeutic and educational activities, and individualize visual activities to enhance their responsiveness and progress. Cases are presented that highlight the functional effects of a range of visual disorders on children's orientation and mobility, activities of daily living, educational progress, and psychosocial well-being.

Background

Historical records from the American Printing House for the Blind (APHB) reported that in 1977 there were 29,403 school-aged children and young adults who met the definition of legal blindness and were therefore eligible for adaptive educational materials from APHB.[1] In 2020, that number almost doubled to 56,866.[2] This increase is due in part to significant advances in medical pre- and post-natal care that increase the chance for survival of premature and/or very sick infants who are born with a wide range of disorders and syndromes. Many of these disorders and syndromes have associated ocular as well as visual abnormalities. Intrauterine infections such

DOI: 10.4324/9781003526841-11

as rubella, syphilis, and cytomegalovirus are frequently associated with significant visual impairment. Genetic syndromes and disorders such as Down syndrome (trisomy 21), Hallermann-Streiff syndrome, Bardet-Biedl syndrome, Crouzon syndrome, and Leber's congenital amaurosis are each associated with a host of ocular and visual disorders. Children born with a history of intrauterine brain ischemia are at greater risk for visual deficits of neurological origin and at greater risk for cerebral visual impairment as well as other visual disorders. Children born to drug- and alcohol-addicted mothers as well as children who suffer the tragic consequences of shaken baby syndrome and other forms of child abuse are often also left with multiple systemic and visual impairments. Surviving infants may also exhibit additional lasting handicapping conditions, such as hearing loss, cerebral palsy, learning disabilities, and developmental disabilities. This trend of increasing numbers of children with disabilities, many of whom have associated vision disorders, is not likely to reverse in the near future.

While medical care is increasingly able to save these children, many still do not receive timely and appropriate vision-related services during the critical first few years of life. This is partly due to the perception that developmentally delayed or sensory-impaired children are unresponsive to traditional measures of vision and are therefore untestable. This misconception is prevalent among some health care providers who are unfamiliar with specialized testing strategies that are used to evaluate visual status in non- or preverbal children. As a result, children with usable vision may be mislabeled as blind because they do not respond to standard vision testing procedures. The key elements in formulating appropriate vision interventions for developmentally delayed and visually impaired children are adequate and accurate information about a child's visual status and visual disorder(s) and avoidance of labels that limit treatment and dampen rehabilitative efforts. The following discussion explores the types and nature of the ocular and vision disorders that are most commonly found in children with physical, developmental, and/or visual disabilities.

Types of Disorders

Refractive Error

Myopia: There is a high correlation between significant refractive error and developmental disabilities (Table 11.1). Premature birth resulting from intrauterine trauma (e.g., preterm premature rupture of membranes), infection, or fetal abnormality[3,4] may give rise to an ocular disorder known as retinopathy of prematurity. Retinopathy of prematurity (ROP) is associated with a number of potential ocular and visual disorders including a high magnitude of myopic refractive error. High myopia often prevents affected children from clearly seeing objects that are located at a distance beyond arm's reach. For example, a child with retinopathy of prematurity and a high myopic refractive error of 10 diopters will clearly see objects located at 4 inches or closer but will experience increasing visual blur at greater distances. Children with high myopia will be unable to see objects located across a room unless an appropriate spectacle or contact lens correction is worn. Although there are conflicting reports in the literature, some studies indicate that there is a greater prevalence of high myopia among children with Down syndrome (trisomy 21) due, in part, to a higher likelihood of refractive error progression with increasing age in children with Down syndrome.[5] High myopia can also occur in other disorders including Stickler syndrome, Noonan syndrome, and Marfan syndrome.[6] It is essential that children with high myopic refractive errors are closely monitored by their eye care provider as they are at increased risk for retinal holes and tears which can progress to retinal detachments. If left untreated, retinal detachment can result in severe visual impairment or total blindness.

Hyperopia: Hyperopic refractive error is a common finding in children with developmental and physical disabilities.[7,8] Children with systemic conditions such as cerebral palsy, fragile X syndrome, hydrocephalus, and brain malformations (e.g., septo-optic dysplasia) frequently manifest hyperopic

Table 11.1

Refractive Error and Developmental Disabilities

Refractive Error	Conditions or Syndromes
Myopia	Retinopathy of prematurity
	Stickler syndrome
	Microcornea
	Marfan syndrome
Hyperopia	Marfan syndrome (in aphakic pupillary sector)
	Microphthalmos
	Spastic cerebral palsy
	Oculocutaneous albinism
Astigmatism	Oculocutaneous albinism
	Keratoglobus
	Congenital pendular nystagmus
	Treacher Collins syndrome

refractive error. Hyperopia is also a common finding in children with oculo-visual disorders such as albinism and microphthalmia. Conditions such as Marfan syndrome that are associated with the displacement of the lens of the eye create a situation where only part of the pupillary region is occupied by the lens. In this type of disorder, significant myopic refractive error may coexist with significant hyperopic refractive error in the same eye. Hyperopia is often found in the area within the eye's pupil that is not occupied by the displaced lens. Children with disabilities who have uncorrected hyperopia may experience visual fatigue, especially after tasks requiring a close viewing distance. A significant uncorrected hyperopic refractive error may also result in strabismus and amblyopia.

Astigmatism: Eye diseases that involve corneal disorders are typically associated with significant amounts of astigmatism. Examples include keratoconus, corneal dystrophies, and microcornea. Any surgical procedure involving the cornea, such as corneal transplantation or removal of a cataract, may result in significant astigmatism. Astigmatism may also be found in children with congenital nystagmus. Congenital nystagmus is associated with ocular disorders such as retinal and optic nerve colobomas, aniridia, albinism, retinopathy of prematurity, as well as Leber's congenital amaurosis. Syndromes associated with significant facial and lid deformities such as Treacher Collins syndrome may also be accompanied by significant astigmatic refractive error.

Aphakia: Surgical removal of cataracts results in a refractive disorder known as aphakia. Congenital cataracts (clouding of the eye's crystalline lens) are associated with intrauterine infections such as rubella and congenital syphilis, chromosomal anomalies which include Down syndrome and Turner syndrome, as well as metabolic disturbances such as homocystinuria. If an aphakic refractive error is uncorrected by a spectacle, contact lens, or intraocular lens correction, the child experiences significant blur both at distance and near. The nature of the aphakic refractive error is typically high hyperopia unless the child had a significant myopic refractive error before removal of the cataracts. In that situation, the child may be mildly myopic or hyperopic depending on the magnitude of the original myopic refractive error. The child with aphakia cannot change focus for varying distances due to the absence of an anatomical lens which, by changing its shape, is able to refocus for a wide range of viewing distances. These children, therefore, typically require bifocals to enable them to view objects at arm's length or closer.

During the course of the evaluation, a frequently asked question is whether to prescribe a correction to a child who exhibits significant developmental disabilities. The impression held by some professionals is that the child with developmental delays will be unresponsive to the visual enhancement provided by the corrective lenses. In many cases, even a child who appears to be totally withdrawn and unresponsive to their environment may, in time, exhibit changes in visual behaviors after adapting to corrective lenses.

Case One

An 8-year-old girl with a history of autism, developmental disability, and degenerative neuropathy presented for evaluation of her visual status. She had previously been examined at other eye care facilities. No ocular pathology had been noted. No corrective lenses had ever been prescribed. During the course of the evaluation, the girl was found to be minimally responsive to any visual or sensory stimuli. She exhibited minimal movement except for occasional head movements. During the refractive component of the evaluation, significant myopia, coupled with a high degree of astigmatism was found. She was prescribed corrective lenses with instructions to slowly habituate her to the correction. When she returned for a follow-up evaluation two months later, the mother reported that the child's teachers had noted improved eye contact and an overall increase in attention. The child's mother also reported that her daughter cried at night when the glasses were removed. During the course of the evaluation, she exhibited measurably improved responses to visual stimuli and the presence of brief visual tracking behaviors which had not been noted previously. This 8-year-old girl had been without an essential correction during a critical time of her visual and overall development with a resultant reduced quality of life due to the mistaken belief that she was too developmentally delayed to benefit from corrective glasses.

Case Two

A 16-year-old girl with a history of developmental disability, hearing impairment, and bilateral retinal colobomas was evaluated at the school for the blind that she attended. Due to her hearing impairment, her teachers communicated with her by signing. They wanted information on how to adapt their signing (position and distance) to ensure that it was appropriate for her visual status. The girl was unresponsive and generally not cooperative for any of the acuity measurement testing procedures that were appropriate for her developmental age. Due to an upper visual field deficit found during testing, her teachers were advised to position their hands in the girl's lower visual field region when signing. During the refraction, a high hyperopic refractive error was measured. Her teachers were uncertain if she would wear corrective glasses due to her significant tactual defensiveness and resistance to wearing her hearing aids. When a trial prescription was placed on her face, the student grabbed the frame and, instead of removing it as had been expected, she pushed it higher up on the bridge of her nose. Her use of vision while walking increased significantly while wearing the correction. Her use of vision was also observed during her workshop activity, which consisted of feeding paper into a shredding machine. With the spectacle correction, she was able to visually guide the paper to the appropriate slot for shredding. Her teachers reported that she had previously performed the same activity solely by touch.

This 16-year-old girl's previously uncorrected refractive error had interfered with her ability to learn, communicate and effectively perform activities of daily living. Corrective glasses were dispensed at a follow-up visit and her teachers reported that, after a short adaptation period, she had adapted well to the new correction.

Visual Efficiency

EYE MOVEMENTS

Children with developmental and visual impairments frequently exhibit abnormalities in eye movements. Children with significant gross and fine motor delays, as is the case in children with cerebral palsy, often manifest eye movements that are choppy rather than smooth when visually following a target.[9] They may also exhibit difficulties maintaining fixation on objects, accurately scanning their environment, and often overshoot or undershoot when reaching for visual targets. It is important to note that overall postural issues frequently have an impact on a neurologically impaired child's visual responsiveness. For example, if a child with cerebral palsy is physically stressed due to lack of postural and head support during a visual activity, that child will manifest more significant impairment in visual skills than if the child is not in postural distress. The occupational therapist's role in ensuring appropriate positioning is, therefore, critical. Overall fatigue, emotional distress, as well as discomfort or illness can also further degrade the efficiency of these children's eye movements.

Children with significant visual field defects will also often exhibit pronounced eye movement disorders. Children with central scotomas (blind spots) resulting from macular degeneration or dystrophy may exhibit frequent losses in fixation as they track a visual target. The losses in fixation may lead to the erroneous diagnosis of intermittent nystagmus. These children's fixation may also be unstable during visual scanning activities, as the visual targets are often obscured by the central scotomas. Children with peripheral visual field constriction may also exhibit frequent losses of fixation when tracking a visual target, especially if the target is moved quickly. They may also have a very difficult time initiating accurate saccadic eye movements (shifts in fixation from one target to another) during visual scanning activities. Children who manifest hemianopic visual field defects will typically have greater difficulty with visual search activities within the defective visual field region.

Neurological defects may eliminate all eye movements or only eye movements in a certain direction. Vertical gaze palsies result in an inability of both eyes to fully look up or down. This may be caused by encephalitis, damage to the midbrain region from tumors or strokes, and degenerative neurological disease. Horizontal gaze palsies result in the inability of both eyes to look to the right or left. The eyes are affected symmetrically, thereby eliminating double vision. These disorders most commonly result from strokes. Children with congenital ocular motor apraxia do not exhibit any restrictions in horizontal eye movements. They do, however, exhibit significant difficulty with the initiation of voluntary saccadic eye movements. This disorder may be caused by brain abnormalities of a sporadic or genetic origin. It may also be associated with neurodegenerative or metabolic syndromes. Children who have these significant eye movement disorders will typically combine head movements with eye movements in order to increase the range and efficiency of their eye movements. Children with restrictions in gaze will often adapt head turns or tilts toward the gaze-restricted area in order to bring their eyes into that visual region.

Case Three

A 7-year-old developmentally disabled girl with a history of head trauma presented for a vision evaluation. In her educational setting, she had been undergoing a vision stimulation program that involved eye movement activities including both vertical and horizontal tracking of objects. Her mother reported that her daughter was very frustrated during these activities and her vision teacher was frustrated by her daughter's lack of cooperation, especially during vertical tracking activities. During the vision evaluation, the child manifested pupillary abnormalities along with a marked vertical gaze palsy that prevented her from initiating and maintaining vertical gaze movements. In school, she had been asked to perform an activity that was impossible for her to successfully accomplish as a result of neurological damage to the midbrain region. These findings from the vision evaluation were shared with the mother and the teacher, and the vertical tracking activities, the source of the child's frustration, were eliminated. It was also recommended that the girl be allowed to use head movements to enable her to carry out vertical tracking and scanning activities more efficiently. This includes placement of objects at the child's eye level whenever possible.

NYSTAGMUS

Nystagmus is an involuntary repetitive eye movement disorder that is most commonly found in children that have a history of neurological diseases such as hydrocephalus, meningitis, and cerebral palsy or in children with congenital visual impairments such as oculocutaneous albinism or achromatopsia. It is also present in children with chromosomal disorders such as Down syndrome. Studies have reported that an estimated 18% to 30% of children with Down syndrome exhibit some form of nystagmus.[10] Nystagmus may be acquired or congenital. A child with congenital nystagmus will experience degradation of visual images due to retinal smearing of visual images associated with the nystagmoid eye movements. The child will not, however, experience any oscillopsia or perceived movement of stationary visual targets due to the nystagmoid eye movements. Symptoms of oscillopsia reported by children are most likely due to acquired nystagmus or a change in the nature of their congenital nystagmus and should be evaluated to rule out an emerging or progressing neurological disease.

Congenital nystagmus of neurological origin most commonly presents as a jerk-type nystagmus, but may also present as a pendular, rotary, or downbeat nystagmus. A jerk-type nystagmus often has a null point. This is the eye position in which the nystagmus is significantly reduced or eliminated, resulting in improved visual function. Some children will adapt a head turn or tilt in order to consistently place their eyes in the null-point position, especially when they are engaged in visually challenging activities. This becomes especially evident during visually challenging activities.

Visual deprivation congenital nystagmus associated with congenital visual impairment is often pendular in central gaze. It may, however, transition to jerk-type nystagmus on lateral, upward, or downward gaze. Pendular nystagmus is typically found in disorders such as oculocutaneous albinism, aniridia, and congenital cataracts. Pendular nystagmus typically does not have a true null point. It may dampen significantly, however, during convergence of the eyes when viewing visual detail located at a reduced viewing distance. If the nystagmus worsens in one direction of gaze, the child will typically turn their head in the direction of the worsening nystagmus to avoid placing their eyes in that position of gaze.

Other forms of nystagmus found in children with developmental disabilities include latent and endpoint nystagmus. Latent nystagmus is only present when one eye is covered. This type of nystagmus may be associated with congenital strabismus or when one eye has a significantly greater reduction in visual acuity due to more severe ocular disease. Children with latent nystagmus will not respond as expected to patching activities, as their visual acuity and efficiency may be significantly degraded by the latent nystagmus. Endpoint or gaze-evoked nystagmus will occur when a child's eyes shift to the limits of their range. This type of nystagmus may be associated with a paretic muscle, with cerebellar or cerebral disorders, or with internuclear ophthalmoplegia. Endpoint nystagmus may also be precipitated by anti-seizure medications. Pharmacologically induced nystagmus will disappear after discontinuation of the medication. Table 11.2 summarizes the most common forms of nystagmus.

CONVERGENCE

Accurate convergence or the ability to align the eyes for near visual targets including pictures, words, or text is necessary for normal comfortable binocular vision including stereopsis (3D vision) as well as for the elimination of either suppression or diplopia (double vision). Convergence insufficiency is an inability to maintain comfortable, single, and binocular vision at reduced viewing distances. Convergence insufficiency can be associated with some forms of strabismus, phorias, and accommodative difficulties and is also seen following concussion. A person's ability to converge their eyes may also be affected by neurological disorders, such as brain trauma and encephalitis that may result in convergence palsy. Another condition that may result in convergence insufficiency is hypertelorism, or abnormally widely spaced eyes, which is typically found in syndromes like Crouzon syndrome that are associated with skull deformity and may also include

Table 11.2

Common Forms of Nystagmus

Type of Nystagmus	Description
Pendular	Horizontal congenital nystagmus that may become jerk-type on extreme lateral gaze
	Dampens on convergence
	Typically does not have a true null point
	Associated with congenital macular and optic nerve abnormalities
Jerk	Horizontal rhythmic jerky eye movements
	Characterized by a slow component in one direction followed by fast component in the opposite direction
Rotary (tortional)	Nystagmus characterized by circular oscillations
Latent	Nystagmus that occurs when one eye is covered
Endpoint	Nystagmus that occurs at the extremes of gaze, typically a jerk-type nystagmus

developmental disabilities. The child with hypertelorism has a greater convergence demand and will be more likely to experience convergence fatigue and diplopia and, as a result, may give up trying to converge for near visual targets or when reading. The child may either adopt a head turn or close one eye as a viewing strategy to eliminate the need for convergence. Medications such as phenobarbital, which are used to control seizure activity, may also decrease convergence. It is essential to identify convergence difficulties in children in order to ensure that proper interventions are implemented so that the child can function effectively during near visual activities.

Case Four

A 4-year-old boy with a history of hyperactivity, hearing impairment, developmental disability, and hypertelorism had a history of reduced visual attention and head turning behaviors when viewing objects located at reduced distances. During the vision evaluation, there was no evidence of gaze restriction; however, he was not able to converge his eyes for objects that were presented at a reduced distance. When asked to look at an object at near, he would turn his head to the right or left of the object to view it monocularly. In order to provide him with binocularity for near targets, bilateral prismatic lenses in a spectacle correction were evaluated. With the prisms, he was able to view the object without any head-turning behaviors. Brief convergence responses were also possible as objects were brought closer to him. He also demonstrated better eye-hand coordination while wearing the correction. A prescription was issued for prismatic corrective glasses with instructions to use the glasses during activities that required a reduced viewing distance.

Table 11.3 summarizes the causes of accommodative and convergence abnormalities.

STRABISMUS

Strabismus or a misalignment of the eyes is often associated with developmental disabilities and is commonly seen in various syndromes. The lack of binocularity when the eyes are not well aligned results in decreased or absent stereopsis. This may negatively affect activities that necessitate accurate eye-hand coordination and compromise the child's safety during mobility-related activities that require accurate depth perception such as negotiating curbs and stairs. While strabismus in a general population has been reported to occur in 1.3% to 4.5% of the general population,[11,12,13] the prevalence of strabismus in children with developmental disabilities is often much higher, depending on the diagnosis.[14] Therefore, a careful assessment of both the motor and

Table 11.3	
Causes of Accommodative and Convergence Problems	
Problem	*Causation*
Accommodation	Medications
	Gross and fine motor delays
	Aphakia
	Visual fatigue caused by significant uncorrected hyperopic refractive error
	Neurological disorders
Convergence	Neurological disorders
	Medications
	Accommodative disorders
	Strabismus
	Hypertelorism

sensory status of the eyes should be attempted in all of these children. Strabismus can occur for a variety of reasons including decreased visual acuity, brain trauma, or damage resulting in conditions such as cortical visual impairment, craniofacial anomalies, poor muscle tone, significant refractive error, or without any specific etiology.

Strabismus Secondary to Decreased Visual Acuity

Strabismus frequently occurs secondary to an early onset long-term reduction of visual acuity in one or both eyes. An example would be congenital cataracts, especially when the cataract is present in one eye only. Even when the cataract is removed and the eyes are optically corrected, there is a very high prevalence of strabismus and rarely is any type of binocularity present.[15–17]

Strabismus Secondary to Poor Muscle Tone

Strabismus is a common feature in conditions in which poor muscle tone is present, such as cerebral palsy. Studies have shown the prevalence of strabismus to be between 31% and 60% in individuals with cerebral palsy.[18–21] The strabismus can be esotropia, exotropia, hypertropia, and/or hypotropia. It can also be variable in nature, changing from exotropia to esotropia periodically. Children with cerebral palsy also show a high prevalence of limitations of gaze ranging from 4% to 18%.[18,21] Both the variability of the strabismus and the gaze paresis make the management of binocular vision anomalies in children with cerebral palsy more challenging.

Strabismus Secondary to Significant Refractive Error

Because children with developmental disabilities and/or some types of visual impairment may have high hyperopia, it is not uncommon for there to be an accompanying accommodative esotropia secondary to the uncorrected hyperopia and the associated need for increased focusing power when viewing visual detail at near. For example, children with albinism are more likely to have significant hyperopic and astigmatic refractive errors[22] which may be one of the factors contributing to the higher prevalence of esotropia in these children.

Strabismus Secondary to Craniofacial Anomalies

Facial structure can contribute to the development of strabismus. An example is hypertelorism, which is an abnormally wide separation between the eyes. This anatomical feature can result in the presence of exotropia, especially at near distances.[23] Crouzon syndrome is an example of the association between hypertelorism and exotropia. A literature review of ocular anomalies associated with craniofacial anomalies found a 46% incidence of exotropia in individuals with this syndrome.[24]

Strabismus of Unknown Etiology

No specific etiology may be associated with strabismus other than its known association with a particular syndrome or condition. An example of this would be Down syndrome in which studies have found the prevalence of strabismus to range from 9.5% to 57%.[5] Fragile X syndrome is another frequently encountered, inherited genetic disorder that results in intellectual disability. It is also associated with strabismus (either esotropia or exotropia) at a higher rate than the general population.[25] Other chromosomal abnormalities are also highly associated with the presence of strabismus including syndromes associated with the duplication, trisomy, and deletion of various chromosomes.[18]

A wide range of developmental disabilities are associated with the presence of some type of strabismus. The type and magnitude of the strabismus are as variable as the presenting condition and the child who is being examined. The prognosis for achieving ocular alignment or normal binocular functioning depends upon many factors, including the type, magnitude, and frequency of the strabismus present, the nature of associated eye disorders, as well as the visual acuity, age, and cognitive functioning of the developmentally disabled child. Most importantly, an accurate assessment of both the child's motor (how the eyes look) and sensory (what the child sees) functioning should be attempted in each case.

CONTRAST SENSITIVITY

A reduction in contrast sensitivity function, or the ability to discern low-contrast visual detail, will compromise a child's ability to see low contrast objects in the environment. Although this aspect of vision is often overlooked during the standard eye examination, it plays a significant role in the use of vision during activities of daily living and mobility, as many objects in the child's environment tend to be of low contrast. A child with a contrast sensitivity deficit will have difficulty seeing low-contrast curbs, stairs, facial detail, or educational materials such as low-contrast drawings or text.[26] Contrast sensitivity deficits may be associated with ocular as well as brain disorders. Any clouding of normally transparent ocular structures arising from internal eye inflammation, cataracts, corneal disease, or vitreous abnormalities can result in reduced contrast sensitivity function. Contrast sensitivity deficits are also associated with damage to the optic nerve or central retina. Cerebral visual impairment associated with hypoxic-ischemic brain damage has also been associated with a higher incidence of contrast sensitivity deficits.[27] Contrast-enhancing strategies such as the use of high-contrast markings on stairs or curbs as well as high-contrast educational materials, such as bold-lined paper and broad-tipped soft graphite pencils, will enhance the use of vision in children with reduced contrast sensitivity. Reduction of ambient glare with anti-reflection coatings and/or tinting of corrective lenses as well as the use of glare-free task lighting will also enhance the contrast of educational materials.

ACCOMMODATION

Accommodative (focusing) disorders in children with developmental disabilities can interfere with their fine motor development as well as with overall learning. There are a number of causative factors for accommodative disorders in children with disabilities as well as children with visual impairments. Significant uncorrected hyperopic refractive error can create visual stress that reduces the efficiency and stability of a child's accommodation. Correcting the refractive error ensures that the visual stress is eliminated, thereby facilitating accommodation. Children with gross and fine motor delays, as is the case in cerebral palsy, will often display inaccurate or poorly maintained accommodation for near visual tasks.[28,29] Children with low vision also have a higher incidence of accommodative disorders. Accommodation may also be adversely affected by systemic medication used to control secretions, seizures, depression, and hyperactivity. Accommodation is totally absent in children with aphakia or pseudophakia who have undergone cataract surgery. It is important to establish the presence of accommodative disorders during the vision evaluation by the eye care provider in order to prescribe appropriate corrective lenses or implement appropriate accommodative therapy.

FLUCTUATIONS IN VISION

Many caregivers, teachers, and therapists report that they are concerned about fluctuating levels of visual attention in children with disabilities, which they interpret to be a result of visual changes. Systemic conditions may cause changes in visual acuities. For example, diabetes and hypoglycemia may create changes in refractive error and instabilities in visual acuity due to fluctuating blood glucose levels. Multiple sclerosis, which is most often found in adults but, although rare, may also be found in children,[30] can also result in fluctuating acuity depending on energy, stress, and even temperature levels.

Medications such as scopolamine, which is given to control oral secretions, may create an accommodative insufficiency that adversely affects a child's ability to see clearly at reduced distances. In some situations, however, mild or focal seizure activity is misinterpreted as changes in visual acuity or attention. It is important to observe if there are consistent changes in facial expressions, ocular deviations, increases in nystagmoid eye movements, or if there are subtle postural changes that may indicate the possibility of seizure-related activity. In such situations, prompt referral to a neurologist is indicated.

Ocular Disorders Associated With Visual Impairment

When working with children who have visual impairments, it is important to note that only a small percentage (approximately 15%) of individuals with visual impairments are functionally or totally blind.[31] The majority of children with visual impairments have residual or low vision and, with visual accommodations, are able to access educational materials and independently perform activities of daily living. It would take an entire textbook to adequately explore all of the conditions that result in low vision. The following discussion will explore some of the more common pediatric ocular and visual disorders as well as their implications for overall visual functioning. Table 11.4 lists the ocular manifestations of syndromes found in children with multiple impairments.

Table 11.4 describes the ocular manifestations of the syndromes that we have encountered in our Special Populations Clinic (SPARC). For a more detailed discussion of both systemic and ocular manifestations of syndromes resulting in multiple impairments, the following texts may be consulted.[45,46]

Table 11.4

Ocular Manifestations of Syndromes With Multiple Impairments

Syndrome	Ocular Manifestation
Aicardi syndrome	Chorioretinitis, microphthalmia, optic disc anomalies
Alstrom syndrome	Pigmentary retinal dystrophy, visual field defects
Apert syndrome	Downward slant of lids, strabismus, exophthalmos, optic atrophy, cataracts, congenital glaucoma, retinal hypopigmentation
Bardet-Biedl syndrome	Pigmentary retinal dystrophy, strabismus, cataract
Cerebral palsy	Optic atrophy, strabismus, refractive error (typically hyperopia), accommodative dysfunction, eye movement abnormalities, nystagmus
CHARGE syndrome	Ocular colobomas, microphthalmia, visual field defects
Cornelia de Lange syndrome	Strabismus, optic atrophy, ptosis, prominent eyebrows
Crouzon syndrome	Optic atrophy, hypertelorism, exotropia, exophthalmos, cataracts, convergence abnormalities
Cytomegalovirus (congenital)	Chorioretinitis, optic atrophy, microphthalmia, cataracts

(Continued)

Dandy-Walker syndrome	Optic atrophy, nystagmus, strabismus, visual field defects, gaze palsies, pupillary abnormalities
Fetal alcohol syndrome	Optic nerve hypoplasia, ptosis, strabismus, refractive error
Fragile X syndrome	Refractive error, strabismus, accommodative abnormalities, convergence abnormalities, amblyopia, ptosis, eye movement abnormalities
Hallermann-Streiff syndrome	Microphthalmia, cataracts, blue sclera, nystagmus
Hydrocephalus	Optic atrophy, strabismus, nystagmus, visual field defects, gaze palsies
Infantile Refsum syndrome	Pigmentary retinal dystrophy, visual field defects, optic atrophy
Joubert syndrome	Pigmentary retinal dystrophy, optic nerve pallor, nystagmus, eye movement dysfunction, visual field defects
Laurence-Moon Bardet-Biedl syndrome	Pigmentary retinal dystrophy, strabismus, cataract, visual field defects
Lowe syndrome	Congenital cataracts, glaucoma, corneal opacity
Marfan syndrome	Lens dislocation, glaucoma, retinal detachment, sectoral myopia in the pupillary area occupied by the lens
Peters plus syndrome	Corneal opacity, cataract, iris adhesions, glaucoma, microphthalmia
Pierre Robin syndrome	High myopia, retinal detachment, strabismus, microphthalmia, cataracts, glaucoma
Reiger's syndrome	Glaucoma, pupillary abnormalities, corneal opacity, microcornea, iris adhesions
Rubella (congenital)	Cataracts, pigmentary retinal dystrophy, microphthalmia, glaucoma, keratitis
Septo-optic dysplasia (de Morsier's syndrome)	Optic nerve hypoplasia, visual field defects, amblyopia
Shaken baby syndrome	Retinal hemorrhages, retinal detachment, optic atrophy, eye movement disorders, pupillary asymmetry, cataracts, dislocated lenses
Spina bifida	Optic atrophy, strabismus, visual field defects, gaze palsies
Spinocerebellar ataxia	Cone rod dystrophy, visual field defects
Stickler syndrome	High myopia, vitreous abnormalities, retinal detachment, glaucoma
Syphilis (congenital)	Chorioretinitis, uveitis, interstitial keratitis, corneal scarring, astigmatic refractive error associated with corneal scarring, optic atrophy, nystagmus
Toxoplasmosis (congenital)	Chorioretinitis, macular atrophy, microphthalmia, cataracts, uveitis, optic atrophy
Trisomy 18	Short palpebral fissures, coloboma, epicanthal folds, ptosis, cataract, microphthalmia
Trisomy 21 (Down syndrome)	Strabismus, nystagmus, keratoconus, cataract, myopia, Brushfield spots (iris flecks), epicanthal folds, downward slant to lids
Treacher Collins syndrome	Downward slanting lids, coloboma of the lower lid, astigmatic refractive error
Turner syndrome	Cataract, ptosis
Usher syndrome	Pigmentary retinal dystrophy, visual field defects, posterior subcapsular cataracts

ACHROMATOPSIA

Achromatopsia (also referred to as rod monochromatism) is a hereditary retinal disorder that is associated with a severe or total loss of color vision. Individuals with the complete form of achromatopsia have no appreciation of color. They can only see black, white, and shades of gray. The absence of color vision in children with this hereditary disorder is due to defects in the cone photoreceptors of the retina that are sensitive to colors in the short, medium, and long wavelengths of light. These photoreceptors are also responsible for processing fine visual detail and facilitating adaptation to brightly illuminated environments. Only the rod photoreceptors are fully functional. Children with this condition tend to be very photophobic and experience significant glare-related discomfort in both indoor and outdoor environments. They experience increased comfort and enhanced vision with a reduction in ambient illumination (hemeralopia) and visual acuity may actually improve under dimmer illumination. Children with this disorder typically have visual acuity in the range of 20/100 to 20/200 and normal visual fields. Retinal and optic nerve appearance is normal in a majority of affected children. Congenital nystagmus is also frequently associated with achromatopsia. Interventions recommended by the low vision rehabilitation optometrist to improve visual functioning include light filtration, magnification, and contrast enhancement, especially for visual targets with poorly contrasting colors. Dark red contact lenses and sunglasses have been found to significantly reduce outdoor light sensitivity and lighter tints are used to reduce indoor glare.

Blue cone monochromacy is also a hereditary disorder that affects color vision but less completely than achromatopsia. In this disorder, only the cone photoreceptors that are sensitive to short wavelength light and the rod photoreceptors are fully functional. The cones that are sensitive to medium and long wavelength light are defective. Children with this disorder are able to appreciate shades of blue but are unable to appreciate colors in the red and green color spectrum. Reduced visual acuity, ranging from 20/60 to 20/200, as well as congenital nystagmus are typically associated with this disorder. Although they are also bothered by glare and sunny environments, their discomfort is typically not as severe as individuals with achromatopsia.

Case Five

A 5-year-old boy with a history of Leber's congenital amaurosis presented for a low vision evaluation. His parents reported that he demonstrated significant difficulty maintaining visual attention, especially outdoors. He tended to keep his head down and held on to someone's hand when walking in brightly lit environments. His parents reported that he preferred dimly lit environments. Examination revealed that his corrected visual acuities were approximately 20/120 and his visual fields were full. Retinal and optic nerve appearance was normal. He exhibited a pendular nystagmus, total color blindness defects, and was very photophobic. Indoors, he demonstrated greater visual comfort when wearing light gray tinted lenses. Follow-up testing with an electroretinogram confirmed the diagnosis of achromatopsia. His parents were educated about low vision rehabilitative options and were advised to return for a magnification evaluation in 1 year when he will transition to first grade. His parents reported during a follow-up telephone conversation that the dark red sunglasses significantly improved his visual attention and his independence outdoors.

ALBINISM

Oculocutaneous albinism is a hereditary disorder that results from the body's reduced or inability to produce the melanin that is necessary for pigmentation of the skin, hair, and eyes. The following are the four most common types of oculocutaneous albinism. Individuals with the full manifestation of this condition, oculocutaneous albinism or OCA 1A, typically have very pale skin as well as white to yellow-white hair. Eye color is typically light blue due to the lack of iris pigmentation and retinal regions also lack pigmentation. OCA 1A is associated with underdevelopment (hypoplasia) of the macular/foveal region of the retina and congenital pendular nystagmus. It is also frequently associated with hypoplasia of the optic nerves. Children with oculocutaneous albinism (OCA 1A) tend to be very sensitive to brightly illuminated environments, as there is minimal pigmentation within the iris to filter out the excess light. Visual acuity in children with OCA 1A typically ranges from 20/100–20/400. Individuals with milder forms of oculocutaneous albinism (OCA 1B, OCA 2, OCA 3, and OCA 4) are able to produce some pigment and may exhibit increased hair, skin, iris, as well as retinal pigmentation. They, however, also exhibit macular/foveal hypoplasia and optic nerve hypoplasia as well as congenital nystagmus. The visual disability as well as the sensitivity to light is less severe in children with these genetic disorders and visual acuity typically ranges from 20/70–20/200. Astigmatic refractive error is common in all four forms of oculocutaneous albinism. Strabismus and lack of stereopsis is also common in individuals with oculocutaneous albinism due to the abnormal crossing pattern of neural fibers at the optic chiasm. This abnormality also increases the prevalence of strabismus in individuals with this disorder.

Some forms of oculocutaneous albinism have associated systemic disorders. Hermansky-Pudlak syndrome is associated with oculocutaneous albinism and is a blood platelet disorder resulting in prolonged bleeding. It is also associated with a gastrointestinal disorder and pulmonary fibrosis. This hereditary disorder has a higher incidence in individuals of Puerto Rican descent but is found in other nationalities as well. Chédiak-Higashi syndrome is associated with oculocutaneous albinism and blood platelet abnormalities, recurrent infections, and increased mortality at a younger age.

Unlike oculocutaneous albinism, the changes associated with another hereditary form of albinism, ocular albinism, are restricted to the eye. Children with ocular albinism tend to have higher levels of vision and more ocular pigmentation. Children with ocular and oculocutaneous albinism respond well to low vision rehabilitation. Interventions typically recommended by the low vision rehabilitation optometrist include large print materials, light filtration and magnification devices, contrast enhancement, assistive technology, as well as ongoing vision services throughout the child's educational program.

Aniridia

Aniridia is a hereditary developmental disorder that results in an absent or rudimentary iris (Figure 11.1). As the iris provides the mechanism for light control in the eye through the constriction and dilation of the pupil, these children tend to be very photophobic. This disorder is typically associated with underdevelopment of the foveal region and congenital nystagmus. It may also be associated with optic nerve hypoplasia, cataracts, glaucoma, and corneal disorders that may result in corneal clouding and reduced contrast sensitivity. Visual acuity is usually between 20/100 and 20/200. No visual field defects are associated with aniridia unless there is secondary glaucoma as a result of an abnormality in the eye's fluid circulation system that causes an increase in fluid pressure within the eye resulting in damage to the optic nerve. In cases of aniridia where there is no previous family history of the disorder, there is an increased chance of developing a metastatic kidney tumor, Wilms' tumor, within the first decade of life. Children with this sporadic form of aniridia must be monitored for this tumor during the first decade of life, as the prognosis is excellent if the tumor is removed during the early stage of its development. Interventions for visual

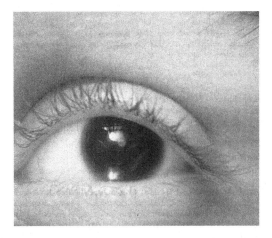

Figure 11.1. Aniridia is a hereditary developmental disorder that results in an absent or rudimentary iris.

enhancement recommended by a low vision rehabilitation optometrist include large print, light filtration glasses or contact lenses, magnification devices, assistive technology, reduced aperture contact lenses, enhanced contrast, and vision services throughout the child's educational program.

CATARACTS

Cataracts are associated with a number of syndromes including rubella, retinopathy of prematurity, Down syndrome, and Hallermann-Streiff syndrome. They are also associated with hereditary eye disorders such as retinitis pigmentosa and aniridia. Cataracts may also be caused by trauma to the child's eye region or by systemic medications, such as cortisone. Cataracts may be associated with congenital glaucoma or present as an isolated finding in children with inherited congenital cataracts. Congenital cataracts typically result in visual impairment and nystagmus unless they are removed early in the child's visual development. Long-standing congenital cataracts result in amblyopia due to significant sensory deprivation during the critical period of the brain's development. The surgical removal of the cataracts results in aphakia. It is necessary to correct the significant refractive error induced by surgical aphakia through the use of corrective spectacle lenses, contact lenses, or intraocular lenses. If the child has an associated visual impairment, intervention consists of magnification, contrast enhancement, and illumination control.

COLOBOMAS

Congenital colobomas are caused by a defect in the early fetal developmental process, resulting in a gap within otherwise intact ocular structures (Figure 11.2). A chorioretinal coloboma results from the absence of normal retinal and choroidal layers in the lower ocular region. This lower retinal colobomatous defect may translate into significant upper visual field loss. Children with this type of defect are prone to injuries from objects such as tree branches, the corners of cabinets, and shelving that are undetected in their defective upper visual field region. If the macula and/or the optic nerve is involved, there is typically also an associated reduction in visual acuity and contrast sensitivity. Children with chorioretinal colobomas are at higher risk for retinal detachments and should be regularly monitored by their eye care provider. Colobomas may also be found in the lens and iris. Iris colobomas will result in a misshaped (typically "keyhole" in shape) or displaced pupil that is poorly or unreactive to light. A child with an iris coloboma may experience glare-related discomfort.

Magnification devices and large print educational materials should be introduced to children with reduced vision. If the child has an upper visual field deficit, a discussion should also occur with the child's caregivers and teachers about repositioning visual targets into the lower field region in order to reduce the child's visual fatigue and enhance visual attention. The child would also benefit from protective photochromic lenses that will reduce the child's risk for eye injuries and increase visual comfort when outdoors in a bright sunny environment. Reduced aperture contact lenses may be used for the correction of a misshaped colobomatous pupil. Children should also

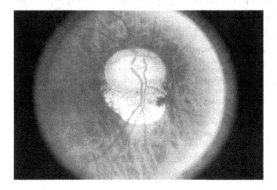

Figure 11.2. Colobomas are developmental disorders that result in the segmental absence of normal ocular structures.

be referred to an orientation and mobility professional who will teach the child how to use their residual vision for travel.

Cone and Cone-Rod Degenerations

Cone and cone-rod dystrophies are typically hereditary disorders. Cone dystrophy is characterized by the progressive degeneration of the retinal cone photoreceptors that are responsible for fine detail central acuity, color vision, and adaptation to light. As a result, children with a progressive disorder of the cone photoreceptors typically have central blind spots, reduced visual acuity, color vision, and contrast sensitivity along with significant light sensitivity. Children who have progressive cone-rod dystrophies also experience a degeneration of the rod photoreceptors later in the course of the disorder. They will develop progressive peripheral visual field loss as well as dark adaptation difficulties. This group of disorders may also be associated with a systemic disorder, spinocerebellar ataxia (SCA7), that results in both visual and progressive neurological impairment. The severity of the visual and neurological impairment increases with each generation of children who have inherited this disorder. Children with cone and cone-rod dystrophies benefit from large print text, magnification devices, contrast enhancement, sunglasses, vision services, and orientation and mobility services. Due to the progressive nature of these disorders, the child may benefit from a learning media assessment performed by a teacher of the visually impaired to determine if and when Braille as well as auditory learning strategies should be introduced.

Case Six

A 6-year-old girl presented to the low vision service with a history of refractive amblyopia. Her mother reported that her daughter was depressed and withdrawn and was having difficulty keeping up with her class. She held books at a very reduced distance and had difficulty seeing the classroom board. She was bothered by glare and bumped into people in a crowded environment. She had been recently seen by her eye care provider who felt that the child was having difficulty transitioning to first grade due to a learning disability and not to changes in her vision or eye health.

The low vision evaluation revealed visual acuity to be 20/250 in each eye with best correction, color vision, and contrast sensitivity deficits as well as peripheral field constriction. Ocular health evaluation revealed macular atrophy and retinal pigmentary changes suggestive of cone-rod dystrophy. She was significantly withdrawn throughout the evaluation. Subsequent genetic testing confirmed that she had progressive cone-rod dystrophy. A report was written to her school with recommendations that included 24-point print text, a video magnification device for reading, high contrast materials, sunglasses, and a learning media assessment by a teacher of the visually impaired due to the progressive nature of her disorder. We also recommended an orientation and mobility evaluation. When she returned for a follow-up visit for the finalization of recommendations for magnification devices, she was an outgoing, talkative, and happy child. She reported that the school provided the recommended large print and video magnification device. She was receiving vision and orientation and mobility services, and her mother indicated that she was keeping up with her class. Most importantly, she loved going to school.

In a discussion with her mother, it became clear that her daughter's previous depression was a result of her perception that people thought she was lying when she complained about her vision problems. After her low vision evaluation, she felt much better because her complaints had been validated. She finally had the magnification devices and accommodations in place that enabled her to visually access her educational materials and keep up with her class.

Glaucoma

Glaucoma is caused by intraocular pressure that is too high to maintain the normal physiology of the eye. The most common outcome of glaucoma is a damaged optic nerve, which results in visual field loss. Visual field loss may initially be isolated to a small area of the visual field but, if uncontrolled, may progress to significant visual field constriction and eventual total blindness. In the late stages of the disease, visual acuity is significantly reduced. Contrast sensitivity is also adversely affected as the damage to the optic nerve progresses. Congenital glaucoma is associated with many syndromes involving developmental disability. Some of these include rubella, trisomy 13, Lowe syndrome, and Pierre Robin syndrome. The associated significant elevation in intraocular pressure present at such a critical time in the eye's development may result in severe corneal opacification, as well as enlargement of the cornea and, possibly, the entire eye. Pharmacological, as well as surgical, interventions are used to reduce intraocular pressure and control the progression of the disease. In cases of severe corneal damage, corneal transplantation may be an option. Interventions to improve visual functioning typically recommended by vision rehabilitation optometrists include field enhancement devices, contrast enhancement, reading guides, as well as vision services, and orientation and mobility instruction.

JUVENILE MACULAR DISORDERS

There are many types of macular disorders. The most common form of these disorders, age-related macular degeneration, typically occurs after age 60. Hereditary juvenile macular disorders, such as Best vitelliform degeneration and Stargardt disease, typically occur during the first two decades of life. Non-hereditary forms of juvenile macular degeneration may be associated with ocular trauma, metabolic disorder, systemic medications, or infectious agents such as toxoplasmosis. While some macular degenerations such as Best's vitelliform degeneration may result in relatively mild central vision loss, the majority of juvenile macular degenerative disorders which include Stargardt disease and cone dystrophies, result in a central blind spot or scotoma and significant central vision loss. In order to compensate for the loss of central vision and the presence of a central blind spot, children with this condition will adopt an eccentric viewing strategy (see the section on central field defects). Children with macular degeneration or dystrophy typically have a difficult time adapting to glare and experience challenges in successfully accomplishing fine detail visual tasks such as reading. As the peripheral visual field area is typically not involved in macular degeneration, children with this group of disorders will not experience difficulty in negotiating crowded visual environments. They may, however, trip or fall when negotiating curbs and stairs due to associated contrast sensitivity as well as depth perception issues. An orientation and mobility evaluation would determine if the child demonstrates any visually based orientation and mobility issues. Interventions to enhance visual efficiency should include magnification provided by symbol/print enlargement and magnification devices, glare reduction, exploration of and instruction in appropriate eccentric fixation strategies (see Chapter Twelve), and overall contrast enhancement. School-age children with macular degeneration should receive vision services throughout their educational program.

LEBER'S CONGENITAL AMAUROSIS

Leber's congenital amaurosis is a hereditary retinal dystrophy associated with severe visual impairment. It affects both the rod and cone photoreceptors of the retina. Keratoconus and cataracts are also frequently associated with this disorder. Children with Leber's congenital amaurosis prefer higher levels of illumination, although they have a difficult time adapting to glare. Mobility is frequently affected because significant peripheral visual field loss is a common finding. Children with Leber's congenital amaurosis with associated peripheral field constriction have very poor awareness of where their eyes are in relation to their visual environment. These children will often have wandering eye movements that do not fall into any particular pattern, unlike the more rhythmic eye movements that are associated with congenital pendular or jerk-type nystagmus. They also typically have a very poor sense of directionality. An early intervention program, involving activities emphasizing basic visual skills enhancement (see Chapter Twelve) provides the best prognosis for developing higher levels of visual functioning in children with Leber's congenital amaurosis and other eye disorders associated with severe visual impairment. If there is significant vision loss, tactile and auditory learning strategies should be considered to enhance the child's access to educational materials.

Children with Leber's congenital amaurosis and other severe visual impairments are more likely to exhibit a behavior called the oculodigital reflex during which they press on the globe or generalized orbital region. Pressing on the globe in this manner may be visually stimulating, as raising the intraocular pressure will precipitate pressure phosphenes or scintillating lights and multicolored visual phenomena. When this behavior is observed, however, it is important to determine the cause. Other possible etiologies for this behavior should be ruled out. These include pain in the orbital region resulting from injury, infection, elevated intraocular pressure, or stress-related factors. If appropriate, behavior modification programs may be implemented to eliminate the problem. Such eye-poking behavior may result in retinal tears or detachments in children with a previous history of detachment, as well as in children with high myopia or other conditions that are highly associated with retinal detachment. It may also cause corneal thinning resulting in keratoconus.

Optic Atrophy/Optic Nerve Hypoplasia

Optic atrophy may be a result of a hereditary disorder, such as autosomal dominant optic atrophy, or may occur due to other causative factors. These include intrauterine infections, intracerebral hemorrhages, ischemia, inflammatory conditions, maternal drug or alcohol abuse, hydrocephalus, as well as congenital structural malformations of the brain. Optic atrophy presents with visual disorders ranging from minor to severe reductions in visual acuity and visual fields. Reductions in contrast sensitivity are also often associated with optic atrophy, as well as color vision defects which are typically red-green in nature. Congenital brain malformations, such as septo-optic dysplasia (de Morsier's syndrome) and holoprosencephaly, are often associated with an underdeveloped optic nerve (optic nerve hypoplasia). Children who are diagnosed with septo-optic dysplasia should be monitored for associated endocrine disorders. Optic nerve hypoplasia manifests in a range of visual disorders. The most common visual manifestations of optic nerve hypoplasia include peripheral visual field contraction and reductions in visual acuity. In its most severe forms, optic nerve hypoplasia is associated with severe to total loss of visual function. Interventions recommended by the low vision rehabilitation optometrist may include magnification, visual field enhancement, contrast enhancement, and recommendations for vision services and orientation and mobility instruction in the case of significant visual field involvement.

Case Seven

A 10-year-old girl presented to the low vision service with a history of optic nerve hypoplasia. She had been monitored for her eye condition since infancy, and her mother had been told that her visual status was stable. Her mother reported that she tended to be clumsy and that she exhibited reduced visual attention while traveling. This resulted in many bumps and bruises incurred during mobility-related activities. Upon questioning, her mother reported that the most typical site of injury was on top of her head or in the forehead region. During the evaluation, visual field testing revealed a constriction in the upper visual field area to approximately 5 degrees above fixation. Such altitudinal visual field defects are not uncommon in optic nerve hypoplasia. The cause for the "clumsiness" was actually an upper visual field impairment. A referral was made for orientation and mobility services, and protective eyewear was prescribed. Her mother reported back to us that her daughter had experienced a significant reduction in her mobility-related injuries after she was taught how to effectively and consistently scan her upper visual field region.

Photophobia

Photophobia is characterized by extreme sensitivity to environmental illumination. Children with photophobia experience significant discomfort when they are in bright indoor or outdoor environments. Photophobia may be caused by retinal disorders such as achromatopsia and cone dystrophies. It may also be caused by conditions such as aniridia and albinism. These hereditary disorders result in an inability of the eyes to adequately screen out excessive light due to inadequate pigmentation or a lack of pupillary light control. Photophobia is also one of the most common side effects of systemic medications used to control seizures and depression. These medications may cause pupillary dilation, which reduces the eye's ability to screen out extraneous light. Children with photophobia benefit significantly from light-filtration devices such as tinted light-absorptive lenses and contact lenses. Children who will not tolerate frames may benefit from head-worn visors.

RETINOPATHY OF PREMATURITY

Retinopathy of prematurity (ROP) is caused by the proliferation of immature blood vessels and capillaries in premature infants who receive high levels of supplemental oxygen. It has also been found to have a strong association with low birth weight.[32,33] Depending on the severity of the disorder, associated findings may include high myopia, scarring of the retina and vitreous, retinal detachment, and cataracts. Visual status ranges from normal vision to no light perception. Children with the advanced stages of ROP may have residual vision but will experience reductions in visual acuity as well as in visual fields. They will frequently also exhibit congenital nystagmus. Interventions by the eye care provider and vision rehabilitation team include magnification, light filtration to control the scatter of light through a cloudy media, correction of significant myopia with spectacles or contact lenses, vision services, and orientation and mobility instruction if there is significant peripheral visual field loss.

RETINITIS PIGMENTOSA AND ASSOCIATED ROD-CONE DYSTROPHIES

Retinitis pigmentosa is a hereditary pigmentary retinal dystrophy that is characterized by the progressive degeneration of the retinal photoreceptors. Initially, the disease affects only the rods, which mediate adaptation to reduced light levels and provide peripheral visual information. At the end stage of this disorder, there is progressive degeneration of the cone photoreceptors as well. The earliest symptom of this disorder is "night blindness" or nyctalopia. Children with retinitis pigmentosa may be temporarily blinded when entering an area of lower illumination from a bright outdoor environment and their adaptation to the reduction in illumination will take much longer than children without the disorder. For these children, vision is optimal in a well illuminated glare-free environment. During the second decade, especially children with the more severe forms of retinitis pigmentosa (x-linked and autosomal recessive) may experience mid-peripheral visual field impairments, which typically present as a "ring scotoma." This ring-shaped blind region will gradually progress to total peripheral visual field loss until they are left with the characteristic visual field constriction associated with retinitis pigmentosa. At this stage, which typically occurs during the adult years, progressive degeneration of the remaining central visual region's cone photoreceptors ultimately leads to profound visual impairment or total blindness. As the retinal degeneration progresses there is an associated reduction in contrast sensitivity function which makes it difficult for the child to see low contrast symbols or text, faces, and mobility-related drop-offs such as unmarked curbs or stairs. Retinitis pigmentosa is also associated with an increased risk of the development of early onset cataracts as well as macular edema and children should be regularly monitored for these disorders.

Retinitis pigmentosa and other related hereditary rod-cone dystrophies may also be associated with neurological and multisystem syndromes. Usher syndrome is a group of inherited disorders (Usher 1–3) that cause both sensorineural hearing loss and retinitis pigmentosa.[34] Usher 1 and Usher 3 also cause vestibular dysfunction. Usher 1 and Usher 2 present with congenital hearing impairment, with Usher 1 exhibiting the most severe vision impairment. Usher syndrome is the most common cause of deaf blindness and has been estimated to affect 18% of individuals with retinitis pigmentosa.[35,36] Children with this disorder experience progressive hearing as well as vision loss. Cochlear implantation, when performed within the first three years of life, has been shown to be most effective in improving hearing, speech, and cognition in children with early onset Usher syndrome.[37] Due to this combination of sensory deficits Braille is frequently a primary learning medium. Other syndromes that are associated with retinitis pigmentosa include Laurence Moon Bardet Biedl syndrome, Joubert syndrome, infantile Refsum syndrome, and Alstrom syndrome.[38] Low vision interventions for enhancing the use of residual vision include field-enhancing devices (prismatic lenses and image minifiers), glare free illumination devices, night vision enhancers, contrast enhancement strategies, vision services, and orientation and mobility instruction.

Neurological Visual Impairment

CEREBRAL PALSY

Cerebral palsy is a disorder of movement and posture resulting from a brain injury that has occurred before the brain has matured or that is due to a nonprogressive developmental abnormality of the brain. The defect in this disorder is in the brain's control of muscle and nerve function and not in the actual nerve and muscle fibers.[39–41] The most common form of cerebral palsy, spastic cerebral palsy, consists of a tightening or stiffening of muscles. Less common forms are dyskinetic cerebral palsy, which consists of uncontrolled movements of arms, legs, and head, and ataxic cerebral palsy, which results in coordination and balance issues.[40] Cerebral palsy may be caused by pre- and perinatal issues, such as intrauterine infections, intracerebral hemorrhages, drug abuse by pregnant women, developmental abnormalities, birth trauma, prematurity, and lack of oxygen. Postnatal causes include severe malnutrition, meningitis, head trauma, and lead poisoning. Ocular defects may include strabismus, nystagmus, and optic atrophy. Eye movements are typically choppy and poorly controlled. Accommodative dysfunction is common.[27,28] Many children with cerebral palsy will have a refractive error, with a greater proportion of children with spastic cerebral palsy demonstrating a hyperopic error.[42]

Cerebral palsy is also highly associated with cerebral visual impairment, which is also referred to as cortical visual impairment (CVI). 60% to 70% of children with cerebral palsy also exhibit CVI.[9] Children with cerebral palsy that have also been diagnosed with periventricular leukomalacia are most likely to have CVI. The most common cause of CVI is ischemic damage to the visual pathway regions of the brain which include the optic radiations and visual cortex located in the occipital lobes.[43] Children with CVI exhibit significant visual processing disorders including visual recognition, cognition, orientation to their environment, seeing multiple targets at one time, and are typically overwhelmed in a crowded visual environment. They may also exhibit hemianopic visual field deficits, reduced contrast sensitivity, reduced visual acuity, eye movement disorders as well as eye-hand coordination deficits. These deficits affect their ability to learn, interact socially, and navigate safely, especially in unfamiliar environments. Children with cerebral palsy and CVI would benefit from a comprehensive visual and ocular health evaluation which would provide information about the child's visual status as well as recommendations for accommodations that will enhance the child's ability to access educational materials.

Visual Field Disorders

CENTRAL VISUAL FIELD DEFECTS

Central visual field defects are most typically associated with macular diseases or disorders. Central defects may present as areas of distortion or metamorphopsia. Metamorphopsia causes bending or warping of visual detail so that it becomes difficult to identify the target. An individual with metamorphopsia who views a grid pattern will notice a bending or bowing of the lines or may notice that a section of the grid may be foggy or missing. Metamorphopsia is commonly present in the early stages of macular degeneration. People with metamorphopsia will complain that words appear to run together while reading. The other type of central visual field defect is characterized by a central scotoma. This is the type of visual field defect found in individuals with toxoplasmosis or with late stage macular atrophy in hereditary disorders such as Stargardt disease or cone dystrophy. The blind spot is typically at visual midline, resulting in an obscuration or deterioration of visual detail in the central visual region. The blind spot corresponds to an area of damaged retina in the affected macular region. Magnification can reduce the portion of the visual detail that is obscured or distorted, by enlarging the image size, thereby placing a greater portion of the image outside of the damaged macular region.

A child with central field defects benefits from an eccentric viewing strategy. This strategy enables them to view with an undamaged retinal area (preferred retinal locus) that is outside of the damaged macular region and enhances their ability to discern visual detail as well as their visual efficiency. Despite societal pressures to "look someone in the eyes" while conversing, the child with macular degeneration should be encouraged to shift fixation to the side of the visual target (eccentric viewing) in order to obtain optimal visual information. Some children may adapt a head turn in order to more easily achieve and sustain a large-angle eccentric viewing position.

PERIPHERAL VISUAL FIELD DEFECTS

Peripheral visual field constriction is most typically associated with retinitis pigmentosa and with end-stage glaucoma. It may also, however, occur in children with shunt-treated hydrocephalus.[44] Children with this type of visual field impairment will have a very difficult time with independent mobility. Children with developmental delays who experience such significant visual field loss may be very fearful of unfamiliar locations. Tactile compensatory behaviors, such as dragging their feet while walking or trailing a wall with their hand, provide essential feedback that reduces the chances of mobility-related mishaps. Children with peripheral visual field constriction should wear protective lenses and receive orientation and mobility services as they are at higher risk for mobility-related accidents and injuries. Specialized sectoral prismatic lenses, used when developmentally and cognitively appropriate, will alert the child to potential mobility related obstacles in their visual periphery.

Hemianopic or hemifield defects associated with brain injury or disease can also significantly compromise mobility-related activities. Individuals with such defects will frequently adapt head turns to the direction of the impaired visual field region. During mobility-related activities, children with hemianopic defects tend to gradually veer toward the intact visual environment. They also attempt to obtain tactile feedback from the missing visual field environment. Children with hemianopic visual field defects will consistently miss objects in the affected visual field region unless they learn to scan their visual environment effectively and efficiently. Orientation and mobility evaluation and instruction are the key to safe and independent mobility for children with peripheral visual field loss. The use of a white cane or auditory biofeedback mobility aids provides essential information about the unseen visual region. Optical devices such as prismatic lenses and mirrors, when developmentally appropriate, provide the visually impaired child with an image of the missing visual environment.

Case Eight

A 7-year-old girl had a long-standing history of bilateral hemianopic lower visual field loss. Her mother reported that her daughter was unable to read or write for extended periods of time. This was due to postural discomfort created by the severe downward head tilt that was necessary for her to see objects in the lower visual field region. Her daughter also experienced significant mobility-related issues, especially with stairs and curbs. Prismatic lenses for reading were evaluated. The upward image shift created by the prismatic lenses significantly reduced the girl's downward head tilt. When the prismatic glasses were coupled with a slant board that raised the position of her educational materials, she was able to achieve a comfortable head position while reading and writing. A prescription was issued for prismatic glasses to be used for reading and writing activities at school and at home. She and her mother were instructed not to wear the prismatic correction when walking as it would make her misjudge the height of curbs and stairs and place her at a higher risk for injuries. Due to her reported mobility issues, the use of a mobility cane was discussed, and the girl was referred for an orientation and mobility evaluation.

Conclusion

Children with visual impairments require specialized services and accommodations to enhance their use of remaining vision for learning, safe mobility, and activities of daily living. These services and accommodations are also essential for children with visual, physical, and developmental disabilities. A collaborative relationship between eye care providers, occupational therapists, teachers of the visually impaired, orientation and mobility specialists, speech and language pathologists, and other rehabilitation professionals facilitates an exchange of critical information about the nature, prognosis, and visual deficits associated with a child's ocular diagnoses. This collaborative approach ensures that all accommodations, as well as therapeutic and educational services, will be appropriately individualized for each child's unique visual capabilities. Chapter Eleven describes the common pediatric ocular and visual disorders seen by optometrists and ophthalmologists specializing in evaluations of children with visual, physical, and developmental disabilities. The chapter also discusses the functional implications of these visual deficits for achieving academic and developmental goals. Chapter Twelve discusses approaches to managing these visual deficits.

Acknowledgments

We would like to thank Marcy Graboyes, LSW, ACSW. Associate Professor, Salus University, Coordinator of Social Services, William Feinbloom Vision Rehabilitation Center, for her valuable insight and contribution to the editing of this chapter.

References

1. Scholl GT. What does it mean to be blind? Definitions, terminology, prevalence. In: Scholl GT, ed. *Foundations of Education for Blind and Visually Handicapped Children and Youth*. New York, NY: American Foundation for the Blind; 1986:23–33.
2. American Printing House for the Blind Inc. *2021 Annual Report*. www.aph.org/app/uploads/2022/04/annual-report-fy2021.pdf.
3. Goldenberg R, Culhane J, Iams JD, et al. Epidemiology and causes of premature birth. *Lancet*. 2008 Jan;371(9606):75–84.
4. Honein M, Kirby RS, Meyer RE, et al. The association between major birth defects and preterm birth. *Matern Child Health J*. 2009 Mar;13(2):164–175.
5. Sun E, Kraus CL. The ophthalmic manifestations of Down syndrome. *Children (Basel)*. 2023 Feb 9;2:341.
6. Marr JE, Halliwell-Ewen J, Fisher B, et al. Association of high myopia in childhood. *Eye*. 2001 Feb;15(Pt 1):70–74.
7. Sauer T, Lawrence L, Mayo-Ortega L, et al. Refractive error and ocular findings among infants and young children with severe problem behavior and developmental disabilities. *J Ment Health Res Intellect Disabil*. 2018;11(4):251–265.
8. Park MJ, Yoo YJ, Chung CY, et al. Ocular findings in patients with spastic type cerebral palsy. *BMC Ophthalmol*. 2016;16:195.
9. Fazzi E, Signorini SG, La Piana R, et al. Neuro-ophthalmological disorders in cerebral palsy: ophthalmological, oculomotor, and visual aspects. *Developmental Medicine & Child Neurology*. 2012;54(8):730–736.
10. Postolache L, Monier A, Lhoir S. Neuro-ophthalmological manifestations in children with Down syndrome: current perspectives. *Eye Brain*. 2021 Jul 21;13:193–203.
11. McKean-Cowdin R, Cotter SA, Tarczy-Hornoch K, et al. Prevalence of amblyopia or strabismus in Asian and non-Hispanic white preschool children. *Ophthalmology*. 2013 Oct; 120(10): 2117–2124.
12. Donnelly UM, Stewart NM, Hollinger M. Prevalence and outcomes of childhood visual disorders. *Ophthalmic Epidemiol*. 2005 Aug;12(4):243–250.
13. Friedman Z, Neumann E, Hyams SW, Peleg B. Ophthalmic screening of 38,000 children, age 1 to 2½ years, in child welfare clinics. *J Pediatr Ophthalmol Strabismus*. 1980;17:261–267.
14. Ciner EB, Macks B, Schanel-Klitsch E. A cooperative demonstration project for early intervention vision services. *Occup Ther Pract*. 1991;3(1):42–56.

15. Gelbart SS, Hoyt CS, Jastrebski G, Marg E. Long-term visual results in bilateral congenital cataracts. *Am J Ophthalmol.* 1982;93:615–621.
16. Maurer D, Lewis TL. Visual outcomes after infantile cataract. In: Simons K, ed. *Early Visual Development, Normal and Abnormal.* New York, NY: Oxford University Press; 1993.
17. Demirkilinc Biler ED, Bozbiyik DI, Uretmen O, et al. Strabismus in infants following congenital cataract surgery. In: *Graefe's Archive for Clinical and Experimental Ophthalmology.* 2015 Oct;253(10):1801–1807.
18. Duckman R. The incidence of visual anomalies in a population of cerebral palsied children. *J Am Optom Assoc.* 1979;50:1013–1016.
19. Wesson MD, Maino DM. Oculovisual findings in children with Down syndrome, cerebral palsy, and mental retardation without specific etiology. In: Maino DM, ed. *Diagnosis and Management of Special Populations.* St. Louis, MO: Mosby; 1995.
20. Ciner E, Appel S, Graboyes M, Kenny E. Testing visual function and visual evaluation outcomes in the child with cerebral palsy. In: Miller F, Bachrach S, Lennon N, O'Neill M, eds. *Cerebral Palsy.* Cham: Springer; 2018:1–26.
21. Scheiman MM. Optometric findings in children with cerebral palsy. *Am J Optom Physiol Opt.* 1984;61:321–333.
22. Sayed KM, Mahmoud Abdellah M, Gad Kamel A. Analysis of the refractive profile of children with oculocutaneous albinism versus an age-matched non-albino group. *Clin Ophthalmol.* 2021 Jan 8;15:73–78.
23. Hwang, JM, Baek RM, Lee SW. Ocular findings in children with orbital hypertelorism. *Plastic and Reconstructive Surgery.* 2012 Oct;130(4):624e–627e.
24. Rostamzad P, Arslan ZF, Mathijssen IM, et al. Prevalence of ocular anomalies in craniosynostosis: a systemic and meta-analysis. *J Clin Med.* 2022 Feb 18;11(4):1060.
25. Hatton DD, Buckley E, Lachiewicz A, et al. Ocular status of boys with fragile X syndrome: a prospective study. *J AAPOS.* 1998 Oct;2(5):298–302.
26. Ciner EB, Appel SD, Graboyes M. Low vision special populations I. In: Brilliant RL, ed. *Essentials of Low Vision Practice.* Boston, MA: Butterworth-Heinemann; 1999:313–333.
27. Fazzi E, Signorini SG, Bova SM. Spectrum of visual disorders in children with cerebral visual impairment. *J Child Neurol.* 2007 Mar;22(3):294–301.
28. McClelland JF, Parkes J, Hill N, Jackson AJ, Saunders KJ, et al. Accommodative dysfunction in children with cerebral palsy: a populations-based study. *Invest Ophthalmol Vis Sci.* 2006;47:1824–1830.
29. Leat SJ. Reduced accommodation in children with cerebral palsy. *Ophthalmic Physiol Opt.* 1996;16:385–390.
30. Brenton JN, Kammeyer R, Gluck L, et al. Multiple Sclerosis in Children: Current and Emerging Concepts. *Semin Neurol.* 2020 Apr;40(2):192–200.
31. Kirschner C. *Data on Blindness and Visual Impairment in the United States.* New York, NY: American Foundation for the Blind; 1985:82.
32. The STOP-ROP Multicenter Study Group. Supplemental therapeutic oxygen for prethreshold retinopathy of prematurity (STOP-ROP): a randomized, controlled trial. I: primary outcomes. *Pediatrics.* 2000;105:295–310.
33. Kennedy KA, Fielder AR, Hardy RJ, et al., for the LIGHT-ROP Cooperative Group. Reduced lighting does not improve medical outcomes in very-low-birth-weight infants. *J Pediatrics.* 2001;139:527–531.
34. Toms M, Pagarkar W, Moosajee M. Usher syndrome: clinical features, molecular genetics, and advancing therapeutics. *Ther Adv Ophthalmol.* 2020 Sept 17;12:2515841420952194.
35. Marazita ML, Ploughman LM, Rawlings B, et al. Genetic epidemiologic studies of early-onset deafness in the United States school-age population. *Am J Med Genet.* 1993;46:486–491.
36. Boughman JA, Vernon M, Shaver KA. Usher syndrome—definition and estimate of prevalence from two high-risk populations. *J Chronic Dis.* 1983;36:595–603.
37. Davies C, Bergman J, Misztal C, et al. The outcomes of cochlear implantation in Usher syndrome: a systematic review. *J Clin Med.* 2021 Jun 29;10(13):2915.
38. Hamel C. Retinitis pigmentosa. *Orphanet J Rare Dis.* 2006 Oct 11;1:40.
39. Ghasia F, Brunstrom J, Gordon M, Tychsen L. Frequency and severity of visual sensory and motor deficits in children with cerebral palsy: gross motor function classification scale. *Invest Ophthalmol Vis Sci.* 2008 Feb;49(2):572–580.
40. Paul S, Nahar A, Bhagawati M, Kunwar AJ. A review on recent advances of cerebral palsy. *Oxid Med Cell Longev.* 2022 Jul 30;2022:2622310.
41. Scheiman M. Assessment and management of the exceptional child. In: Rosenbloom A, Morgan M, eds. *Principles and Practice of Pediatric Optometry.* Philadelphia, PA: JB Lippincott; 1990:388–419.
42. Park MJ, Yoo YJ, Chung CY, et al. Ocular findings in patients with spastic type cerebral palsy. *BMC Ophthalmol.* 2016 Nov 8;16(1):195.
43. Philip SS, Dutton GN. Identifying and characterising cerebral visual impairment in children: a review. *Clin Exp Optom.* 2014; 97:196–208.
44. Rudolph D, Sterker I, Graefe G, et al. Visual field constriction in children with shunt-treated hydrocephalus. *J Neurosurg Pediatr.* 2010 Nov;6(5):481–485.
45. Nelson LB, ed. *Harley's Pediatric Ophthalmology.* 6th ed. Philadelphia, PA: WB Saunders; 2013.
46. Maino DM, ed. *Diagnosis and Management of Special Populations.* St. Louis, MO: CV Mosby; 1995.

Chapter Twelve

Management of Vision Disorders in Children With Disabilities

Elise B. Ciner, Sarah D. Appel, and Marcy Graboyes

Children with disabilities experience a high rate of vision disorders that can interfere with development and learning. A comprehensive vision evaluation is therefore necessary to diagnose and treat any vision disorders in these children. The consequent management plan by eye care providers specializing in pediatrics and/or low vision rehabilitation should include the impact the child's vision disorder(s) may have within the framework of the medical, functional, and educational needs of the child. Occupational therapists often see children with disabilities on a regular basis through the child's school, early intervention program or privately. They therefore play a critical role in facilitating and implementing the individualized vision management plan that has been developed for the child during the comprehensive vision evaluation. This chapter emphasizes those management recommendations where the occupational therapists' engagement can likely have the most impact in the co-management of vision problems for children with disabilities.

Background

The pediatric population with disabilities encompasses a wide range of health conditions, with each child having their own unique profile of visual, educational, and rehabilitative needs. As vision is a fundamental component of development and learning for children, a comprehensive vision evaluation by eye care providers (optometrists or ophthalmologists) who specialize in pediatrics and/or low vision rehabilitation becomes an essential component of a child's health care management plan. The consequent development and implementation of an individualized management plan that addresses each child's vision issues is based upon information collected before, during, and after the actual vision evaluation. Information may be gathered from sources that include the child's parent/caregiver, educational and rehabilitation teams, as well as health and eye care specialists. The following are examples of information that can be elicited during the case history: Observations and concerns related to vision raised by family and team members; historical information regarding the child's ocular (eye) and systemic (general) health; developmental status; educational and rehabilitation plans and goals. This information is combined with visual data that are gathered and analyzed during the evaluation to develop an appropriate management plan. The plan should include the impact of the child's vision disorder(s) within the framework of the medical, functional,

DOI: 10.4324/9781003526841-12

and educational needs of the child. Occupational therapists accompanying the child and parent(s) to the visual examination may provide valuable information including optimal positioning, the child's best viewing distance and preference for color, sounds/songs or objects that can enhance the child's responsiveness during testing. As occupational therapists often see children with disabilities on a regular basis either through the child's school, early intervention program or privately, they play a critical role in facilitating any additional appointments or referrals and ensure that appropriate care is received in a timely manner. The management plan that is developed during the comprehensive vision evaluation typically includes a series of recommendations and/or interventions by the eye care provider that addresses the individualized needs of each child.

Eye Health Recommendations

Eye health recommendations closely mirror those made during any routine eye exam. They may include treatment for common pediatric eye health disorders such as conjunctivitis or chronic blepharitis (inflammation of the eyelids). If more complex disorders are found, referral to other eye health care providers for co-management including retinal, glaucoma or neuro-eye specialists, pediatric ophthalmologists, or neurologists could also be indicated. Additional evaluations may also be warranted, such as visual field testing, optical coherence tomography (OCT) or electrodiagnostic testing (e.g., visual evoked potential [VEP] or electroretinogram [ERG]) to aid in determining the general etiology of the child's vision loss (e.g., retinal vs cortical), level of functional vision and the specific visual diagnosis. It is important for the occupational therapist to understand why a referral is being made and how soon the child needs to be seen.

Functional Recommendations

Functional recommendations relate directly to the child's developmental needs, including the implementation of communication devices and appropriate visual interactions in an educational, therapeutic, or residential environment. A typical comprehensive vision evaluation report might state that the child has normal ocular health, good eye alignment, minimal refractive error, and 20/80 visual acuity. Functional recommendations, however, often go significantly beyond this data in meeting the visual needs of children with developmental disabilities. For example, it is not only important for the therapist to know that a child sees 20/80 but also how efficiently that child is using their level of vision during educational and/or rehabilitative programs. Children with reduced visual acuity often need to use print that is larger than the actual level measured during an exam. It is important for the therapist to also understand what 20/80 means at various distances and under various levels of illumination. Excessive or reduced lighting can impede functional use of best visual acuity, depending on the child's ocular disorder. Of equal importance is the type of visual acuity testing that was administered. Single pictures or letters on a chart that are *uncrowded* and therefore free of clutter or visual distractions are easier to recognize and may overestimate a child's functional visual acuity than the same pictures or letters presented with *crowding* bars. Children with amblyopia or cortical visual impairment (CVI) are known to have more difficulty with crowded symbols or letters. The latter are considered the *gold standard* for accurately measuring visual acuity both clinically and in research studies and are more reflective of the visual clutter that is often present in a home or classroom setting (Figure 12.1).

Case in Point A: A child with a history of a retinal disorder achieved a visual acuity of 20/60 when tested with single symbols. When tested with crowded symbols, however, the child could only achieve a visual acuity of 20/100. The latter is a better representation of the child's functional visual acuity. This is because reading continuous text print or identifying a field of symbols on an augmentative communication device may involve significant visual clutter that

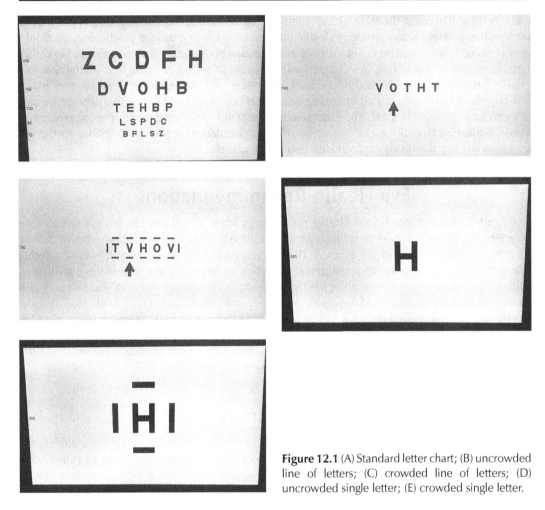

Figure 12.1 (A) Standard letter chart; (B) uncrowded line of letters; (C) crowded line of letters; (D) uncrowded single letter; (E) crowded single letter.

could result in greater visual instability when compared to reading single letters or symbols on flash cards.

Beyond the actual description of a child's functional level of vision, recommendations may be made regarding prognosis for improvement of vision, strategies to adapt the learning environment with respect to the child's visual needs, as well as guidelines for how appropriate vision stimulation programs should be developed and implemented. The following is a discussion of functional vision recommendations that might be made depending on the results of the evaluation and the individual needs of each child.

Lenses and Low Vision Magnification Device Recommendations

An eye care provider's prescription of various types of lenses and low vision magnification devices for a child with disabilities is often the most common, wide ranging, and easily implemented intervention. The decision to prescribe glasses is made by the eye care provider with input from the child's parents as well as other members of the educational and rehabilitation team. This can include, for example, consideration as to whether the child has the ability to use the lens or devices effectively and how sensory issues may impact a child's ability to tolerate wearing a frame. The occupational therapist can then be helpful in assessing any sensory challenges, and behavioral or functional changes demonstrated by the child when these treatments are implemented. Some of the types of lenses that may be prescribed are as follows:

LENSES FOR CORRECTION OF REFRACTIVE ERROR

It is well known that significant refractive errors (myopia, hyperopia, astigmatism, and/or anisometropia) are common visual problems in children with disabilities.[1–11] The presence of a refractive error, however, does not automatically necessitate prescribing glasses. When recommended, lenses that are more impact-resistant and provide protection for outdoors (e.g., polycarbonate or Trivex) should always be used for children to avoid injury from the lenses or falls, and to shield the eyes from glare-related discomfort and the sun's ultraviolet rays. Children with reduced peripheral vision who are mobile are at increased risk for ocular injuries and should be prescribed protective lenses regardless of the magnitude of the refractive error. Occasionally for non-mobile children, glasses may be contraindicated if the child is tactually defensive or has a limited visual field, which might be further impeded by the presence of a frame. For all children, frames that are too small or have rims that are too thick may interfere with their ability to fully scan the surrounding visual environment. There are several factors that eye care providers consider when deciding when and how to prescribe.[12–18] These include the following:

Age of the Child

The chronological age of the child is one of the first factors that should be considered. This is because the presence of moderate or even high refractive error may be normal at certain ages and can often change (increase or decrease) throughout a child's lifetime. This is especially true during the first few years of life when refractive error is often present.[19–24] An example is astigmatism, which is very common during infancy, but often decreases or disappears by age 3 or 4 years.[24–27] An exception would be in young children with nystagmus where the astigmatism tends to persist, warranting early correction.[28] In general, the younger the child, the more common it will be to find a significant refractive error and the more likely it will be that the eye care provider may want to monitor it for a period of time before correction. There are, however, several instances in which the refractive error may be corrected as early as possible. In general, this would occur in a child who has a very high magnitude of refractive error, beyond that typically seen for their age or in the presence of an eye misalignment (e.g., esotropia) that improves with the application of lenses. The presence of aphakia (where the lens of one or both eyes has been removed due to early or congenital cataracts), which may leave a child with a very high amount of hyperopia and significantly blurred vision, is another reason to prescribe at a very early age as soon as the cataract is removed. It is important to understand that each type of refractive error has its own developmental timeline, which impacts the decision as to how and when to prescribe. The eye care provider who is aware of these changes can discuss them with the child's parents, and the educational and/or rehabilitative team.

Magnitude of Refractive Error

The amount or magnitude of refractive error present is the next consideration when prescribing. Although it is very common for children with a developmental disability to have some refractive error, in many cases the magnitude is low, is considered within a normal range, and has no impact on the child's clarity or other visual skills. An example of this is low astigmatism or low hyperopia, both of which are common during the preschool years and are often not necessary to correct unless there are accompanying deficits in visual acuity or binocular vision. In contrast, when a moderate to high amount of refractive error is present, glasses and sometimes contact lenses may be important to optimize visual acuity, binocularity, and the child's ability to focus at near. The correction of these refractive errors may have a profound effect on the attention level of children with developmental disabilities.[3,29] It is important to always consider prescribing for even moderate amounts of refractive error as it is not always known in advance what impact corrective lenses will have on the child's responsiveness to their environment, rehabilitative, and/or educational program. For example, a child with low vision who requires a reduced viewing distance to achieve magnification should wear a hyperopic correction even if moderate. The decision to prescribe, however, depends not only on the child's age and magnitude of the refractive error, but on several other factors as well.

Level of Visual Impairment

The decision to provide optical correction also depends on the type and degree of visual impairment of the child. In general, there are three levels of visual impairment that can be considered when prescribing.

No Light Perception. In these cases, the child is not responding to any type of illuminated objects under any conditions. It is unlikely that any level of refractive correction would provide improved ability to see lights. Protective lenses are, however, indicated to reduce the likelihood of eye injuries.

Light Perception Only. If the child is responding only to illuminated targets, correction of moderate or low refractive errors would be unlikely to provide better light perception or to allow patterned vision. Unless the refractive error is exceedingly high, it is often advisable to hold off on prescribing until the child becomes more visually responsive through a vision stimulation program. Prescribing glasses in these cases may give parents or caretakers a false sense of hope that glasses will cure the vision loss. Exceptions to this guideline may include children who are sensitive to glare, those showing self-stimulatory behaviors such as *eye poking* or for those working on independent mobility. In the latter two cases, protective lenses with the prescription should be prescribed to prevent eye injury.

Pattern Vision Present. When the child shows even a minimum level of responsiveness to pattern vision (e.g., 20/1200 or one of the widest black and white stripes with forced choice preferential looking [FPL] acuity) and a high amount of uncorrected refractive error is present, a trial period with lenses is often attempted as long as the child can learn to tolerate frame wear. When a child has higher levels of visual acuity (e.g. 20/400 or better with FPL), moderate amounts of refractive error may be corrected in order to improve visual acuity, provide magnification, reduce the effort to sustain focus at near, and optimize the level of visual functioning. If a child's level of pattern vision is within a normal range for their age (e.g., 20/60 or better with FPL or a recognition acuity such as LEA or HOTV), consideration can be given to correcting milder amounts of refractive error that may be causing blurred vision, difficulty focusing, or visual discomfort at near.

Developmental Age

The child's developmental age is another important factor when prescribing glasses for refractive error correction. Specific areas that must be considered are the child's cognitive level, communication abilities, and educational needs. This includes the type of communication device, educational and rehabilitation materials being used or considered, and the child's working distances at which these will be implemented.

Case in Point B: A child with a moderate amount of hyperopia is functioning at a 6-month developmental level and is only responding to large, illuminated objects. Corrective lenses may not be indicated because this child's visual demands are not likely to be at a sufficiently high level to benefit from correction. In contrast, a child functioning at a level where they are learning to use a communication device (requiring sustained visual attention at near) would likely benefit from correction of a similar moderate amount of hyperopia. In the latter case, corrective lenses would allow the child to see detailed objects at a near distance with decreased accommodative (focusing) effort and increased comfort. Correction of hyperopia or farsightedness has the further advantage of providing additional magnification to make near viewing easier. Any child going through a vision stimulation program should periodically have their refractive error re-evaluated especially when there are improvements in visual responsiveness. This is especially important in children of all developmental ages who are taking anti-secretion medication associated with significant accommodative (focusing) deficits.

Refractive Error and Other Aspects of Vision

While the eye care provider's decision to prescribe glasses may initially be based on facilitating optimal clarity of vision (visual acuity) for distance viewing, other visual skills are also factored in. These can include the effect of refractive error on near visual acuity, eye coordination (eye alignment and binocularity/stereopsis), accommodation (focusing), image size (magnification), and/or visual fields (peripheral or side vision).

Case in Point C: A child with a low degree of hyperopia, aligned eyes, good stereopsis, and normal visual acuity at both distance and near would not typically be prescribed glasses by many eye care providers. A child with an intermittent esotropia (one eye periodically drifts inward) or a large esophoria (tendency for one or the other eye to drift inward without an actual eye turn) would, however, benefit from correction of lower amounts of hyperopia to improve eye coordination and binocularity.

Case in Point D: If a child has a moderate to high amount of hyperopia and would benefit from a prescription to improve clarity of vision and focusing but also has either an exotropia (outward eye turn) or exophoria (outward eye drift), the actual prescription can be reduced in order to provide optimal visual acuity without causing the eye to turn out more as a result of the corrective lenses.

Case in Point E: A child has cortical visual impairment resulting in significantly reduced visual acuity and is using their vision primarily for close viewing. If this child is found to have a mild to moderate amount of myopia, corrective lenses may be contraindicated. This is because the presence of low to moderate myopia allows the child to be naturally focused for near working distances without optical correction (depending on the magnitude of the prescription). Wearing glasses would therefore result in a greater accommodative (focusing) demand at near along with a minification of the image. Both of these effects would place more demand on the child's visual system, making it more difficult for them to sustain focus at near through the lenses. The result might be a child who either refuses to wear the glasses or who is less attentive for near tasks where much of learning often takes place. The child may, however, benefit from the myopic prescription when engaged in distance viewing activities or outdoors.

SUNGLASSES AND TINTS

It is not uncommon for some children with disabilities to have enhanced sensitivities to external stimuli, including photosensitivity or photophobia in brightly lit rooms and/or outdoors. Photosensitivity may be a result of medications that cause pupillary dilation or heightened sensitivity to glare. Photosensitivity is also associated with certain congenital ocular disorders, such as rod monochromatism, congenital cataracts, albinism, and aniridia. If photosensitivity or photophobia is reported during the history or observed during the examination, the eye care provider may prescribe various filters or absorptive lenses (Figure 12.2). Recommendations can include an anti-glare/reflection coating, polarized lenses, photochromatic lenses, and/or a tint with a specified color and percentage of light transmission. The addition of side or top shields to prescribed sunglasses or the

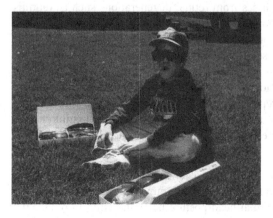

Figure 12.2. Various filters or absorptive lenses used by the optometrist for light sensitivity. (Photograph by Ron Davidoff.)

use of a visor or cap can help filter stray light that escapes into the eyes from the side (even with glasses on) and cause glare or discomfort. In addition, a tactually defensive child may not tolerate a frame at all but may accept a visor that can provide relief from a glare-filled environment.

Case in Point F: A 5-year-old child with oculocutaneous albinism is currently wearing glasses from an eye care provider that corrects a moderately high amount of nearsightedness and astigmatism in each eye. The child is very sensitive to the sun and glare. When asked about outdoors during daylight, the parent showed a pair of store-bought pink children's sunglasses with diamonds and dark tint but without a correction. The child reportedly switches to these from their prescriptive lenses when outside. The child will be entering a full-day kindergarten program in just a few months. The mother reports that it is unlikely the child, even with the help of teachers, will reliably switch back and forth between the glasses when going outdoors. A new pair of glasses with an updated prescription and XTRActive lenses (lenses that become darker than traditional photochromatic lenses outdoors) was prescribed to allow the child to keep their glasses on throughout the day, providing maximum acuity, enhanced comfort, and reduced glare. The slight tint that is retained in the lenses indoors will also be of benefit by reducing glare from indoor lighting and windows.

Prism Lenses

Prisms can be incorporated into most prescriptions. Prisms function by bending light and moving the image onto a specific part of the retina (see Chapter Seven). An eye care provider might prescribe prism for several reasons as described below.

Prism to Improve Binocularity

Prism may be prescribed in order to allow a child with a strabismus to achieve fusion and stereopsis. Low amounts of prism can be ground into the actual lenses of the child's glasses when they are made and are included on the written prescription. Higher amounts of prism can make the lenses too thick. Alternatively, removable Fresnel or press-on prisms may be recommended instead (see Chapter Seven).

Case in Point G: A child with cerebral palsy (CP) who also has an eye that intermittently turns inward may have poor ability to control the eye drift due to reduced muscular control associated with the CP. The application of a small amount of prism might be enough in this case to allow the child to avoid double vision (diplopia) and attain more comfortable binocular vision on a regular basis without the need for surgical intervention.

Prism to Improve Visual Fields

Another reason prism may be prescribed is to allow greater access to all areas of the visual environment for children with peripheral visual field loss. This type of prism functions as an enhancer of peripheral field awareness. Visual field disorders that respond well to Fresnel prism intervention include hemianopic and altitudinal visual field defects that arise from brain injury as well as concentric constriction that typically arises from retinal degenerations such as retinitis pigmentosa and optic nerve damage resulting from glaucoma (see Chapter Eleven).

Case in Point H: A Fresnel prism is placed on a segment of a spectacle lens that corresponds to the missing visual field area. When the child scans into the region where the prism is placed, visual information is shifted from that region onto the child's undamaged visual area so that those previously unseen images become visible. Without the prism, the child would have to initiate extreme eye and head movements in order to reposition visual targets on a retinal location that corresponds to an area of residual vision. This strategy is, however, only used with children who have sufficient cognitive ability to learn to use these sectoral prisms safely and efficiently.

Prism to Improve Head Posture and Balance

Prism can also be useful to improve a head turn or tilt secondary to an extraocular muscle palsy that has caused a child to position their head in a manner that moves the viewed image into the visual field of the affected muscle. The abnormal head posture helps the child to reduce the incidence of diplopia that might otherwise occur. Yoked (ambient) prisms (Chapter Seven) have also been used to improve a head turn or tilt in a child with a visual field loss and have been used to alter visual space for children with autism and thereby affect their behavior.[30] The occupational therapist can provide valuable insights as to whether a child with disabilities is showing significant and consistent head turns or tilts or exhibits behaviors that might warrant a trial of yoked or other prisms. Once prescribed, the occupational therapist's observations are critical to monitoring compliance and efficacy of these types of glasses.

Case in Point I: The strategic placement of a prism for a child with an extraocular muscle palsy could move the image so that the child is able to achieve binocularity in spite of the paretic muscle. This would allow them to continue to use the vision from each eye and avoid diplopia.

Case in Point J: A child responds to a missing lower field by adapting a downward head tilt during activities such as eating, typing, or viewing a communication board. This allows visual scanning to occur more efficiently in the lower visual field region. Placement of a vertical prism in front of each eye would have the effect of raising the images in the lower visual field so that the child will not have to assume the awkward and uncomfortable downward head tilt. Full-field vertical prism in this case would not be appropriate for mobility-related activities as the prisms shift the position of potential obstacles such as stairs or curbs and may confuse a child who must maneuver safely around them. (The white cane is the most effective traveling tool for children with significant inferior visual field defects. Use of the cane while in motion enables the child to maintain a normal head posture while detecting obstacles efficiently and effectively.)

Occupational Therapy Evaluation of Lens Effectiveness

Once lenses or devices are prescribed, it is important for the occupational therapist to communicate with the eye care provider in order to understand the purpose and function of the glasses as the occupational therapist can play an important role in determining the effectiveness of the corrective lenses. This is most easily accomplished by answering a number of questions and reporting this information back to the eye care provider:

1. Are the glasses being worn by the child on a regular basis?
2. Are the glasses sitting comfortably on the child's face?
3. Does the child seem annoyed with the glasses?
4. Are there marks on the child's nose, temples, or behind the ears when the glasses are removed indicating a need for adjustment?
5. Are the glasses cleaned regularly and free of smudges and smears, which can reduce clarity and increase glare?
6. Are the glasses sitting flush against the face or do they slide down the child's nose?
7. Does the child seem to look over the top of the glasses to view?
8. Does the child seem more attentive, smile more, or make better eye contact with the glasses on?
9. Does the child appear to see better with the glasses?
10. Do the child's eyes appear more aligned with the glasses?
11. Does the child hold their head straighter or more upright?
12. Is the child more or less aware of peripheral objects while wearing the glasses?
13. Are the child's facial muscles more relaxed with the glasses?
14. Is the child's mobility and/or orientation to the environment better with the glasses?
15. Does wearing the glasses make the child seem less irritable?
16. Is the child squinting more or less with the glasses?
17. Do the glasses make the child seem more confident and self-assured?
18. Does the child seem happier when wearing the glasses?
19. Are there other changes in behavior noted when the child wears their glasses?

LOW VISION MAGNIFICATION DEVICES—NEAR VIEWING

Children with visual impairment may benefit from magnification devices for enhancement of vision during near viewing activities. Juvenile disorders associated with macular degeneration result in a central blind spot that significantly interferes with the identification of small targets. Magnification increases the image size of small targets sufficiently so that the child with a visual impairment is able to identify them. The magnification requirements depend on the difference between the child's visual acuity and the visual requirements of the activities in which they are involved. Children respond well to a variety of stand magnifiers that are placed directly on pictures or letters. They especially enjoy dome stand magnifiers, as they can easily incorporate the magnifier into playtime activities as a "crystal ball" that magically makes things easier to see (Figure 12.3). When determining the type of magnification device that may be helpful it is important to consider the child's developmental level and motor function.

Case in Point K: A child with visual impairment may be viewing objects at a very reduced distance, as close as 1 to 2 inches from their eyes. This extremely near viewing distance magnifies the image of the object on the retina. Long-term viewing of visual targets at such a reduced distance can, however, result in visual and postural fatigue. Use of a magnifier will enlarge the visual target so that the child can view it at a greater, more comfortable distance.

Children can also be introduced at an early age to desktop or handheld video or digital magnification devices previously referred to as a closed-circuit television (CCTV). These devices provide high contrast, reverse contrast and variable magnification, as well as an enhanced field of view and comfortable viewing distances. They also have glare reduction capabilities by changing the color of both the text and the background (e.g., white letters on black background) for children who experience significant glare-related discomfort (Figure 12.4). Technologies that provide screen magnification options as well as text-to-speech capability are also of significant value when developmentally appropriate. Magnification can also be introduced by enlargement of print and

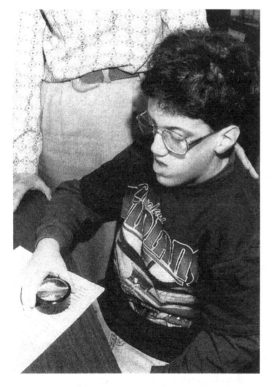

Figure 12.3. A dome stand used to enlarge the visual target so that the child can view at a greater, more comfortable distance.

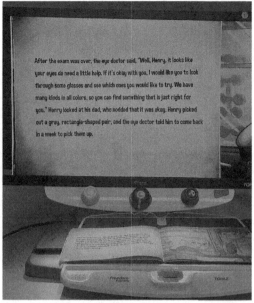

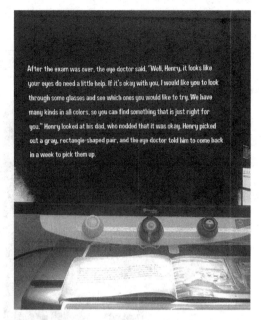

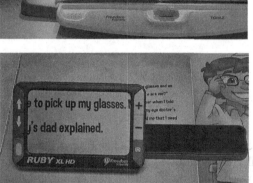

Figure 12.4. Desktop and handheld video magnifiers provide variable contrast and magnification as well as an enhanced field of view. (A) desktop high contrast magnification; (B) desktop reverse contrast magnification; (C) handheld video magnifier.

visual targets. It is also essential to discuss nonvisual reading options such as braille or speech output devices when the child's visual status is so compromised that visual reading will interfere with educational progress. In these situations, the child may choose to use vision for short-term reading and nonvisual educational media for extended reading tasks. Recommendations may be made for a learning media assessment, which is performed by a teacher of the visually impaired (also referred to as a teacher of students with visual impairments) who will evaluate the child's use of sensory channels to determine if print, braille, pictures and objects, auditory strategies, or combinations thereof would be best for accessing and creating information most efficiently. Further considerations for appropriate lighting, high-contrast lined paper, and writing implements as well as the use of reading stands and other non-optical devices will further facilitate the use of vision with or without recommended devices.

LOW VISION MAGNIFICATION DEVICES—DISTANCE VIEWING

Children with visual impairment may also enjoy looking through monocular or binocular telescopes that magnify distant objects on a television screen, other side of the room, or across the street (Figure 12.5). These telescopic devices magnify visual targets without requiring a reduced viewing distance. Telescopic devices may also be mounted onto spectacle lenses so that the child's hands are free for other activities. Lens mounted telescopes significantly reduce fatigue during prolonged viewing sessions. Such devices are ideal for long-term stationary visual activities, such as

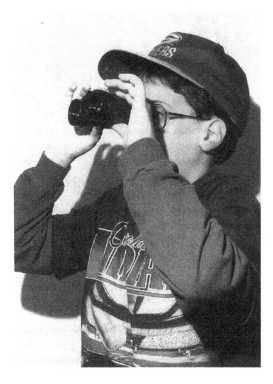

Figure 12.5. Low-powered telescope binoculars that magnify distant objects on a television screen, other side of the room, or across the street.

watching a movie or television. Transportable video magnifiers can also be helpful in a classroom setting to help children see the board at a normal viewing distance (Figure 12.6). The key is to make visual activities fun so that the child is motivated to use the magnifier. For all magnification devices, rehabilitative instruction in the use of the device(s) by a certified low vision therapist or teacher of the visually impaired is critical to ensure proper usage and facilitate adaptation.

Binocular Vision Recommendations

The high prevalence of binocular vision disorders in children with disabilities[1,2,6,9–11,31–34] presents a unique challenge and opportunity for occupational therapists to work closely with eye care providers during rehabilitation. There are several strategies for treatment of strabismus and other binocular vision disorders including convergence insufficiency.[35] Children with limited cognitive and communication skills, however, are often unable to describe or communicate what they are seeing and may be unable to participate in standard therapeutic interventions such as home- or office-based vision therapy programs. While this may narrow the various approaches, there are treatments that can be considered. These include but are not limited to the following.

Surgery for Binocular Vision Disorders

Surgery is performed by an ophthalmologist and involves a procedure whereby one or more extraocular muscles are tightened, loosened, or repositioned to prevent the eye from physically turning in or out independent of the other eye. Surgery may be successful in providing cosmetically aligned eyes and is often recommended when the eye turn is either constant or very large. When a child has an eye turn (e.g., esotropia or exotropia) and is nonverbal, the therapists, educators, and family members may not always be able to determine if the child is visually *on task* during rehabilitative or other activities as each eye may be intermittently or constantly *pointing* in a different

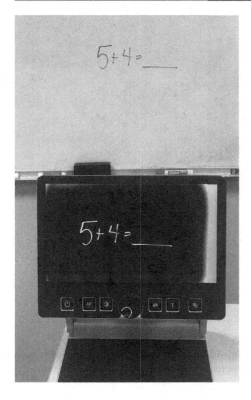

Figure 12.6. Transportable video magnifier for classroom use.

direction. Surgically aligning the eyes may allow for a better understanding as to when the child is visually attending and encourages increased eye contact with the child. While surgery has benefits for children with disabilities and may result in better ocular alignment, there is not necessarily an accompanying improvement in functional binocular vision and stereopsis (3D vision).[34] This is especially true when there is amblyopia or poor vision in one eye or the eye turn was constant for an extended period at a young age prior to surgery.

REFRACTIVE CORRECTION FOR BINOCULAR VISION DISORDERS

As mentioned earlier, correction of refractive error may result in a change in a child's binocular vision along with a change in visual acuity. Correction of hyperopia when the eye is turned in (eso) may result in better alignment of the eyes, while correction of hyperopia when an eye is turned out (exo) may result in an increase in the deviation. Similarly, correction of myopia when the eye is turned in (eso) may result in an increase in the deviation, while correction of myopia when the eye is turned out (exo) may result in better alignment of the eyes. The eye care provider often considers eye alignment as a factor in determining when and how much to prescribe.

PRISMATIC CORRECTION FOR BINOCULAR VISION DISORDERS

Application of prism can result in an improvement in eye alignment, allowing for increased binocularity and stereopsis. Prism is also sometimes prescribed in order to allow for a better cosmetic appearance of the eyes even though no improvement in binocularity is expected.

PARTIAL OCCLUSION FOR BINOCULAR VISION DISORDERS

Partial occlusion/patching in the form of bitemporal or binasal occlusion is sometimes used to provide the child with feedback about eye alignment. An example is a child with an intermittent exotropia. Application of partial occlusion to the temporal aspect of each lens might increase the child's visual awareness of when the eye actually drifts outward (Figure 12.7).

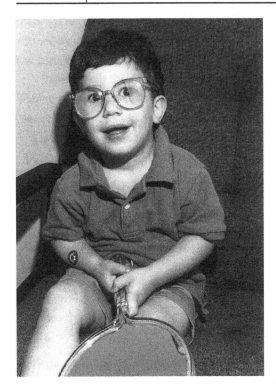

Figure 12.7. Bitemporal occlusion used with intermittent exotropia.

VISION THERAPY FOR BINOCULAR VISION DISORDERS

Vision therapy or orthoptics has been shown to be effective in the treatment of binocular vision disorders[35] in addition to amblyopia, accommodative, and ocular motor and visual processing disorders. Generally, vision therapy is a plan developed by the eye care provider based on the results of the vision assessment. It is conducted at the eye care provider's office using specially developed lenses, prisms, anaglyphic, polarized, and/or computerized equipment. In-office therapy is often supplemented with short periods of home-based exercises each day that may also be computerized. Ideally, a child would need to be at a cognitive level of approximately 5 years of age in order to benefit from in-office therapy, although decisions always need to be made on an individual basis. There are times when in-office therapy is not practical or possible. For example, a child who is developmentally delayed may not be able to tolerate a therapy program for more than a few short minutes at a time throughout the day or may not be able to understand the instructions. In the former case, the occupational therapist, teacher, and other members of the rehabilitation team can be invaluable in providing a more limited type of vision therapy program through more frequent and regular rehabilitation sessions. Providing this type of therapy can also alleviate the burdens on the parent or caregiver who is often already overloaded with day-to-day responsibilities associated with caring for a child with disabilities. The following are examples of the types of therapies that can easily be administered by an occupational therapist in a school or rehabilitation setting.

Convergence Therapy

Short periods of convergence therapy each day can be helpful for children with either convergence insufficiency or intermittent exotropia. In either case, the child has difficulty converging their eyes for objects at near viewing distances such as learning materials and communication boards. The objective of convergence exercises is to increase and maintain eye alignment and convergence of the eyes to the near object of regard. As a detailed object is brought close to the eyes, one eye actually drifts outward (temporally), and double vision may be reported or aversion to near viewing may be observed. The occupational therapist can generally administer convergence exercises when prescribed by an eye care provider in the rehabilitation setting. The following procedure can be used by occupational therapists to assist with convergence therapy.

Example 1: Convergence Therapy. Several appropriate targets of high interest to the child are used based upon the results of the vision exam and recommendations of the eye care provider. Targets will be a specified size, such as 1-inch stickers or 2-inch finger puppets, and there may be recommendations for optimal color, contrast, and luminance. Appropriate targets are typically as small and detailed as possible, yet large enough so the child can see them. Scratch-and-sniff stickers are often ideal because they provide visual as well as olfactory input to the child. Hold the target in front of the child along the midline and begin approximately 20 inches from the eyes. Slowly move the target in toward the child's eyes along the midline and watch for equal movements of both eyes toward the nose. The endpoint occurs when one or both eyes are no longer fixating on the target or when one eye appears to drift outward. Record the closest distance at which the child is able to converge. Repeat several times. Change targets as needed or when the child loses interest (Figure 12.8).

Anti-Suppression Therapy

This type of therapy can be useful for children who have the ability to develop normal binocular vision but who are unable to do so because they are actively suppressing the information from one eye. Anti-suppression therapy is useful in certain cases of amblyopia or intermittent strabismus. This type of therapy should only be instituted upon the recommendation of the eye care provider. The use of anti-suppression therapy with children who do not have the potential to develop normal binocular vision could result in the development of untreatable and permanent double vision. Anti-suppression therapy can be either active, whereby the child is engaged in a game, or passive, whereby the child is simply made aware that the eyes are not working together in unison without engaging in an actual task or interactive activity. In both cases, the child wears anaglyphic glasses which have a red filter over one eye (usually right eye) and a green filter over the other eye. The objective is to increase awareness of when the two eyes are not working together as a team.

Example 2: Active Anti-Suppression Therapy. When viewing non-illuminated red and green objects, the right eye (with the red filter) will see the objects that are red in color while the eye with the green filter will see the objects that are green in color. If the vision from one eye is suppressed or not being used (due to an eye drift), the objects seen by that eye will darken and appear black. The goal of this activity is therefore to sort objects by color into piles of red, green, and black. Red, green, and black blocks, balls, pick-up sticks, beads, craft bears or other similar objects (of an appropriate developmental level size and task), or edibles such as red, green and brown M&Ms can be used (Figure 12.9).

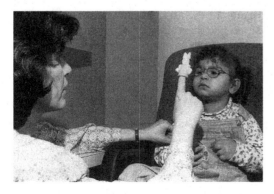

Figure 12.8. Convergence exercise is performed by slowly moving the target in toward the eyes until one eye no longer fixates on the target or one eye appears to drift outward.

Example 3: Passive Anti-Suppression Therapy. Red and green acetate filters are placed side by side (touching, but not overlapping) directly onto a screen (e.g., TV/computer or iPad). The child simply watches the screen while wearing anaglyphic glasses (red filter over one eye and green over the other). If one eye is not being used, half of the screen will darken. With illuminated targets or screens *red sees red* and *green sees green*. If the side of the screen with the red filter darkens, then the eye with the red filter is not being used. If the side of the television with the green filter darkens, then the eye with the green filter is not being used (Figure 12.10).

Computer-Based Vision Therapy

There are several computer-based vision therapy programs available to treat binocular vision disorders (and also eye tracking, accommodative and visual processing deficiencies and amblyopia) that are designed for use in the home.[35,36] These programs can also be incorporated into rehabilitative or educational settings by the occupational therapist with guidance from the eye care provider. As with other types of vision therapy, the child's eye care provider will determine when and if this type of vision therapy program would be of benefit and work with the occupational therapist to determine optimal setting, positioning, and on-task time for the child.

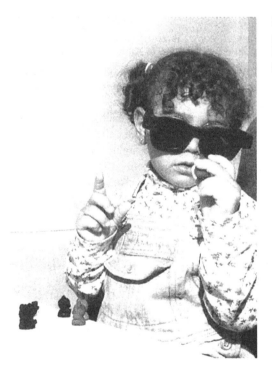

Figure 12.9. Active anti-suppression therapy. The goal of this activity is to sort the small craft "bears" by color into piles of red, green, and black while the child wears anaglyphic red/green glasses.

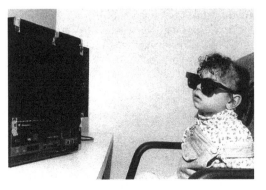

Figure 12.10. Passive anti-suppression therapy. An acetate sheet that is half red and half green is placed directly over the TV screen while the child wears anaglyphic red/green glasses.

Amblyopia Recommendations

Eye care providers often prescribe various treatments for amblyopia (lazy eye) for children with disabilities. This can include children who have a loss of vision in one eye only due to a constant unilateral strabismus or significant unequal refractive errors including unilateral aphakia. Bilateral amblyopia can occur when there is a high magnitude of refractive error in both eyes due, for example, to high bilateral hyperopia or bilateral aphakia. Management of amblyopia includes prescription of glasses to correct significant or unequal refractive error[37-40] as well as some type of occlusion therapy for unilateral amblyopia.[41,42] While patching is not contraindicated when ocular disease or macular scarring is present, the prognosis for success may be much more guarded in these cases. This type of therapy can often be implemented by the occupational therapist under the guidance of the eye care provider. Traditional therapy for unilateral amblyopia requires simply patching the good eye for a specified period of time each day in order to force the weaker, amblyopic eye to be used. Consideration needs to be made by the eye care provider in consultation with the educational and rehabilitation team as to whether the possible benefit of improved vision for a poorly seeing eye after several hours of daily patching outweighs the loss of educational and rehabilitative time they would have gained by using their better seeing eye. When patching is recommended, the following need to be kept in mind.

CHOOSING THE APPROPRIATE PATCH

For children with developmental disabilities, the eye care provider often consults with parents and members of the rehabilitation team who interact with the child on a daily basis. The main goals are to determine the type of patch that will be tolerated by the child and allow full occlusion without *peeking* and the amount of patching and associated activities that are most likely to result in improvements in vision. There are many choices for patches available, among them pirate type patches with a strap, decorative bootie patches that slide over the glasses, and adhesive patches that can either be placed directly over the eye or on the glasses (Figure 12.11). In some children, the patch may also be in the form of a *fogging lens* in front of the better seeing eye which may be more tolerated by a child and can also be recommended when a latent nystagmus emerges upon total occlusion of the better seeing eye. Fogging can be achieved by either prescribing a high-power lens, which in effect blurs out any useful visual information, or by the application of a Bangerter filter[43] (translucent, plastic filter that is applied to the glasses), which have the same effect. At times, the use of a contact lens occluder may be implemented to achieve compliance. This contact lens, which is worn only in the non-amblyopic eye, is either a very high-powered lens that blurs the vision in that eye or a lens with the center blackened to prevent any significant light from reaching that eye while it is worn.

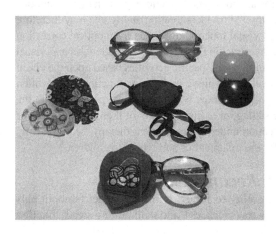

Figure 12.11. Various forms of patches used for occlusion with amblyopia. Clockwise from top: Fogging cling patch/Bangerter filter; clip-on patches; slip-on patch; adhesive patches; (center) strap patch.

MONITORING EFFECTIVENESS AND COMPLIANCE WITH PATCHING

Effectiveness of patching can be accomplished jointly by both the occupational therapist and eye care provider. The latter will periodically measure actual changes in visual acuity and other visual functions during amblyopia therapy using Teller Acuity Cards, matching Lea Symbols, HOTV letters, or standard Snellen Charts. The occupational therapist can provide valuable information of behavioral changes noted during therapy sessions. Signs of effective patching include decreased resistance to wearing the patch, increased alertness when the patch is on, greater ability to detect objects in the environment with the patch on, and improved awareness of depth and enhanced eye-hand coordination skills with the patch off. The occupational therapist co-managing care can help assess whether there is compliance with patching both at school and at home. Based upon these observations, eye care providers can make further recommendations for either an increase or decrease in patching time, changes in the type of patch worn, as well as modifications in the actual activities performed during patching or amblyopia therapy.

Indications of noncompliance include the following:

- A child who is agitated and upset when the patch is applied and continues to be upset with the patch on but does not object if the other eye is patched.
- A child who is constantly trying to remove the patch or turning their head to one side when wearing the patch. The latter often indicates that the child might be peeking out of the side of the patch.

DROPS AS AN ALTERNATIVE TO PATCHING

Dilating the pupil of the better seeing eye with drops used only on the weekends but lasting throughout the week is an effective alternative to wearing a patch.[43–45] This type of *penalization therapy* with atropine drops works by preventing the better seeing eye from focusing at near. This forces the use of the amblyopic eye for reading and near activities while the better seeing eye continues to view clearly at a distance. This alternative to patching is contraindicated in some children, especially those with disabilities who may have increased sensitivity or adverse reactions to the drops. If this strategy is used for children with visual impairment in the poorer seeing eye due to retinal or optic nerve issues, it is essential that educational and rehabilitative materials are sufficiently magnified for their level of visual acuity. The occupational therapist can be helpful in observing any side effects or other difficulties the child has due to the drops. Since one eye is dilated, the child may also experience reduced depth perception which can impact mobility and eye-hand coordination tasks. In addition, there may be increased sun sensitivity and photophobia which often necessitates the use of sunglasses outdoors.

ACTIVE THERAPY FOR AMBLYOPIA

An amblyopic eye has both reduced visual acuity and poor visual functioning and it may be important to include perceptual learning in amblyopia therapy.[46] Providers treating amblyopia may therefore design a treatment program to work on all aspects of visual functioning. Aside from optical correction and patching, activities to improve visual skills, such as tracking, focusing, visual attention and visual processing may be equally beneficial when treating amblyopia. Specific activities based upon the visual skill level of the amblyopic eye and the child's level of cognitive and motor functioning are often recommended and can be accomplished through in-office therapy with an eye care provider, with the occupational therapist in a school, or rehabilitative setting, or at home. Many of these are the same or similar to activities that are discussed in the next section under eye movement therapy. More recently iPad-based binocular therapy has shown promise for the treatment of amblyopia in children.[47,48]

Eye Tracking and Visual Attention Recommendations

Eye tracking or ocular motilities include the ability to follow a moving target (smooth pursuits), shifting eye gaze between two stationary objects (saccades), and maintaining steady fixation on an object of regard (e.g., fixation and visual attention). These are often challenging for some children with disabilities. Deficiencies in eye tracking skills can impede communication and learning. The eye care provider often recommends pursuit, saccades, and searching and/or scanning exercises for children with poor skills in one or more of these areas. The actual size, color, and luminance of the targets used will depend on the visual and cognitive skills of the child and can be determined by the eye care provider with input from the occupational therapist. Tracking exercises can be done in conjunction with amblyopia therapy (described above) or as a primary vision therapy activity. For children who are reading text or engaged in acquiring early literacy skills, the use of a typoscope (an aid with a viewing window for tracking lines of text) with or without a colored filter may be beneficial. For video magnifiers, settings include lines (underline) and blinds/masks/shadow masking (one line or section of print visible) (Figure 12.12).

Example 4: A child is learning to use a communication device that has an Eyegaze detector incorporated into it. This is an infrared device that tracks a child's eye movements. The device verbally communicates those pictures or icons that the child fixates their eyes on for a specified period of time. A child who is nonverbal and relies on eye movements to learn and communicate may benefit from tracking therapy to help them use their device more effectively.

The following are examples of activities that are useful for children with disabilities who have eye tracking challenges or amblyopia in one eye. These may need to be modified to meet the individualized needs of each child and may not be applicable in all situations.

ACTIVITY 1—FOLLOW THE FLASHLIGHT
Objective
The objective is to work on the development of accurate and smooth pursuit eye movements of the amblyopic eye.

Equipment Needed
- Two flashlights with a colored filter over one light
- Eye patch over the better seeing eye (if amblyopia is present)

The therapist holds one flashlight, and the child, if able, holds the other. Room illumination is initially kept to a minimum but is sufficient enough for the therapist to watch the child's eyes. If a child is unable to hold a flashlight, they can be encouraged to simply follow the therapist's light with their eyes. Positive reinforcement in the form of verbal praise or other behavior-motivating techniques should be used to encourage attention to the task. The therapist shines the light in various and random patterns on the wall, ceiling, and floor. The child is to keep their projected beam

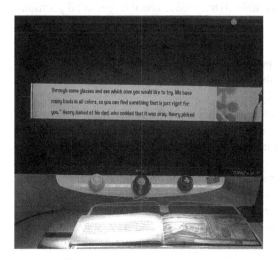

Figure 12.12. Video magnifier with masking.

of light on the therapist's beam as much as possible. Using colored lights that mix such as blue and yellow to create a green light when the child is successful may help maintain or improve attention. Once this is easily achieved, a second method is to have the child keep the light a specified distance (e.g., about 1 or 2 feet) behind the leading light as they *follow the leader.*

Activity 2—Lollipop Licks Tag
Objective
The objective is to facilitate the development of accurate pursuit eye movements (or one eye in amblyopia).

Equipment Needed
- One lollipop in a flavor the patient enjoys and of a size they are able to see
- Eye patch over the better seeing eye (if amblyopic)

A lollipop or other food is held approximately 15 inches in front of the child's eyes. The child is encouraged to keep their eyes on the lollipop at all times. The therapist slowly moves the lollipop back and forth and up and down at a speed the child is able to visually follow. Periodically allow the child to lick the lollipop as positive reinforcement for maintaining fixation and visual attention.

Activity 3—Figure Ground Play Activity
Objective
The objective is to help develop age-appropriate perceptual skills.

Equipment Needed
- Assorted objects of a size that can be seen by the seeing (or amblyopic) eye
- Eye patch over the better seeing eye (if amblyopic)

Assorted objects of interest are placed in front of the child on a table or tray. Examples of objects include a favorite picture, toy, or food (such as Cheerios). Depending on the visual acuity and developmental level of the child, the background upon which the objects are placed can be either high- or low-contrast relative to the objects. The child is encouraged to find the objects one at a time. If the high-interest object is food, and the child has the motor skills to reach for and grab, they can be allowed to eat it for further reinforcement. The objects are *shuffled* when the child is not looking, and the activity is repeated.

Activity 4—Smooth Pursuit Tracking
Objective
The objective is to encourage the child to maintain fixation on a visual target to all positions of gaze (e.g., right, left, up, and down).

Equipment Needed
- Lights, glowing objects, mirror, large hand puppet, small finger puppet, or colorful, various size stickers, depending upon the visual skills of the child (Flickering lights should be used with caution in children with known seizures.)

For children with severe visual deficits, initial targets often are a flickering light, glow worm, flashlight, or hand puppet. Horizontal tracking is often initiated first. Place the target at approximately 15 inches from the child's eyes and move it back and forth slowly. Keep in mind that many children with developmental disabilities may show a time delay in their visual responses. If a flickering light or flashlight is used, periodically turn the light off and then on again in order to enhance the child's interest in the task. If the child enjoys music, it may also be helpful to initially use a tape recorder or pleasing sounds coupled with the moving objects. Reinforcement using auditory or tactile feedback is also recommended. This can be done by using objects such as a shining ball, a bell, or a tactually pleasing toy. Eventually, the child should be able to initiate visual tracking without any other sensory reinforcement. The goal is to bring about a consistent and repeatable visual tracking response in the absence of sound.

ACTIVITY 5—VISUAL SCANNING ACTIVITIES
Objective
The objective is to develop the child's ability to search for important and useful visual information in the environment.

Equipment Needed
* Objects and toys of interest
* A flashlight

Several objects of high interest are placed in front of the child. These can be favorite toys, pleasing food, or other special objects. The child should be asked to look from one object to another in the horizontal plane initially, and then vertically and diagonally. Positive reinforcement and motivating targets are essential for success. Training techniques can also include shining a flashlight on various objects in a visual area close to the child and encouraging them to look at each object as it is illuminated. This can be done starting in a dimly lit room in order to eliminate other visual distractions and to emphasize the contrast between the illuminated target and the background.

ACTIVITY 6—VISUAL REACH ACTIVITIES
Objective
The objective is to encourage the child to begin to tactually interact with objects in their environment using appropriate eye-hand coordination skills.

Equipment Needed
* Objects and toys of interest and finger foods when appropriate

Visual reach activities are especially important when working with children who have been diagnosed with severe visual impairment. Place a favorite toy, object, or food just beyond the child's reach and encourage them to find it, first with their eyes and then with their hands. This should be done in different quadrants of the visual space around them. When doing this exercise, it is important to initially use toys or objects with high contrast that do not visually *blend* into the background. For example, placing a red ball on a white rug or a vanilla cookie on a black felt background improves contrast and enables the child to see and grasp the object or food more readily. Initially, these activities may be coupled with sound to motivate visual attention (e.g., swatting at a ball that chimes when hit), although the goal is for the child to be able to reach without associated sounds.

ACTIVITY 7—PERIPHERAL AWARENESS THERAPY
Objective
The objective is to increase the ability to detect and then look at objects in the peripheral visual field.

Equipment Needed
* Toys and objects with bright colors and high contrast that are of interest to the child; these items should not have any sounds associated with them
* Light-up objects or toys that do not cast a significant glow

This type of therapy is most useful for children who are unaware or neglectful of surroundings due to neurological and/or visual disorders such as visual spatial neglect or peripheral visual field deficits. Begin with lights or toys that are easy to see and gradually change to objects that are smaller and of lower contrast (Figure 12.13). An example of the order of presentation of objects is as follows: flickering lights (e.g., flickering bulb); glowing toys (e.g., Glow Worm); large, high-contrast hand puppets; large, low-contrast hand puppets; small, high-contrast finger puppets;

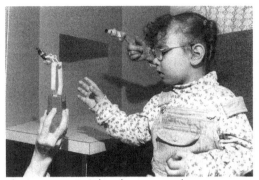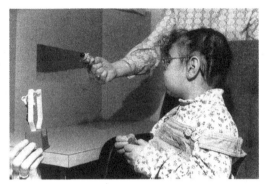

Figure 12.13. Peripheral awareness therapy.

and small, low-contrast finger puppets. The child's gaze should be directed straight ahead at an appropriate high-interest target, such as the television or video or a friendly face (parent) that is positioned directly in front of the child at the beginning of this exercise. A toy or object is slowly and quietly brought in from the periphery until the child indicates that they can detect it by either initiating a head turn, looking at it, or indicating with some other type of behavioral response that they see it (e.g., grabbing or smiling). Positive reinforcement is essential for optimal performance.

Contrast Awareness and Enhancement Recommendations

Contrast sensitivity deficits are associated with many eye disorders, including cortical visual impairment. A reduction in contrast sensitivity can have a significant impact on independent mobility, as well as on visual tasks relating to activities of daily living. Poor contrast awareness can also reduce visual responsiveness during educational activities. A dual approach should be used to compensate for reduced contrast sensitivity. The following strategies are used to both enhance the contrast of targets in the child's environment and increase the child's awareness of poorer contrast targets as long as they are within the limits of their contrast sensitivity as measured clinically.

ENHANCEMENT OF CONTRAST IN THE ENVIRONMENT

The following environmental modifications will increase contrast:
* High-contrast stripes, tape, or markings on stairs, curbs, and other areas of drop-off that impact mobility
* Bold contrasting primary colors or black-on-white figures for all visual targets
* Use of contrasting backgrounds to offset the visual target (e.g., use of a white plate on a black placemat at mealtime)
* Reducing ambient, discomfort, and disabling glare as much as possible by using task lighting that is directed toward the visual target and not toward the child's face, covering windows and shading lights
* Use of anti-reflection coatings and/or tints in eyeglasses
* Exploring the use of colored filters to enhance contrast (e.g., evaluate the use of yellow filters for printed materials to improve contrast
* Use of high-contrast educational materials such as bold-lined paper, broad-tipped soft graphite pencils, black gel erasable pens, or black markers for writing activities

ACTIVITY 8—ENHANCING REDUCED CONTRAST AWARENESS
Objective
The objective is to increase the child's awareness of reduced contrast using visual targets.

Equipment Needed
- High-contrast meaningful visual symbols or pictures appropriate for the child's developmental level
- Reduced-contrast visual symbols or pictures identical in size and shape to the high-contrast symbols that are within the contrast threshold of the child
- High-contrast border of identical size and shape to be placed around the lower contrast symbols (this can be created by cutting out the symbol from contrasting construction paper); symbol sizes should be appropriate for the child's level of visual acuity based upon the results of the vision evaluation

High-contrast symbols or pictures placed before the child who is asked to point to each or make a match with a duplicate. If successful, low-contrast symbols or pictures are then placed before the child who is asked to point to the named symbols or picture or match to a duplicate one of high contrast. If the child is unable to find the symbols or picture, the contrasting borders are placed on the lower contrast symbols, and the child is asked to point to the named symbols or make a match to another high-contrast sample. The contrasting borders are then removed, and the child is again asked to point to the named symbols. The child is then asked to participate in a *scavenger hunt* for specific low-contrast symbols or pictures. These can be scattered throughout the visual environment on backgrounds of varying contrast. The child is rewarded for bringing back the symbols or pictures.

Central/Eccentric Fixation Recommendations
This type of therapy is useful for children who are not using fixation strategies that are appropriate for their visual status. It is designed to increase the ability to efficiently and accurately identify targets in the visual environment.

ACTIVITY 9—CENTRAL FIXATION THERAPY
Objective
The objective is to improve fixation in children without ocular pathology or central visual field defects who will only respond to targets that are presented eccentrically and who have poor central fixation strategies.

Equipment Needed
- Targets consisting of toys or objects with bright colors and high contrast that are visually stimulating
- High- and low-contrast pictures that are developmentally age-appropriate
- Frames with lenses
- Construction paper cut out in the shape of the lenses
- A 5 mm diameter round aperture cut from the construction paper template at the anatomical pupillary distance of the child. The construction paper template is taped onto the spectacle lenses, and the frames are placed on the child.

This technique is only for children who inappropriately view objects at an eccentric viewing angle. It is not for children with central macular disorders who need to eccentrically fixate as a compensation strategy in order to obtain optimal visual information about the environment. It is also not suitable for children with a diagnosis of strabismus and a small angle of eccentric fixation. Children should be positioned so that visual targets are presented at the postural midline. Avoid any head turns during visual activities that enable them to view the target eccentrically. Present varying targets at midline and ask the child to touch or grab for the targets. Present pictures of varying contrast and size and ask them to identify the pictures. If the child enjoys watching television, have them wear the glasses while watching a favorite show.

ACTIVITY 10—ECCENTRIC FIXATION THERAPY
Objective

The objective is to embed an appropriate eccentric viewing strategy in a child with a recent-onset visual impairment who has not yet adopted an eccentric fixation strategy.

Equipment Needed

- Targets consisting of toys and objects of varying sizes and with bright colors and high contrast are visually stimulating. Some targets should have auditory output capability. Children should be able to focus at the testing distance either through corrective lenses or by accommodation.

- The size of the visual target and the viewing distance must be appropriate for the child's decreased visual acuity. That information as well as the clinically observed eccentric fixation position may be obtained from the low vision rehabilitation optometrists working with the visually impaired child.

A child with central vision loss will typically benefit from using retinal points eccentric to the damaged macular region while fixating on visual targets. Such eccentric fixation strategies, when combined with magnification of the target, will enhance the visual image. Many children with long-term central vision defects develop eccentric fixation strategies on their own. The child's fixation should be oriented toward a large, high-contrast target that is presented at postural midline. They may, for example, be told that the puppet is expecting visitors, and they should say or indicate when the visitors are first seen. The child is asked to look at the puppet. A different puppet that the child can identify is then brought in from behind the child in a wide arc until they are able to identify it. The child is then asked to look at the visiting puppet and ask if the puppet looks the same. In the presence of a central scotoma, central fixation, especially on a smaller target, should significantly reduce visual detail. The activity is continued in the other three visual quadrants (parts of the visual field) to determine if the child is able to identify the incoming targets more easily or more consistently at these other eccentric viewing positions. Activities are then concentrated in the best eccentric viewing angle that provides optimal visual discrimination. Visual targets are placed at the appropriate visual angle, and the child is asked to identify them while looking straight ahead. Always allow the child to fixate centrally on the target in order to demonstrate that vision is reduced when a central fixation strategy is employed. The optimal eccentric viewing strategy is always determined by the eye care provider based on the vision exam results. Once determined, the occupational therapist can incorporate this activity into the child's rehabilitative program.

Educational Recommendations

The eye care provider will be able to assess whether the child is considered to be legally blind. Legal blindness is referred to as statutory blindness by the Social Security Administration. In the Social Security Act of 1935, statutory blindness was defined as a visual acuity of 20/200 or less in the better seeing eye with the use of a correcting lens or if the residual visual field diameter in the better seeing eye is 20 degrees or less.[49,50] This definition, however, was revised and the most recent wording of that statute (Social Security Administration 2017) indicates that an inability to see any letters on the 20/100 line of an ETDRS or Bailey Lovie Visual Acuity Chart meets the definition of statutory blindness[51] (Figure 12.1 (A)).

The guideline for visual impairment that is not considered to be legal blindness is a visual acuity of 20/70 to 20/100 in the corrected better seeing eye. A child with this level of visual impairment is considered to have a moderate visual impairment or low vision and is also eligible for educational vision services. For children, a diagnosis of visual impairment, including blindness, signifies an impairment in vision that, even with correction, adversely affects their educational performance and for which they may be eligible for vision services. The term includes both low vision and blindness. Each state or school district may have additional guidelines for providing services for children with visual diagnoses.

The eye care provider is often also asked to provide input to assist in determining recommendations, such as educational placement and learning adaptations, based upon the results of the visual evaluation. The occupational therapist can be helpful in this process by documenting behavioral observations and by preparing a list of questions to be brought to the vision evaluation. The following are examples of possible questions that can be presented to the low vision or pediatric optometrist or ophthalmologist with expertise in evaluating children with disabilities:

- What is the appropriate level of lighting?
- Does the child have increased sensitivity to glare or brightness?
- What level of contrast should materials have?
- What is the appropriate positioning of the child that will maximize visual responsiveness?
- What size materials will the child best respond to?
- Where in the visual field should objects or materials be placed?
- Are there any colors that the child is most responsive to or is adverse to?
- Is there a need for clutter reduction in the work area?
- Does visual information need to be spaced in any particular way?
- What is the child's level of visual processing?
- Is the level of visual skills presenting potential concerns for mobility and orientation?

Case Studies

Case One

A 7-year-old girl presented with a history of encephalocele and developmental delays. She had a wide bridge and an ocular diagnosis of hypertelorism (a wider than typical distance between the two eyes). Her occupational therapist and teachers noticed that she would turn her head to one side whenever she was required to look at objects up close (Figure 12.14). A vision evaluation indicated that she had an intermittent alternating exotropia that was only present at distances closer than approximately 15 inches. Her visual acuity was 20/30 with preferential looking in each eye and she demonstrated poor tracking and scanning skills.

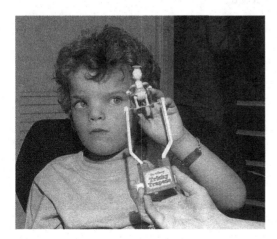

Figure 12.14a. The child turns her head to one side whenever she looks at objects up close.

INTERDISCIPLINARY VISION MANAGEMENT PLAN

1. Eye care provider treatment: Glasses prescribed with base-in prism binocularly to decrease the demand on convergence
2. Occupational therapy intervention: Convergence exercises; visual search, tracking and reaching activities to improve scanning and grasping
3. Teacher of the visually impaired: Functional vision assessment
4. Educational compensation techniques: Reduce visual clutter in the classroom; holding material no closer than 15 inches

OUTCOME

- Improved ability to maintain eye alignment
- Decreased head turning at near (Figure 12.14b)
- Increased visual attention for near objects
- Vision follow-up—she continues to do well with prism and able to view without head turn at near

Case Two

A 6-year-old was born at 27 weeks of gestation with a history of retinopathy of prematurity and cerebral palsy. The child had 20/100 in the right eye and 20/80 in the left eye with reduced contrast sensitivity. They were receiving occupational therapy and vision stimulation from a teacher of the visually impaired. The school recommended a vision evaluation to obtain further information regarding the child's vision and wanted to understand how they interpreted what they observed.

INTERDISCIPLINARY VISION MANAGEMENT PLAN

1. Eye care provider treatment: Small stand magnifier that can be used to view small pictures in books; portable desk-top video magnifier for distance board work; eyeglasses to correct a moderate amount of hyperopia to improve clarity and decrease focusing effort; in-office visual perceptual therapy to address weaknesses
2. Occupational therapy intervention: Fine motor coordination techniques; school-based visual perceptual therapy (see Chapter Five)
3. Teacher of the visually impaired: Functional vision assessment and learning media assessment and facilitates use of video magnifier in classroom
4. Educational compensation techniques: Decrease clutter; enlarge educational materials; allow child to walk up to the board at school when needed

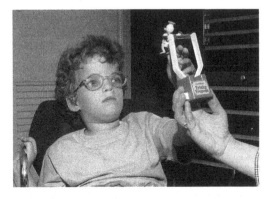

Figure 12.14b. Decrease in head turning at near with prism glasses.

OUTCOME OF TREATMENT

- Increased ability to find visual objects in the classroom, in books and on paper
- Significant increase in visual perceptual skills
- Improved reading skills in school

Case Three

A 4-year-old boy was diagnosed with Treacher Collins syndrome. In this rare syndrome, lid and ear deformities, along with hearing impairment, are present. The specific lid malformation is a downward slant of the eyelids. He had been previously diagnosed with moderate myopia in both eyes by another eye care provider but never wore corrective lenses due to the difficulty in finding appropriate frames that would fit over his ears. The primary concern of his parents and therapists was that he required a very close working distance for all his visual activities, including signing he used to communicate. He also exhibited a significant head tilt and had difficulty with indoor and outdoor glare. The new eye care provider evaluation indicated a high amount of astigmatism corresponding to the orientation of his eyelids and no myopia. Visual acuity was reduced to 20/100 in each eye, and he had a tendency to move his head, rather than his eyes, in order to view objects. He was also sensitive to sunlight.

INTERDISCIPLINARY VISION MANAGEMENT PLAN

1. Eye care provider treatment: Glasses to fully correct the astigmatism with special frames adapted for his ears; sunglasses or photochromatic lenses recommended for outdoors
2. Occupational therapy intervention: Tracking and scanning exercises to reduce head movement
3. Teacher of the visually impaired: Functional vision assessment and learning media assessment including recommendations for maximizing use of vision in the classroom and at school; expanded core curriculum assessment to identify content necessary for him to learn with further evaluation by an orientation and mobility instructor
4. Educational intervention: Total communication program geared toward vision, speech, and language stimulation.

OUTCOME OF TREATMENT

- Increased attentiveness
- Developing better communication skills
- Holding books at a comfortable working distance
- Improved awareness of his surroundings

Conclusion

Vision plays a key role in the education and rehabilitation of children with disabilities. The management of these visual needs can be a rewarding experience when the low vision or pediatric optometrist or ophthalmologist with expertise in evaluating children with disabilities, low vision rehabilitation professionals (e.g., certified low vision therapists, teacher of the visually impaired, certified orientation and mobility specialists), other rehabilitation and health care specialists, and occupational therapists work together as a team. The areas of vision that were discussed, the techniques described, and the case studies presented in this chapter are only a few examples of how this cooperative effort can benefit the child with special needs. Most important is that each professional provides the knowledge and expertise of their respective discipline and collaborates as a team for the benefit of each child. The eye care providers, whose knowledge lies in a complete understanding of the visual system, can guide the occupational therapist in providing the most appropriate services in education and rehabilitation settings along with the type of vision services that are needed for each child.

Acknowledgments

We would like to thank Kerry S. Lueders MS, COMS, TVI, CLVT, Associate Professor, Director, Low Vision Rehabilitation Program Salus University, for her help creating the photos of the video magnifiers and for reviewing and providing input with respect to the role of the teacher of students with visual impairments in this chapter.

Suggested Resources for Children With Visual Impairment

American Council of the Blind: Organizational listing of resources for parents and teachers of children who are blind and visually impaired.

American Foundation for the Blind: Resources on issues related to children with visual impairment, such as publications and local agencies.

Family Connect: Part of the American Printing House for the Blind (APH), it provides a supportive forum for families of children with blindness and low vision from birth to adulthood as well as professionals to share and obtain resources.

National Organization for Parents of Blind Children (division of the National Federation of the Blind): Offers many programs, services, and resources for parents of blind children.

National Library Services for the Blind and Print Disabled Library of Congress: Resource for parent of blind and low vision children.

Prevent Blindness: Mission is to prevent blindness and preserve sight. It includes the National Center for Children's Vision and Eye Health whose statement of need is a call to action to improve children's vision and eye health in the United States.

References

1. Ciner EB, Macks B, Schanel-Klitsch E. A cooperative demonstration project for early intervention vision services. *Occup Ther Pract.* 1991;3(1):42–56.
2. Zambone A, Ciner EB, Appel S, Graboyes M. Children with multiple impairments. In: Silverstone B, Llang M, Rosenthal B, Faye E, eds. *Interaction of Vision Impairments With Other Disabilities and Sensory Impairments. The Lighthouse Handbook on Vision Impairment & Rehabilitation.* New York, NY: Oxford University Press; 2000:451–468.
3. Maino D. *Diagnosis and Management of Special Populations.* St. Louis, MO: Optometric Extension Program Foundation; 2001.
4. Das M, Spowart K, Crossley S, Dutton GN. Evidence that children with special needs all require visual assessment. *Arch Dis Child.* 2010 Nov;95(11):888–892.
5. Kaur G, Thomas S, Jindal M, Bhatti SM. Visual function and ocular status in children with disabilities in special schools of Northern India. *J Clin Diagn Res.* 2016 Oct;10(10):NC01–NC04.
6. Menacker SJ, Fernandes A, Ward L. Prevalence of visual impairment, ocular pathology, and ability to achieve a thorough examination in an eye clinic for patients with disabilities. *J AAPOS.* 2019 Oct;23(5):274.e1–274.e5.
7. Holhos LB, Coroi M, Hainarosie AI, Holhos T, Lazar L. Children with disabilities/special health needs and ocular refractive disorders. *Maedica (Bucur).* 2021 Jun;16(2):255–260.
8. Holhoş LB, Coroi MC, Lazăr L. Observations on refractive status and risk factors for visual impairment in children with disabilities. *Medicina (Kaunas).* 2021 Apr 22;57(5):403.
9. Salt A, Sargent J. Common visual problems in children with disability. *Arch Dis Child.* 2014 Dec;99(12):1163–1168.
10. Haseeb A, Huynh E, ElSheikh RH, et al. Down syndrome: a review of ocular manifestations. *Ther Adv Ophthalmol.* 2022 Jun 30;14:25158414221101718.
11. Ljubic A, Trajkovski V, Stankovic B. Strabismus, refractive errors and nystagmus in children and young adults with Down syndrome. *Ophthalmic Genet.* 2011;32:204–211.

12. Ciner EB. Management of refractive error in infants, toddlers and preschool children. *Problems in Optometry*. 1990;2(3):204–219.

13. Wutthiphan S. Guidelines for prescribing optical correction in children. *J Med Assoc Thai*. 2005 Nov;88(Suppl 9):S163–169.

14. Donahue SP. Prescribing spectacles in children: a pediatric ophthalmologist's approach. *Optom Vis Sci*. 2007 Feb;84(2):110–114.

15. Chukwuyem EC, Musa MJ, Zeppieri M. *Prescribing Glasses for Children*. Treasure Island, FL: StatPearls Publishing; 2023.

16. Leat SJ. To prescribe or not to prescribe? Guidelines for spectacle prescribing in infants and children. *Clin Exp Optom*. 2011 Nov;94(6):514–527.

17. Leat SJ, Mittelstaedt A, McIntosh S, et al. Prescribing for hyperopia in childhood and teenage by academic optometrists. *Optom Vis Sci*. 2011 Nov;88(11):1333–1342.

18. Morrison AM, Kulp MT, Ciner EB, et al. Prescribing patterns for paediatric hyperopia among paediatric eye care providers. *Ophthalmic Physiol Opt*. 2023 Jun 19.

19. Mutti DO, Sinnott LT, Lynn Mitchell G, et al. Ocular component development during infancy and early childhood. *Optom Vis Sci*. 2018 Nov;95(11):976–985.

20. Ehrlich DL, Braddick OJ, Atkinson J, et al. Infant emmetropization: longitudinal changes in refraction components from nine to twenty months of age. *Optom Vis Sci*. 1997 Oct;74(10):822–843.

21. Schein Y, Yu Y, Ying GS, Binenbaum G. Emmetropization during early childhood. *Ophthalmology*. 2022 Apr;129(4):461–463.

22. Zadnik K. The Glenn A. Fry Award Lecture (1995). Myopia development in childhood. *Optom Vis Sci*. 1997 Aug;74(8):603–608.

23. Jones-Jordan LA, Sinnott LT, Manny RE, et al. Early childhood refractive error and parental history of myopia as predictors of myopia. *Invest Ophthalmol Vis Sci*. 2010 Jan;51(1):115–121.

24. Wen G, Tarczy-Hornoch K, McKean-Cowdin R, et al. Prevalence of myopia, hyperopia, and astigmatism in non-Hispanic white and Asian children: multi-ethnic pediatric eye disease study. *Ophthalmology*. 2013 Oct;120(10):2109–2116.

25. Gwiazda J, Scheiman M, Mohindra I, Held R. Astigmatism in children: changes in axis and amount from birth to six years. *Invest Ophthalmol Vis Sci*. 1984;25:88–92.

26. Dobson V, Fulton AB, Sebris SL. Cycloplegic refractions of infants and young children: the axis of astigmatism. *Invest Ophthalmol Vis Sci*. 1984 Jan;25(1):83–87.

27. Howland HC, Sayles N. Photorefractive measurements of astigmatism in infants and young children. *Invest Ophthalmol Vis Sci*. 1984 Jan;25(1):93–102.

28. Wang J, Wyatt LM, Felius J, et al. Onset and progression of with-the-rule astigmatism in children with infantile nystagmus syndrome. *Invest Ophthalmol Vis Sci*. 2010 Jan;51(1):594–601.

29. Bader D, Woodruff ME. The effectiveness of corrective lenses on various behaviors of mentally retarded persons. *Am J Optom Physiol Opt*. 1980;57:447–459.

30. Kaplan M, Edelson SM, Seip JL. Behavioral changes in autistic individuals as a result of wearing ambient transitional prism lenses. *Child Psychiatry and Human Development*. 1998;29(1):65–76.

31. Harcourt B. Strabismus affecting children with multiple handicaps. *Br J Ophthalmol*. 1974 Mar;58(3):272–280.

32. Sandfeld Nielsen L, Skov L, Jensen H. Visual dysfunctions and ocular disorders in children with developmental delay. II. Aspects of refractive errors, strabismus and contrast sensitivity. *Acta Ophthalmol Scand*. 2007 Jun;85(4):419–426

33. Ciner E, Appel S, Graboyes M, Kenny E. (2018) Testing visual function and visual evaluation outcomes in the child with cerebral palsy. In: Miller F, Bachrach S, Lennon N, O'Neil M, eds. *Cerebral Palsy*. Cham: Springer; 2018:1–26.

34. Collins ML. Strabismus in cerebral palsy: when and why to operate. *Am Orthopt J*. 2014;64:17–20.

35. Scheiman M, Kulp MT, Cotter SA, Lawrenson JG, Wang L, Li T. Interventions for convergence insufficiency: a network meta-analysis. *Cochrane Database Syst Rev*. 2020 Dec 2;12(12):CD006768.

36. Huston PA, Hoover DL. Treatment of symptomatic convergence insufficiency with home-based computerized vergence system therapy in children. *J AAPOS*. 2015 Oct;19(5):417–421.

37. Cotter SA, Pediatric Eye Disease Investigator Group, Edwards AR, et al. Treatment of anisometropic amblyopia in children with refractive correction. *Ophthalmology*. 2006 Jun;113(6):895–903.

38. Cotter SA, Edwards AR, Arnold RW, et al. Treatment of strabismic amblyopia with refractive correction. *Am J Ophthalmol*. 2007 Jun;143(6):1060–1063.

39. Writing Committee for the Pediatric Eye Disease Investigator Group, Cotter SA, Foster NC, et al. Optical treatment of strabismic and combined strabismic-anisometropic amblyopia. *Ophthalmology*. 2012 Jan;119(1):150–158.

40. Moseley MJ, Neufeld M, McCarry B, et al. Remediation of refractive amblyopia by optical correction alone. *Ophthalmic Physiol Opt*. 2002 Jul;22(4):296–299.

41. Levi DM. Rethinking amblyopia 2020. *Vision Res*. 2020 Nov;176:118–129.

42. Wu C, Hunter DG. Amblyopia: diagnostic and therapeutic options. *Am J Ophthalmol*. 2006 Jan;141(1):175–184.

43. Pediatric Eye Disease Investigator Group Writing Committee, Rutstein RP, Quinn GE, et al. A randomized trial comparing Bangerter filters and patching for the treatment of moderate amblyopia in children. *Ophthalmology*. 2010 May;117(5):998–1004.e6.

44. Repka MX, Kraker RT, Beck RW, et al. Treatment of severe amblyopia with weekend atropine: results from 2 randomized clinical trials. *J AAPOS.* 2009;13(3):258–263.

45. Scheiman MM, Hertle RW, Kraker RT, et al. Patching vs. atropine to treat amblyopia in children aged 7 to 12 years: a randomized trial. *Arch Ophthalmol.* 2008;126(12):1634–1642.

46. Levi DM, Li RW. Perceptual learning as a potential treatment for amblyopia: a mini-review. *Vision Res.* 2009 Oct;49(21):2535–2549.

47. Manny RE, Holmes JM, Kraker RT, et al. A randomized trial of binocular Dig Rush game treatment for amblyopia in children aged 4 to 6 years. *Optom Vis Sci.* 2022 Mar 1;99(3):213–227.

48. Kelly KR, Jost RM, Dao L, et al. Binocular iPad game vs patching for treatment of amblyopia in children: a randomized clinical trial. *JAMA Ophthalmol.* 2016 Dec 1;134(12):1402–1408.

49. Koestler F. *The Unseen Minority: A Social History of Blindness in the United States.* New York, NY: American Foundation for the Blind; 2004.

50. US Social Security Administration. Disability Evaluation Under Social Security. 102.00 Special Senses and Speech—Childhood. https://www.ssa.gov/disability/professionals/bluebook/102.00-SpecialSensesandSpeech-Childhood.htm.

51. US Social Security Administration. Program Operations Manual System (POMS). http://policy.ssa.gov/poms.nsf/lnx/0426001005.

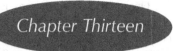

Chapter Thirteen

Using an Interprofessional Collaborative Approach for the Successful Care of the Person

Amber Fessler and Alicia Reiser

Overview

Interprofessional collaborative practice is well known and well researched to support efficient, patient-centered care while optimizing health-related outcomes.[1] As discussed in Chapter One of this book, several similarities exist between optometry (OD) and occupational therapy (OT) that support a collaborative relationship between these professions. While optometrists strive to identify and remediate vision deficits that impact an individual's performance in daily tasks, occupational therapists have a more scoping view, taking into account many performance skills and client factors (including vision skills), the context of environment, and performance patterns of roles and routines. One of the most evident similarities is the shared emphasis on participation and performance in daily living tasks to enhance the person's quality of life. Even though obstacles exist that can challenge team development, several factors are present that can foster successful interprofessional collaboration. As such, this chapter is designed to provide a more in-depth view of both optometry and occupational therapy scopes of practice and the theories and frames of reference guiding the two professions. Additionally, this chapter will highlight a variety of OD/OT collaborative approaches as well as the factors that can enable or impede rewarding collaborative relationships. Finally, two case studies are presented to offer an example of OD/OT collaboration leading to successful client outcomes.

Optometry Scope of Practice

Optometry's scope of practice includes:

> *the prevention and remediation of disorders of the vision system through the examination, diagnosis, treatment, and/or management of visual efficiency and eye health as well as the recognition and diagnosis of related systemic manifestations, all of which are designed to preserve and enhance the quality of our lives and environment.[2]*

DOI: 10.4324/9781003526841-13

Optometric vision therapy is used primarily for those with acquired injuries, like concussion or stroke, or individuals with learning problems. The American Optometric Association's (AOA) position paper *Optometric Care of the Patient With Acquired Brain Injury*[3] describes the role of optometrists as a consultant to the rehabilitation team, providing both remediation and guidance. Optometric evaluation for acquired brain injury (ABI) includes an eye and vision examination, sensorimotor evaluation, visual information processing assessment, low vision evaluation, visual field assessment, and electrodiagnostic testing. Treatment includes remediation of any visual inefficiencies identified within the evaluation. Additional treatment may also include counseling the patient and consulting with other members of the team, as mentioned prior.

Like their role in the management of visual deficits in the acquired brain injury population, optometrists serve as valuable members of the multidisciplinary team managing care in individuals with learning delays.[4] *Optometric Care of the Patient With Learning Related Vision Problems*[4] describes the role of the optometrist as three-fold: Evaluation for accurate diagnosis, remediation, and education of other members of the multidisciplinary team. Evaluation of learning-related vision problems includes a vision examination to rule out visual integrity concerns and an assessment of the visual efficiency skills of accommodation, vergence, and ocular motility. Additionally, the optometrist assesses visual information processing including visual-spatial skills, visual perception, and visual motor integration. Optometric intervention is directed at remediating those visual deficits identified in the evaluation to minimize the impact on the student's learning. To further support their client and the multidisciplinary team, the optometrist's findings and care management strategies should be relayed to other team members.

In addition to the vision examination, a large part of the optometrist's evaluation is the identification of visual efficiency skill dysfunction, namely accommodation and vergence deficits. The *Optometric Care of Accommodative and Vergence Dysfunction*[5] illustrates the complexity of these vision challenges and guides the optometrist in evaluation and remediation. In the evaluative process, optometrists consider the patient history, symptomatic complaints, ocular examination, and visual integrity, along with several components of accommodation and vergence functions to thoroughly assess these skill areas. Intervention may include the use of prescriptive lenses, prisms, and/or optometric vision therapy to improve school or work performance and relieve symptomatic complaints.

Each of these clinical guidelines is consistent with established processes for evaluation and treatment regardless of age or mechanism of dysfunction. The Three Component Model of Vision, as discussed previously in Chapters Three, Four, and Five, serves as a frame of reference for a comprehensive and evidenced-based approach in the evaluation and management of remedial vision deficits. Additionally, models for evidence-based practice have been proposed to supplement these guidelines. In Peachey's[6] suggested model, the authors advocate for the use of strategies to ensure patient-centered interventions that are goal-oriented while in collaboration with other team members. Furthermore, this model promotes working with each client's "zone of proximal development," or just-right challenge, a strategy familiar to occupational therapists as well.

Occupational Therapy Scope of Practice

The *Occupational Therapy Practice Framework*[7] defines occupational therapy as "the therapeutic use of everyday life activities (occupations) with individuals or groups for the purpose of enhancing or enabling participation in roles, habits, and routines in the home, school, workplace, community, and other settings." The domain of "occupations" includes participation in activities of daily living, instrumental activities of daily living, health management, education, work, play, leisure, and social interactions. All of these domains can be impacted by concussion, acquired brain injury, or developmental deficits and may be improved or restored through skilled occupational therapy interventions.

Berryman and Rasavage[8] agree that occupational therapists are key contributors to addressing visual impairments in the acquired brain injury population. Additionally, Bodack[9] identified occupational therapists as valued members in supporting a child's participation in vision exams, educating parents and teachers, and executing intervention recommendations. Areas assessed and treated by occupational therapists on an interprofessional team include visual efficiency skills, visual motor skills, visual perception, and their impact on participation in "occupations." This can be done through a basic vision screening, formal assessment, and observation during functional activity. The justification for occupational therapists to detect and help manage vision disorders is guided by occupational therapy models and frames of reference.

Occupational Therapy Models and Frames of Reference

Whether clearly articulated or unspoken, any well-conceived and successful intervention in practice is typically grounded in a theory.[10] The domain of occupational therapy practice complements the World Health Organization's (WHO) conceptualization of participation and health articulated in the International Classification of Functioning, Disability and Health.[11] Occupational therapy incorporates the basic constructs of ICF, including environment, participation, activities, and body structures and functions, when providing interventions to enable full participation in occupations and maximize occupational engagement.[12] Both occupations and activities are used as interventions by practitioners. Participation in occupations is considered the end result of interventions, and practitioners use occupations during the intervention process as the means to the end.[7] By using these two ideologies, one can support the use of both an occupation-based model as well as a performance-based model to achieve anticipated outcomes of returning to desired occupations, symptom-free, when working with clients with vision disorders.

PERSON-ENVIRONMENT-OCCUPATION-PERFORMANCE MODEL

The Person-Environment-Occupation-Performance (PEOP) model relates best to the aims set forth within an occupation-based model.

> *Occupational therapists are trained to identify factors that may limit the person's capacity to engage in their occupations by observing the person, the environment, and the task to determine what contributes to and what limits successful performance. The occupational therapy evaluation process must include documentation of person factors that limit overall performance.[13]*

These client factors include cognitive, motor, psychological, linguistic, and sensory aspects, all impacted either after an acquired event or with developmental delays. Within the *Occupational Therapy Practice Framework*, 4th edition (OTPF-4), the body function of vision is part of the sensory aspect that should be screened as a possible limitation when addressing occupational performance.

As the PEOP model has developed over time, the main construct that performance is central to the interaction of person, environment, and occupation remains consistent.[14] When addressing the person, the intrinsic qualities, noted above, are aspects to be considered. Environment incorporates social supports, the natural environment, economics, and culture. Roles, tasks, and salient activities are addressed within the occupation concept, while performance incorporates the ability to engage in those responsibilities.[10,15] These four defining components of PEOP are addressed throughout the entire rehabilitation process in stages.

By using these stages, which include narrative, assessment and evaluation, interventions, and outcomes[16] within the PEOP model for occupational therapy process, one can link theory to practice in the treatment of both developmental and acquired vision disorders.

DYNAMIC SYSTEMS THEORY

In addition to the PEOP model, the foundation of occupational therapists providing vision remediation is also supported by dynamics systems theory. While using an occupation-based model for treating vision disorders is well supported, as noted above, dynamic systems theory and motor learning can bridge any remaining gaps. "A systems model suggests that movement results from the interaction of multiple systems working in synchrony to solve a motor problem."[17] This is relevant when treating acquired and developmental vision disorders as it supports the treatment of visual efficiency problems that affect reading, looking from near to far, and participating in life's occupations. One must acquire a skill, learn it, and enhance it to perform an activity. This is accomplished by using massed practice and feedback, techniques used in occupational therapy and justified within the OTPF-4 and scope of practice documents.

Like PEOP, this model similarly looks at the person, the environment, and the task. The person must be addressed in terms of roles, motivation, and cognitive ability, all of which are impacted when a person sustains a concussion-related vision disorder or has a developmental delay. Roles can be addressed through return-to-learn, return-to-work, and return-to-play protocols, while pediatrics can focus on their role of learning through play and exploration. Concurrently, the individual must be motivated and insightful of limitations, requiring possible adaptations along the way.

Addressing the environment is integral in both pediatric and concussion rehabilitation due to hypersensitivities and the interplay with psychosocial exacerbations, like increased anxiety or depression. Accommodations at work and school may need to be established due to overstimulating environments and difficulty with sustained near visual tasks or alternating near-far activities like looking from the board to desk to write notes. The treatment environment should be both predictable and unpredictable to improve performance and occupations within the natural setting.

Lastly, performance skills, based upon task characteristics, stages of learning, practice conditions, and feedback can improve concussion-related vision disorders, as evidence-based research within optometry has shown.[18] Performance skill improvement allows for increased ability to perform occupations interrupted by concussion- related or developmental vision disorders, like reading, screen time tasks, and hobbies. By remediating these foundational performance skills, one can improve performance in occupation and resume premorbid or developmentally desired occupational roles.

It is imperative to use theory as a basis for evaluation and treatment. For occupational therapists, occupation is key, as "occupational performance is a term unique to the profession of occupational therapy to describe how a person functions in his or her environment."[15] By using both motor learning/dynamic system theory, a performance-based model, and PEOP, an occupation-based model, one can justify the need for screening and treating aspects of acquired and developmental vision disorders, with the collaboration of optometry, within the occupational therapy profession.

Interprofessional Collaboration

The benefits of interprofessional collaboration far outweigh any obstacles and barriers experienced by individual professionals. Ultimately, it is the patient who benefits the most from these interactions. Collaboration between occupational therapists and optometrists can be carried out in a variety of ways. In some eye clinics, the occupational therapist is part of the vision therapy team providing a separate but integrated service. In others, the OT may be the practitioner providing the vision therapy services under the direction and license of the optometrist. Optometrists are also branching out into Rehabilitation Hospitals where they are part of the rehabilitation team. Alternatively, OTs and ODs may have separate practices but collaborate for their patient's care through close communication, referrals, progress updates, treatment planning, etc. In some cases, the practitioners share or have conjoined offices, while maintaining separate businesses, which can minimize the challenge of communication. No matter the structural setup, the barriers and factors for success remain constant.

Factors for Successful Collaboration

Many factors play a role in the success of a multidisciplinary collaborative approach. In 2016, the Interprofessional Education Collaborative (IPEC) board released a report of core competencies needed for safe and quality patient and family-centered care.[1] The American Occupational Therapy Association and the Association of Schools and Colleges of Optometry have adopted these competencies. This framework has not only supported a large number of research studies but has been the cornerstone of many successful team collaborations across various settings and professions. IPEC's four core competencies include: "roles and responsibilities," "communication," "values and ethics," and "teams and teamwork."[1] These competencies are further supported and interwoven in the factors identified in research of the collaborative efforts of optometry and occupational therapy teams.

Professional boundaries, or understanding and respecting each other's roles and responsibilities, were identified as a critical factor for team success in teams of optometrists and occupational therapists.[19] Gaining a gross understanding of each profession's scope of practice, through material such as this book, can provide a starting point for developing professional boundaries. However, further communication is needed to support a more refined understanding of each professional and their competencies. Not every optometrist addresses vision from a functional performance and participation viewpoint. Additionally, those optometrists who do function in this manner use a variety of practice programs (i.e., in-office vision therapy, home-based vision therapy with office follow-up, etc.) and tools. Likewise, OTs have a variety of treatment approaches and areas of proficiency that need to be communicated to team members as well. Simply sharing your treatment approaches and patient updates with the optometrist can foster a team-based approach while supporting their understanding of the OT's role. This approach fosters respect for each other's values and ethics while developing a trusting relationship.

Another factor identified in this study as a fundamental piece to successful collaboration was communication.[19] Clear and concise communication between practitioners is critical for patient care as well as for maintaining an ongoing collaborative relationship between team members. Communication should include each practitioner's capabilities and limitations to determine the most beneficial course of care for each patient in addition to team-based problem-solving and therapeutic planning. The proximity of the professionals can certainly ease contact between practitioners; however, working in separate locations should not deter close communication. Maintaining a patient-driven model supports positive communication as well as promoting ethical professional relationships. Working together to find the most efficient form of communication between the OT and OD is key to developing a good team approach and promoting excellent outcomes.

Other factors are inherently present that can impede successful collaboration as well.[19] Overlap between the two professions has caused blurred boundaries resulting in a negative view of each other's profession in some cases. Some occupational therapists use the verbiage of "vision therapy" in their practice, which causes discord for some optometrists providing optometric vision therapy services. Alternative terms such as "functional vision training or rehabilitation" may be more appropriate for occupational therapists to use.[20] Credentialing and insurance billing challenges are also an obstacle to collaboration, particularly in co-located and integrated practices.

Understanding and acknowledging the factors that both facilitate and impede collaborative efforts among optometrists and occupational therapists can be a catalyst in developing mutually respected and successful professional relationships. Exercising humility and valued appreciation for each other's professional roles, while maintaining close communication, allows for the preservation of a client-centered focus. Using these strategies when approaching interprofessional collaborative relationships ensures compliance with all four of IPEC's core competencies resulting in efficient and effective patient outcomes. Considering the research provided and the shared values and ethics between optometrists and occupational therapists, these two professions are natural partners for collaborative care when treating vision disorders for functional improvement.

The following are two brief case studies highlighting the benefits of a collaborative approach to patient care.

Case One

Ava is a 2-year-old child presenting with developmental delays as a result of cerebral palsy. Her family's goals include independent walking and participation in purposeful play activities appropriate for her developmental level. Throughout play interactions, the OT observed Ava's difficulty in the accuracy of visual motor tasks, postural challenges, and an intermittent eye turn. Her OT referred Ava to an optometrist who prescribed corrective lenses. During subsequent weekly OT visits, her OT observed improved skills in accuracy of reach and persistence in play activities such as completing a ring stacker with the use of glasses. At her six-week follow-up with the optometrist, a new lens prescription was provided. In the following therapy visits, her OT noted regression in her performance skills. In particular, Ava demonstrated poor accuracy in reach with an over-reach when attempting to place a ring on the stacker, over-reach when grasping a toy or object from a family member, decreased visually guided movements, and limited participation with increased frustration during play. Additionally, her OT noted more hesitancy with standing marked by a hunched, forward-leaning posture. During a phone conversation with her optometrist, the OT reported these concerns. Through this collaborative conversation, the OD reported the use of yoked prism presentation in a different plane than previously prescribed that likely contributed to these changes in her performance. Without this collaborative relationship and open communication with mutual respect, the patient would likely have had ongoing motor challenges that negatively impacted her goal achievement with the continued use of these glasses. Following this conversation, Ava returned to the OD to adjust the lens prescription. Upon receipt of her new lenses, she returned to her prior level of function with regard to visual motor skills and persistence in play and began independent walking shortly after.

Case Two

Karla is a 53-year-old female who sustained her first concussion at age 16 when falling off the back of a moving vehicle resulting in a loss of consciousness. No medical treatment was sought at that time and at age 18, she developed vertigo. Ten years ago, she was involved in a motor vehicle accident, sustaining both whiplash and a diagnosed concussion. Last year, she was struck in the head by a student who ran into her while at work, which resulted in persistent symptoms of dizziness, nausea, and double vision. She was referred by an optometrist for vision remediation with a trained occupational therapist with a diagnosis of convergence insufficiency and post-concussion syndrome. She reported dizziness, difficulty with sustained near tasks, decreased memory, decreased depth perception, decreased screen tolerance, decreased mobility on uneven surfaces, trouble focusing with both attention and with her eyes to fixate on an object, headaches, a numb feeling in her head, and was unable to walk straight when bowling. Karla had been making slow steady improvements with objective measures on the Binocular Vision Assessment (BVA), reporting increased tolerance for attending music concerts, bowling, and performing roles as a teacher, but continued to report that she felt like her left eye was always drifting in. Base right yoked prisms were trialed in the clinic by the specifically trained occupational therapist with immediate relief of her persistent nausea and dizziness that she had experienced for the past 37 years, stating, "I'm in heaven!" This information was communicated to the optometrist who then prescribed a permanent yoked prism for everyday use, due to the patient not creating a permanent response from continued remediation. She is now able to complete her daily activities without nausea or dizziness, her biggest symptom resolution.

Summary

The ability of occupational therapy and optometry to work collaboratively versus independently has been established in this chapter. The scope of practice of each profession differentiates them from each other, but indicates, when working together in a collaborative approach, that truly the patient will benefit from a comprehensive, whole-person approach. This can be done by integrating visual, sensory, and cognitive systems in order to improve overall functional performance whether the vision disorder is developmental or acquired. The ultimate goal of both of these services is to improve the patient's quality of life.[5,7] With optometry at the helm of visual dysfunction and occupational therapy at the helm of activities of daily living and resuming life roles, it is believed these two disciplines working together can fill the gap of improving occupation and function sooner than current models.

References

1. Interprofessional Education Collaborative. *Core Competencies for Interprofessional Collaborative Practice: 2016 Update*. Washington, DC: Interprofessional Education Collaborative; 2016.
2. Cohen AH. *The Effectiveness of Vision Therapy in Improving Visual Function: A Report by the American Optometric Association*. St. Louis, MO: American Optometric Association; 1988.
3. American Optometric Association. Optometric care of the patient with acquired brain injury. http://stage.aoa.org/Documents/optometrists/acquired-brain-injury.pdf.
4. Garzia RP, Borsting EJ, Nicholson SB, Press LJ, Scheiman MM, Solan HA. *Optometric Clinical Practice Guideline: Care of the Patient With Learning Related Vision Problems*. St. Louis, MO: American Optometric Association; 2000. https://www.aoa.org/AOA/Documents/Practice%20Management/Clinical%20Guidelines/Consensus-based%20guidelines/Care%20of%20Patient%20with%20Learning%20Related%20Vision%20Problems.pdf.
5. Jeffrey S, Cooper JS, Burns CR, et al. *Optometric Care of Accommodation and Vergence Dysfunction*. St. Louis, MO: American Optometric Association; 2011. https://www.aoa.org/AOA/Documents/Practice%20Management/Clinical%20Guidelines/Consensus-based%20guidelines/Care%20of%20Patient%20with%20Accommodative%20and%20Vergence%20Dysfunction.pdf.
6. Peachey GT, Peachey P. Optometric vision therapy for visual deficits and dysfunctions: a suggested model for evidence-based practice. *Vis Dev and Rehab*. 2015;1(4):290–339.
7. American Occupational Therapy Association. *Occupational Therapy Practice Framework: Domain and Process*. 4th ed. In: *Am J Occup Ther*. 2020 August; 74(Supplement 2):7412410010p1–7412410010p87. https://doi.org/10.5014/ajot.2020.74S2001.
8. Berryman A, Rasavage KG. The interdisciplinary approach to vision rehabilitation following brain injury. In: Suter PS, Harvey HL, eds. *Vision Rehabilitation: Multidisciplinary Care of the Patient Following Brain Injury*. Boca Raton, FL: CRC Press; 2011:31–44.
9. Bodack MI. Eye and vision assessment of children with special needs in an interdisciplinary school setting. *Optom Vis Dev*. 2011;42(4).
10. Taylor RR. The role of theory in occupational therapy. In: Taylor RR, ed. *Kielhofner's Research in Occupational Therapy: Methods of Inquiry for Enhancing Practice*. 2nd ed. Philadelphia, PA: FA Davis Co; 2017:78–85.
11. World Health Organization. *How to Use the ICF: A Practical Manual for Using the International Classification of Functioning, Disability and Health (ICF)*. Exposure draft for comment. Geneva: WHO; October 2013.
12. American Occupational Therapy Association. Occupational therapy scope of practice. *Am J of Occup Ther*. 2021;75(Supplement 3):7513410020.
13. Perlmutter MS, Gronski MP. Identifying person factors that impact occupational performance assessment. In: Law MC, Baum CM, Dunn W, eds. *Measuring Occupational Performance: Supporting Best Practice in Occupational Therapy*. 3rd ed. SLACK Incorporated; 2017:59–68.
14. Bass JD, Baum CM, Christiansen CH. Person-Environment-Occupation-Performance model. In: Hinojosa J, Kramer P, Royeen CB, eds. *Perspectives on Human Occupation: Theories Underlying Practice*. 2nd ed. Philadelphia, PA: FA Davis Co; 2017:161–182.
15. Law MC, Dunn W, Baum CM. General measures of participation across the lifespan. In: Law MC, Baum CM, Dunn W, eds. *Measuring Occupational Performance: Supporting Best Practice in Occupational Therapy*. 3rd ed. SLACK Incorporated; 2017:115–151.
16. Law MC, Baum CM. Measurement in occupational therapy. In: Law MC, Baum CM, Dunn W, eds. *Measuring Occupational Performance: Supporting Best Practice in Occupational Therapy*. 3rd ed. SLACK Incorporated; 2017:1–16.
17. Muratori LM, Lamberg EM, Quinn L, Duff SV. Applying principles of motor learning and control to upper extremity rehabilitation. *J Hand Ther*. 2013;26(2):94–103.
18. Thiagarajan P, Ciuffreda KJ. Accommodative and vergence dysfunctions in mTBI: treatment effects and systems correlations. *Optom Vis Perf*. 2014;2(6):539–554.
19. Fessler A, Kruemmling B, Scheiman M. A worthwhile collaboration: integrating optometry and occupational therapy in the treatment of children. *Vis Dev Rehab*. Published online 2020;6(3):221–236.
20. Erhardt RP, Duckman RH. Optometry and occupational therapy collaboration in vision therapy. In: Gentile M, ed. *Functional Visual Behavior in Children: An Occupational Therapy Guide to Evaluation and Treatment*. 2nd ed. Bethesda, MD: American Occupational Therapy Association; 2005:231.

Chapter Fourteen

OT Management of Eye Movement and Visual Information Processing Disorders
Occupation-Based Remedial Vision Rehabilitation

Alicia Reiser and Amber Fessler

Overview

As occupational therapists, the therapeutic use of everyday occupations is core to our profession. Occupational therapy (OT) practitioners use their unique skill set to address the relationships between the client, the client's engagement in meaningful activities, and the environment to create occupation-based interventions.[1] Psillas and Stav[2] outline four constructs that can guide the development of occupation-based therapy approaches to maximize clients' outcomes and satisfaction. The four constructs include authentic occupation, meaningful and purposeful value, therapeutic intent, and engaged participation; all of which can be employed to varying degrees to support occupation-based intervention. "Authentic occupation" is the act of doing or participating in the specific occupation while "meaningful and purposeful value" incorporates the consideration of the client's personal values when choosing activities. Additionally, the selection of goal-directed activities ("therapeutic intent") and collaboration between the therapist and the client throughout the process of participation ("engaged participation") rounds out the four constructs needed to collectively support occupation-based intervention. Psillas and Stav[2] also identify four factors that serve as facilitators and/or barriers that may influence an occupation-based therapeutic approach. These include system factors (reimbursement, documentation requirements, time), physical environment factors (location, supplies), client factors (complexity of health status and client roles), and influential factors (practitioners' roles and experience). The barriers of resources (equipment, budget, and time), education (of medical providers, family, and team members), and evidence (lack of treatment protocol) were also noted by therapists treating concussion-related vision disorders in Reiser's[3] survey when looking at current occupational therapy practice patterns. The intentional use of these constructs, while considering the facilitators or barriers, can guide an occupational therapist in selecting occupation-based activities to support the development of vision skills for clients. Ultimately, these guiding constructs for occupation are then applied to treating the specific person and adapting the environment so that the performance is optimal, no matter what the root cause of the visual inefficiency may be, adhering to the PEOP model and the *Occupational Therapy Practice Framework*, 4th edition (OTPF-4).

DOI: 10.4324/9781003526841-14

This chapter is meant to establish a general guideline for occupational therapists to use remedial vision techniques, based on the profession's strength of activity analysis, within an occupation-based therapeutic approach. As occupational therapists, it can be hard to isolate visual efficiency skills from visual information processing within a task. Therefore, the activities that follow in this chapter may incorporate both of these performance skill areas with attempts to emphasize either the dominant skill required or the skill intended for remediation. Furthermore, the activities used in the subsequent examples are modified from the tasks discussed in Chapter Seven to incorporate the PEOP model and OTPF-4, which are specifically designed to include occupation-based, client-centered aspects to give an idea of how occupation can be incorporated into the vision remediation treatment plan. While the described activity itself relates to the occupation factor of PEOP and OTPF-4, the strategies following the activities take into consideration the person/client factor and environment/context that can support the performance of the occupation within a just-right challenge for each patient. These occupation-based tasks are intended solely to provoke thought on how to incorporate saliency into an occupational therapist's activity or task selection, ensuring client-centered care when treating vision disorders, as all clients have varying occupations and performance patterns that cannot be accounted for in this chapter.

The Occupational Domains of Education and Work

Education

Successful participation in the core occupation of school is paramount to a child's development, learning, and overall well-being. Students spend approximately 75% of their day with vision directed tasks such as reading and writing.[4] These tasks rely heavily on efficient and accurate eye movements and eye teaming, visual spatial skills, visual information processing, and visual motor integration. Deficits in any one of these client factors can negatively impact a child's success and achievement. Common complaints related to reading include eye strain, blurry vision, omitting or skipping words, skipping lines, poor fluency, and/or comprehension. Common complaints related to visual deficits and handwriting include inconsistent spacing between letters and words, difficulty with line and/or letter orientation, as well as letter and number reversals.

CASE ONE

Allison is a 9-year-old third-grade student presenting with delays in reading and handwriting. When reading, Allison reportedly omits small words, skips lines, and has poor accuracy and comprehension when reading. Additionally, when writing, she exhibits irregular-sized letters, poor spacing between letters and numbers, reversals, and she writes large for her age/grade, and has difficulty with near-point and far-point copy tasks. Allison's optometry evaluation revealed convergence insufficiency, accommodative insufficiency, and deficiency in oculomotor skills. Her occupational therapy evaluation indicated inaccurate pursuits and saccades particularly when crossing the midline of her body, delays in visual motor skills, frequent confusion of left and right directions, as well as decreased endurance for handwriting and reading tasks. Occupational therapy intervention began with the use of occupation-based activities to support her accuracy of eye movements as well as the visual-spatial skills of laterality and directionality.

Occupation-Based Visual Efficiency Activity: Hart Chart

The Hart Chart activity, as outlined in Chapter Seven, p. 142, can be used as a remedial activity allowing the student to practice the performance skill of visual saccades, or eye jumps, between different static fixation points. While this rote activity, in its intended form, can be beneficial for teaching a specific performance skill, modifying the activity to be occupation-based can support the client in their role as a student. Adapting this activity to create a "Battleship" game supports the development of eye movements while rehearsing spelling or sight words.

OBJECTIVE

The objective of Battleship Hart Chart is to increase the accuracy and speed of saccadic eye movements while engaging in a meaningful task pertaining to the student's learning.

EQUIPMENT NEEDED
- Battleship Hart Chart sheet (Figure 14.1a)
- Paper and pencil
- Eye patch

DESCRIPTION AND SETUP

Place the Battleship Hart Chart (Figure 14.1a) within the student's workspace, allowing the child to use motor support to build accuracy of saccadic fixations while engaging in near-point copying. Using the child's current sight words or spelling words, write the coordinates for each letter from the Battleship Hart Chart on the spare paper. Occlude the student's left eye with an eye patch and instruct them to locate the letter at the coordinates of B10 to initiate spelling the

	1	2	3	4	5	6	7	8	9	10
A	G	L	P	E	X	B	M	R	A	S
B	N	F	O	U	W	Z	C	J	Y	T
C	A	O	W	J	P	I	T	E	D	G
D	M	B	V	C	S	F	J	P	K	O
E	D	E	C	R	G	V	T	H	N	U
F	P	M	O	N	I	U	V	Y	C	R
G	A	S	L	K	D	F	J	H	G	S
H	W	P	E	O	R	I	T	U	Y	L
I	Z	M	X	N	C	B	V	G	J	D
J	E	F	H	Y	G	N	Q	M	S	O

Figure 14.1a. Battleship Hart Chart Sheet used to treat the accuracy and speed of saccades while performing with a function based near/far transitional task.

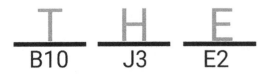

T   H   E
B10   J3   E2

Figure 14.1b. Battleship Hart Chart sight word practice.

word "the" as in the example (Figure 14.1b). After locating the letter, the child should write it above the corresponding coordinates. Continue until the word is completed and instruct the child to read the word. Feedback regarding the accuracy of eye movements is provided if the word is spelled correctly. Continue the activity, switching to the right eye after a set number of words, depending on the child's individual skill and attention level. Once the student has demonstrated accuracy without the use of motor input within near space, transition the Battleship Hart Chart to the wall at approximately 5 to 10 feet from the student to simulate copying from the board.

ENDPOINT
Consider discontinuing this activity when the student can perform the task accurately and efficiently within multiple contexts.

ADDITIONAL GRADING STRATEGIES TO CONSIDER
Grading for Client Factors and Performance Skills:
- Use large eye jumps first as they are easier than small eye jumps, which require a greater amount of control and accuracy.
- Use motor input (such as finger touching, pointing, flashlight, or laser pointer) to help guide the eyes to develop accuracy. Work towards completing with eye movements only.
- First address accuracy before working on increasing speed.
- Utilize targets that are meaningful for the student.
- Use alternative writing lines (i.e., boxes, graph paper, lined paper, notebook paper) to support the student in visually organizing the writing space to promote line or letter orientation and spacing.
- Advance the task with cognitive demands or balance challenges through the use of balance boards, tandem stance, etc. to facilitate automaticity of accurate saccadic eye movements. Placing the Battleship Hart Chart behind the student, so that they must turn in their chair to view, facilitates vestibular stimulation while adding cognitive demands such as working memory and visual memory.

Grading for Environmental Factors:
- Decrease distractions within the student's immediate environment.
- Decrease ambient lighting using a flashlight or lamp to draw visual attention to the target.
- Advance to performing the activity in a busy background or the student's classroom setting.

Occupation-Based Visual Information Processing Activity: Visual Motor Activity Sheet

The directional arrows task, as outlined in Chapter Seven, p. 154, is designed to target the performance skill of directionality by asking the student to identify the left and right sides of inanimate objects. This is a performance skill that can directly impact handwriting and reading fluency. Without the ability to identify the left/right and top/bottom sides of objects in our external space, it will be difficult for the child to discern the difference between similar letters such as b, d, p, and q. Adapting this activity using a directional arrows grid can support the student in acquiring the specific skill of directionality while engaged in near-point copying, typical for the child's learning environment.

OBJECTIVE
The objective of this activity is to assist the student in developing directionality strategies to support the acquisition of underlying performance skills needed for reading and writing.

EQUIPMENT NEEDED

- 5×5 grid of directional arrows, stimulus grid (Figure 14.2a)
- 5×5 grid, blank (Figure 14.2b)
- Multiple square "game pieces" with arrows matching that of the stimulus grid

DESCRIPTION AND SETUP

Level One

Place the stimulus directional arrows grid (Figure 14.2a) within the student's workspace in an orientation typical for near-point copy. Instruct the student to manipulate a game piece to match the direction of the arrow in the top left corner of the stimulus grid and place it on the blank grid (Figure 14.2b). Continue until the child has completed their grid.

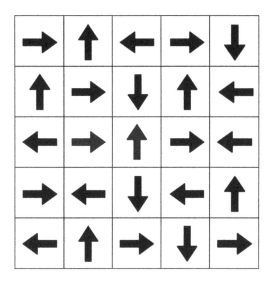

Figure 14.2a. Directional arrows, stimulus grid used to develop directionality strategies required for reading and writing.

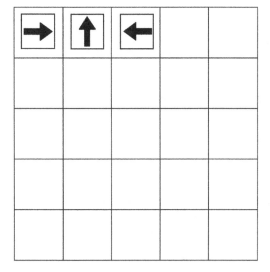

Figure 14.2b. Directional arrows, blank grid, and game pieces.

Level 2

Set up the game the same as in Level One. Ask the child to call out the direction of the arrow as they place it on their grid. It is imperative to stop the child every few squares and ask the student to relay the strategy they used to determine if the arrow is pointing to the left or right, such as, "I write with my right hand and this arrow is pointing to that hand."

Level 3

In this advanced level, show the child how the arrows may correspond to a letter. For example, if the arrow points to the left, it may be similar to a "d" as the semi-circle points to the left on this letter. For up and down arrows, have the child visualize a letter that is "tall" or "fall/goes below the line." Once the education has been provided, instruct the child to follow the arrow chart and write a letter corresponding to the direction of the arrow in each box.

ENDPOINT

The patient can consistently and accurately identify the direction and strategy used without a great deal of thought, matching the patterns and/or writing corresponding letters with accuracy.

ADDITIONAL GRADING STRATEGIES TO CONSIDER

Grading for client factors and performance skills:

- Address the foundation skill of laterality if the child is demonstrating difficulty and/or frustration with this task.
- Use small grid patterns to make this activity easier.
- Print or draw arrow game pieces on a clear plastic sheet allowing the student to place the arrow directly on the stimulus grid to focus on the skill of directionality before including the additional demands of near point copy and visual discrimination.
- Progress to placing the stimulus grid on a wall approximately 5 to 10 feet from the child to simulate far-point copy tasks.
- Advance this activity to include diagonal arrows on the stimulus grid. Alternatively, use colored directional arrows on the stimulus and game pieces to facilitate cognitive demand and visual discrimination skills.

Grading for environmental factors:

- Begin in an uncluttered space with minimal distractions.
- Advance to completing the activity within the classroom setting.

Work

An important role of the brain-injured adult is financially providing for themselves and their family as an employee or worker. It is estimated that 5% to 20% of individuals are unable to return to work 1 to 2 years after mild traumatic brain injury (mTBI).[5] Therefore, it is vital that occupational therapists assist with providing return to work interventions that are specific to the worker's occupation by performing an in-depth activity analysis in regard to visual demands. This should incorporate client limitations involving activity tolerance, balance and pain, environmental demands such as noise, screentime and lighting, and the cognitive demands required for specific duties within their occupation.

CASE TWO

Joe is a 26-year-old male who was rear-ended while stopped at a red light, pushing his car into the stopped vehicle in front of him, sustaining his eighth concussion. He works as a financial advisor, which requires the use of dual monitors, scanning documents on the screen and on paper for information and entering into spreadsheets, interacting with clients across a desk, and driving to and from work located in an office setting. He reports feeling foggy, having headaches and eye fatigue, with eye blurriness and strain after 20 minutes on the computer. Joe acknowledges increased difficulty with recalling information, word finding, and sustained attention. He also reports decreased visual memory with mental math and sensory overwhelm while in the grocery store. When fixating on an object, images tend to move and disappear with time. He also reports issues with depth perception in terms of differentiating foreground and background. He falls off the line when he reads and has limited recall. His spelling has also declined, indicating deficits in visual memory. Joe's optometry evaluation revealed esophoria and paresis of accommodation with a previous diagnosis from his seventh concussion of convergence insufficiency, which had resolved. His occupational therapy evaluation indicated a high score on the Convergence Insufficiency Symptom Scale (CISS) of 31/60 for sustained near work, demonstrating slowed saccades with cancellation testing due to blurriness and decreased fixations on the page, causing a headache. While being screened with the Binocular Vision Assessment (BVA), his screen time was limited and he needed to take frequent breaks after each subtest, indicating poor visual endurance required for his job. Occupational therapy intervention began with the use of occupation-based activities to support the accuracy of eye movements when alternating from screen to screen, as well as the visual information processing skill of visual memory required for mental math and recall of printed information.

Occupation-Based Visual Efficiency Activity: Letter Tracking

The Letter Tracking/Ann Arbor activity, as outlined in Chapter Seven, p. 144, can be used as a remedial activity allowing the worker to practice the performance skill of visual saccades, while dual tasking with attention and sequencing. This activity can be graded in multiple ways to ensure a client-centered, occupation-based, and just-right fit for each client as highlighted by PEOP theory in order to perform their job duties symptom-free. Below, the tracking was changed from letters to numbers to integrate number sequencing, visual memory, and mental math.

OBJECTIVE

The objective of the Number Tracking activity is to increase the speed and accuracy of saccadic fixation while crossing off the numbers in sequential order.

EQUIPMENT NEEDED

* Pencil
* Computer with spreadsheet document function
* Number Tracking activity page or a 1–100 Number Pocket Chart (Figures 14.3 and 14.4)
* Eye patch

DESCRIPTION AND SETUP

Place the computer on the tabletop, centrally located to allow for fixations in a comfortable reading position, about 18 inches away. Place the tracking sheet (Figure 14.3) to the side, as the worker would place paper materials needed for information retrieval prior to data input in the work environment. Occlude the patient's left eye with an eye patch and instruct them to start in the upper left-hand corner and find the first number of the cancellation sequence, in the example pictured, the number 11, and circle it. Have the patient then fixate to the right and left of that number and mentally add the two numbers in those locations. This answer is then transferred over to the spreadsheet on the computer and entered into column 1. If the targeted sequence number is on the end, then the patient uses cognitive flexibility of rule following and only enters the one number. Again, for the example pictured in Figure 14.3, the client would enter 45. For the target sequenced number of 12, they would enter 80. Continue finding the numbers in sequential order, in this case 11–39, and alternating with the mental math portion until the sheet is completed. When all numbers are found in the given sequence, switch to a new tracking sheet, this time occluding the right eye,

11	45	98	17	72	12	8	52	81	3
64	13	21	49	56	5	15	14	1	37
15	14	29	16	93	36	44	82	17	16
46	58	18	2	19	27	61	57	18	20
16	47	68	21	19	22	23	70	12	54
35	24	38	52	99	76	35	25	27	50
49	88	26	9	11	24	27	85	93	28
29	27	33	63	30	54	49	5	31	33
76	22	53	32	31	33	44	34	51	75
83	35	56	91	36	27	37	83	38	10

Figure 14.3 Number Tracking worksheet designed to improve saccadic accuracy and speed while cognitively sequencing the numbers in order, developing visual motor integration with cancellation strokes.

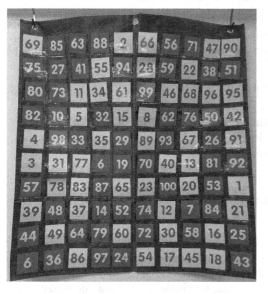

Figure 14.4. 1–100 Number Pocket Chart used to perform saccadic fixations via column jumps or to use from board to table transitions with copying.

repeating the occupation in the same manner, only this time putting the answers to the mental math problems in the second column on the spreadsheet. Complete the new sequence of cancellations. Finally, remove all occlusion and perform with a third tracking sheet, entering the answers in the third column. To conclude the task, have the patient mentally add the three numbers across row 1 in the new spreadsheet they have created and place the answer in column 4.

ENDPOINT

Consider discontinuing this activity when the worker can perform this task accurately and without symptoms of brain fog, headache, eye fatigue, or strain within multiple contexts.

ADDITIONAL GRADING STRATEGIES TO CONSIDER

Grading for client factors and performance skills:

- Use various font sizes on the tracking sheet or on the computer to make the activity easier or more challenging.
- Use motor input (such as finger touching, pointing, pencil, or laser pointer) to support guiding the eyes first to develop accuracy to then completing with eye movements only.
- First work accuracy and then speed of sequencing.
- Eliminate the computer portion and just have the worker call out the math problem solution verbally to avoid multiple steps of sequencing.
- Utilize numbers that are appropriate for the worker on paper and on screen.
- Decrease the challenge by using a line ruler or highlighting the columns on the spreadsheet with color.
- Advance the task with the use of a metronome, additional cognitive demand of naming the number aloud, or perform in standing to facilitate automaticity of accurate saccade in various situations of sit or stand based on job duties.
- Use a 1–100 Number Pocket Chart (Figure 14.4) on the wall, reversing the process described, going from far to near vs near to far, to simulate copying from a white board or work meeting presentation if such a demand is required for working.

Grading for environmental factors:

- Decrease distractions within the worker's immediate environment.
- Encourage the worker to move the paper as needed for clarity of vision.
- Decrease ambient lighting using a desk lamp to draw visual attention to the target.
- Adjust the screen brightness to meet the tolerance of the worker.
- Advance to performing this skill in a busy environment, adding additional distractions including music, conversations as able.
- Enlarge the Number Tracking sheet and place it on the wall for jobs that require wide scanning of shelves, landscapes, or whiteboards.
- Modify number tracking to incorporate visual targets that are pertinent to what the worker needs to scan for at work, adding additional demands of symbols, product, verbal commands, and distractions in open and cluttered environments.

Occupation-Based Visual Information Processing Activity: Design Blocks

The design blocks task, as outlined in Chapter Seven, p. 164, is designed to target the importance of the eye leading the hand for visual motor integration while incorporating visual information processing performance skills of figure ground, form constancy, and spatial relations. Without the ability to transition between tasks after fixating on visual information, the worker may struggle with tasks like data entry, visual memory of what was seen, and transitioning from task to task or from near to far. Adapting the activity by using a design block game, like Rush Hour, this task also incorporates cognitive demands of executive functioning, including working memory, frustration tolerance, planning and organizing, and goal-directed persistence required for any type of work occupation.

OBJECTIVE
The objective of the design blocks task is to have the eye lead the hand to integrate vision and motor functional components. Additionally, the worker becomes aware of the relationship between objects, and their relation to each other, as they place the car pieces on the board to follow the pattern to start the occupation, which also improves central vision.

EQUIPMENT NEEDED
*   Rush Hour game (Figure 14.5)

DESCRIPTION AND SETUP
Level One
Place the Rush Hour game board (Figure 14.5) centrally on the table with the pattern card in the designated holder within the game. Have the worker note that there are different size vehicles (cars and trucks) within the pattern. Have the worker set up the pieces following the given pattern. This in itself allows for pattern recognition, form constancy, and visual motor integration. The object of the activity is to drive the designated car out of the curb cut located on the right side of the game board. Each vehicle piece must stay in its lane. Gameplay includes moving vehicles either up or down for a vertical saccade, or side to side for a horizontal saccade, integrating executive functioning and cognitive demands. The activity has four levels built into the game for increased difficulty, from beginner to advanced.

Level Two
Place the card to the side for alternating fixations side to side or on the wall for near and far functional transitions.

Level 3
Start with an advanced level. On the back of every card is the solution in a coded fashion giving sequenced moves by color and movement description (up, down, left, right) and how many

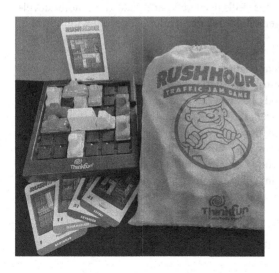

Figure 14.5. Rush Hour game used for the integration of eye-hand movement, saccades, pursuits, pattern following and form constancy, working memory, sustained visual attention, and frustration tolerance.

spaces. Use the solution on the back to decode the movements required to be successful in moving the designated car out of the curb cut.

ENDPOINT
Consider discontinuing the activity when the worker can solve levels in under 5 minutes symptom- and frustration-free.

ADDITIONAL GRADING STRATEGIES TO CONSIDER
Grading for client factors and performance skills:
- Consider if the worker is demonstrating difficulty and/or frustration with this task and chunk the activity into timed sections, alternating it with another task.
- Use beginner card patterns to make this activity easier and slowly advance levels.
- Progress to placing the pattern card on a wall approximately 5 to 10 feet from the worker to simulate far-point copy tasks.
- Advance this activity to include naming the color of the vehicle and if they are moving it up, down, left, or right to enforce laterality, in addition to how many spaces the move contains; for example: blue truck, down 2.

Grading for environmental factors:
- Begin in an uncluttered space with minimal distractions.
- Adjust the lighting from ambient to overhead to increase tolerance for brightness.
- Perform the task in standing vs sitting or on foam to integrate additional demands of standing tolerance while at work and dynamic balance.
- Advance to completing the activity within a distractible setting with noise and conversation.

The Occupational Domains of Play and Social Participation

Play
Play, a fundamental occupation for children, has an integral role in the development of many performance factors including sensorimotor, cognition, and social-emotional skills. As an occupation, play can be highly dependent on the intrinsic motivation of each child. It is not uncommon for children to seek gross motor play activities such as riding a bike or playground play where safety can often be a concern. In addition to the performance skills needed for adequate gross motor development, visual skills support a child's safe engagement in this occupation alone and with others.

CASE THREE
Brody is a 7-year-old boy attending outpatient occupational therapy services with an overall focus on praxis development. He enjoys large-muscle activities such as riding his bike, playing with friends at the park, and climbing. While Brody has worked hard in occupational therapy sessions to develop foundational skills of muscle strength, postural stability, bilateral coordination, and motor planning, he continues to fall frequently during his gross motor play. More specifically, Brody's parents report that he stumbles often, runs into objects and peers, and seems unable to avoid obstacles when riding his bike. Recently, Brody participated in a functional vision evaluation with an optometrist who identified deficits in binocular vision (convergence insufficiency), eye movements, and visuospatial skills. The optometrist prescribed lenses with partial occlusion to support Brody's binocular vision skills. With the information shared by the optometrist, occupational therapy sessions will continue using occupation-based play activities focused on building visual efficiency and information processing skills with the goal of safety during play.

Occupation-Based Visual Efficiency Activity: Flashlight/Laser Tag

Flashlight tag, as outlined in Chapter Seven, p. 148, is a simple procedure often used to improve the speed and accuracy of visual pursuits. Visual pursuits are a critical skill for activities in which the visual target is moving or the person is moving, as well as fundamental in the development of visually guided movements. This activity can be tailored from the original presentation, to simulate movement-based play activities with peers and environmental obstacles.

OBJECTIVE

The objective of flashlight tag is to develop accuracy of visual fixation and pursuit eye movements needed for safety during engagement of gross motor play activities.

EQUIPMENT NEEDED

* Two flashlights or laser pointers (used under careful observation of therapist)
* Eye patch

DESCRIPTION AND SETUP

Level One

The patient should start with a flashlight and an eye patch on one eye. The therapist holds the other flashlight and moves it in front of and toward the child. The child is encouraged to follow the path of the therapist's flashlight with their flashlight, jumping out of the way of the light when it is moved towards the child. Switch the patch to the opposite eye after a short period of time or set number of trials.

Level Two

Using the same setup as in Level One, the patient is encouraged to walk around an open and uncluttered space while avoiding the flashlight held by the therapist. Encourage the child to continue to follow the light as they move around the room.

ENDPOINT

Discontinue this activity when the child can accurately follow all patterns presented by the therapist as well as move their body to avoid the light as it moves towards them.

ADDITIONAL GRADING STRATEGIES TO CONSIDER

Grading for client factors and performance skills:

* Use small eye movements first as they are easier than large eye movements, which require a greater amount of control and accuracy.
* Use slow, predictable movements before increasing speed and randomizing movements.

Grading for environmental factors:

* Begin in uncluttered space with minimal distractions.
* Advance this activity to an outdoor environment where balance is challenged due to surface changes.

Occupation-Based Visual Information Processing Activity: Floor Map (Laterality)

Visual spatial awareness is critical for a child to accurately discern the location of objects in relation to their own body as well as other objects. Laterality, the internal awareness and identification of the right and left sides of one's body, arises from postural stability and bilateral coordination skills.[6] Laterality then gives way to directionality, or the projection of spatial concepts within the child's environment. These skills are integral to safely navigating one's environment during play.

Using concepts from the floor map activity, outlined in Chapter Seven, p. 153, one can support a child's development of laterality within the occupation of play.

OBJECTIVE

The objective of this activity is to develop spatial concepts as the child moves through their environment.

EQUIPMENT NEEDED
- Outside: Playground or park
- Inside: Objects to create an obstacle course

DESCRIPTION AND SETUP

Setup of this activity will be dependent on location. If possible, choosing a local park or school playground provides a more authentic context. However, if access to this context is a factor, simulating a play area inside with the use of an obstacle course can be used. If a child and therapist are playing inside, both individuals should work together to create an obstacle course utilizing various objects for the child to step on, jump to, and climb through, over, or under. The therapist should support the child in constructing the obstacle course to include multiple 90 degree turns. As the child navigates the course or playground, instruct the child to call out the direction they are turning. Support the child in identifying a strategy for labeling the direction correctly. For example, "I write with my right hand and, therefore, I am turning right."

ENDPOINT

Consider increasing the challenge of this activity to support directionality once the child can accurately navigate the obstacle course or playground, correctly identifying right and left sides as well as relaying their strategy.

ADDITIONAL GRADING STRATEGIES TO CONSIDER

Grading for client factors and performance skills:
- Consider using other senses to support the learning of the right and left sides of the body:
  - Tactile prompting using touch, vibration, bracelets, etc.
  - Proprioceptive prompting by encouraging the child to hold their arm out and point in the direction of the turn, squeeze a ball in the hand, or stomp their foot
  - Visual prompting using "R" and "L" on stickers placed on corresponding hands

Grading for environmental factors:
- Use an indoor obstacle course to provide greater control over the child's environment to support learning laterality concepts before moving outdoors where additional distractions may occur.
- Use familiar playgrounds before novel environments.
- Invite peers, friends, or family members to provide distractions and support social participation.

Sport as Play and Social Participation

As humans age, the idea of play remains within us. Play is just as vital for adults to partake in as it is a necessary requirement for children to learn. Play after childhood allows for physical, psychosocial, and emotional benefits and habits. Sports like football, hockey, and soccer are naturally found within this domain of play and performed within a group setting, allowing for social participation with others. Unfortunately, sport is also where many acquired brain injuries can manifest due to its very nature of aggressive contact, impacting visual efficiency skills required to be intact by medical providers for return to play clearance. "About 3.8 million concussions occur each year in the U.S. from sports-related injuries. The Center for Disease Control estimates that 5–10% of athletes will experience a concussion in any given sports season."[7] Without the remediation of visual inefficiencies, a premature return to sport can put the athlete at risk for additional injury, or even worse, second impact if the body is not fully healed, which can result in death.

CASE FOUR

Curtis is a 21-year-old male athlete who was seen for an occupational therapy evaluation 4 years after sustaining his initial injury. While diving for a baseball, another player's shoulder slid into his stomach and he had a positive loss of consciousness. No initial concussion diagnosis was given. Due to the nature of his injury with additional comorbid physical injuries, he was home-schooled for his junior year in high school. With attempts to return to in-person learning for his senior year, Curtis experienced bouts of mood disturbances, learning difficulties causing him to drop all of his AP courses, and environmental noise sensitivities. It was at this time he was diag-nosed with a concussion, only to have the COVID-19 pandemic shut down all opportunities for therapy. Curtis continued to struggle on and off with learning-related issues and anxiety, eventu-ally dropping out of his junior year in college and not playing on the baseball team for which he had a scholarship. He also started to isolate socially. It was at this point that he was referred to a developmental optometrist who diagnosed him with convergence insufficiency. Curtis pushed through all symptoms and lacked interoception and kinesthetic awareness to even know how to control his eyes, despite being seen for vision therapy a year prior with unsuccessful results. He struggled with fight or flight, causing an immediate sympathetic response of sweating when his visual system was challenged with any functional transition from near to far or with saccades and pursuits. With game play, his batting average had significantly decreased, yet he denied having any depth perception issues.

Occupation-Based Visual Efficiency Activity: Hart Chart (Column Jumps)

Saccades and pursuits are vital to being successful in sport. Athletes are constantly transi-tioning from player to player or player to ball and need to be able to accurately perceive visual information in order to respond motorically. Pursuits are used in order to follow a moving player, or to hit, catch, or kick the ball, incorporating eye-hand or eye-foot gross motor control. To develop this skill of fast and accurate fixations during a saccade that may be lacking after an acquired brain injury (ABI), one can adapt the Hart Chart task, described in Chapter Seven, p. 142, with words instead of letters, to improve the accuracy and speed of fixations while incorporating gross motor movements required for dual tasking during sport play.

OBJECTIVE

The objective of this activity is to increase the speed of saccades and accuracy of saccadic fixations and respond motorically to the task described.

EQUIPMENT NEEDED
- Large chart with sport-specific activities (Figure 14.6)
- Eye patch

DESCRIPTION AND SETUP

Place the Sport Hart Chart (Figure 14.6) about 5 to 10 feet from the player. Occlude the player's left eye with the eye patch and have the patient perform column jumps in row 1, fixating on columns 1 and 6. To do this, the player will call out the movement and then perform the task. They then move on to row 2, still fixating on columns 1 and 6, repeating through row 6. Complete

	1	2	3	4	5	6
1	Grounder	Throw	Swing	High Knees	Grounder	Pop Fly
2	Throw	Swing	Burpee	Back Pedal	Slide Right	5 Steps Forward
3	Slide Left	Jump Up	Back Pedal	High Knees	Grounder	Burpee
4	Grounder	Slide Left	5 Steps Forward	Throw	Steal Ready	Pop Fly
5	Bunt	Burpee	Jump Up	Grounder	Back Pedal	Swing
6	High Knees	Pop Fly	Swing	High Knees	Burpee	Steal Ready

Figure 14.6. Sport Hart Chart used as a Visual Motor Activity Sheet, to improve visual motor integration and processing speed based on the activity that is described.

the whole chart with the left eye occluded, jumping from columns 2 to 5, and 3 to 4. Repeat this activity with the right eye occluded and, finally, without patching.

ENDPOINT
Discontinue this technique when the player can complete columns 1 and 6 in 30 seconds with no errors and all of the internal columns within 4 minutes without error or symptoms of headache or visual discomfort.

ADDITIONAL GRADING STRATEGIES TO CONSIDER
Grading for client factors and performance skills:
- Increase the number of repetitions of each activity as the activity tolerance of the athlete improves; for example, five burpees instead of one.
- Add additional balance demands, including foam and bosu balls to increase the challenge.
- Add a metronome to keep pace with alternating fixations, adjusting the pace for faster speeds.
- Add multiple charts with different tasks and place them to the right or left of the player, on the wall above or below eye level, on the ground or behind the player to add additional head turns with fixations, adding a vestibular component. This also incorporates alternating attention and recall as to where the player left off when they transition from chart 1, to 2, to 3.

Grading for environmental factors:
- Perform in an actual training center with other players or on a field if it is available, or go outside to simulate sun and light demands and uneven surfaces that occur during a game.
- Add further distractions like crowds cheering or music to simulate warmups to add an auditory component.
- Use actual equipment including gloves, balls, bats, and weighted bats instead of just mimicking the movement.

Occupation-Based Visual Information Processing Activity: Visual Motor Sheets and Decoding

As discussed previously, visual motor integration is crucial to sport. The athlete must see the object in play in order to respond to it physically. This fast eye-hand or eye-foot coordination is part of what makes a good player even better. Additionally, many sports teams also use visual signs from the coach to tell the player what to do, requiring both the skill of decoding and visual memory to recall what the sign means. By using the Laterality Coding Chart, as described in Chapter Seven, p. 156, the athlete can integrate using fast fixations while incorporating VIP skills of visual memory and visual motor components in a fun and remedial way in order to return to play.

OBJECTIVE

The objective of this activity is to have the player demonstrate their understanding of right and left, dissociate arm and leg movement, cross midline, and perform fast fixations while processing visual information that is encoded in symbol formatting to move their body appropriately through space.

EQUIPMENT NEEDED

*   Sport Laterality Coding Chart (Figure 14.7a)
*   1–100 Number Pocket Chart with numbers scattered randomly in non-sequential order (Figure 14.4)
*   Number tiles 0–9 placed on the floor

DESCRIPTION AND SETUP

Place the Sport Laterality Coding Chart (Figure 14.7) to the left of the 1–100 Number Pocket Chart (Figure 14.4). Scatter the number tiles 0–9 on the floor in front of the player. The athlete will start in the upper left-hand corner of the coding chart and identify the desired movement, in the case

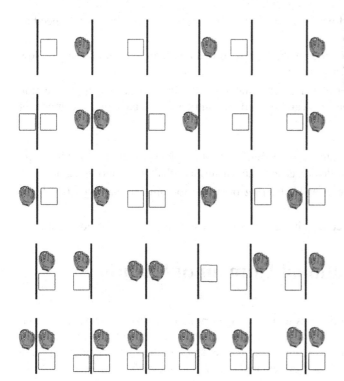

Figure 14.7a. Sport Laterality Coding Chart used to treat directionality, upper and lower extremity dissociation, visual motor integration and decoding based on the picture presented.

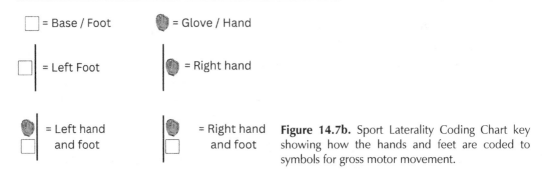

Figure 14.7b. Sport Laterality Coding Chart key showing how the hands and feet are coded to symbols for gross motor movement.

of Figure 14.7, right foot. They will then transition to the 1–100 pocket chart and quickly find the number 1. Based on the movement described, they will either tap out the number on the floor with their foot or on the 1–100 pocket chart on the wall with their hand. They will then return to the coding chart and identify movement number 2, transition to the pocket chart and find the number 2 and again perform the desired movement pattern, in the case of Figure 14.7, left hand tapping the pocket chart. This sequence will continue on the 6×5 coding chart until completed, alternating between all of the steps in the sequence. More complex movements are added as the chart progresses, going from one movement pattern to two, to three, and finally all four extremities responding to movement.

Endpoint
The player can consistently, and without a great deal of effort, identify right and left and accurately perform the desired motor task, alternating with fast and accurate fixations.

Additional Grading Strategies to Consider
Grading for client factors and performance skills:
- Have the player call out the desired movement (right foot) while scanning for the number on the 1–100 pocket chart.
- Add a metronome to fixate and perform the movement on the beat, increasing the speed as the player improves.
- Perform a vertical saccade on the coding sheet or perform a box search pattern mixing up low and high demand gross motor performance.
- Start at a different number other than 1 or have the athlete count by 2s or use multiplication factors. Additionally, the therapist can call out random numbers to add an auditory component for processing speed.

Grading for environmental factors:
- Perform in an actual training center or on a field with other players if it is available, or go outside to simulate sun and light demands and uneven surfaces that occur during a game.
- Add additional distractions like crowds cheering or music to simulate warmups to add an auditory component.
- Add further steps to simulate a coach giving an additional sign at a farther fixation point.

The Occupational Domain of Leisure

Leisure
Leisure, as an occupation, is defined as a "non-obligatory activity that is intrinsically motivated and engaged in during discretionary time."[1] Leisure activities can include a variety of hobbies such as outdoor play, arts and crafts, games, and music, among others. Engagement in these meaningful activities supports a child's self-esteem and overall well-being.[8]

CASE FIVE

Sara is a 7-year-old girl who was referred to an outpatient occupational therapist as recommended by her classroom teacher. Sara has begun to fall behind her peers in writing and math. Additionally, she is easily frustrated in class and has difficulty managing her emotions. At home, her mom shared that she becomes upset regularly when participating in preferred activities such as painting, Lego construction kits, and board games. During these times, she requests help from her mom often and is easily discouraged. Sara's occupational therapy evaluation uncovered mild to moderate delays in manual dexterity skills, oculomotor accuracy, and visual motor integration. Her mom would like Sara to be able to enjoy leisure activities at home by independently participating in these preferred tasks without becoming frustrated and giving up. Occupational therapy began using meaningful leisure activities to target the specific performance skills of fine motor control, visual pursuits, and visual motor integration while grading the task for a just-right challenge to also support her self-esteem.

Occupation-Based Visual Efficiency Activity: Rotating Board

The rotating board task is a visual pursuit activity using a rotating peg board and golf tees. Following the guidelines set forth in Chapter Seven, p. 146, one can alter this activity using the commercial game "Let's Go Fishing" to support the skills targeted in this task. Utilizing this game allows the child to build visual pursuit skills while engaging in the common leisure activity of board games, while also supporting the occupation of social participation.

OBJECTIVE

The objective of this game is to improve the accuracy of visual fixation and pursuit eye movements.

EQUIPMENT NEEDED

- Let's Go Fishing game (Figure 14.8)
- Eye patch

DESCRIPTION AND SETUP
Level One

Set up the "Let's Go Fishing" game (Figure 14.8) within the child's workspace with 3 to 5 different colored fish placed in the gameboard. Using an eye patch for monocular presentation,

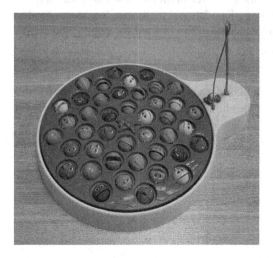

Figure 14.8. Let's Go Fishing game used as a rotator to improve the accuracy of visual fixation and pursuit eye movements. This game includes red, blue, green, yellow, purple, and turquoise colored fish.

instruct the child to find a specific color of fish and hold the fishing pole over the fish following it as it moves around the board. Continue with the other fish on the game board identifying a specific color before the child attempts to catch the fish. Repeat with the other eye occluded.

Level Two

Set up the Let's Go Fishing game (Figure 14.8) in the same manner as above. Direct the child to follow a specific color of fish as it rotates around the board for two to three rotations before attempting to catch the fish.

Level Three

Play the game as intended, placing all of the fish on the game board before play. Remind the child to choose one fish and follow it until they can catch it.

ENDPOINT

Consider mastery of this leisure-based activity when the child can efficiently follow and catch the fish without much effort.

ADDITIONAL GRADING STRATEGIES TO CONSIDER

Grading for client factors and performance skills:

- Consider modifying the fishing pole to support the child's current fine motor skills and/or to decrease frustration in early participation in this game.
- Small pursuit eye movements are easier than larger movements. Therefore, place fish near the center of the game board initially before moving fish to the outer edge.
- Consider adding a visual color pattern or sequence (corresponding to the colors of the fish) for each player to follow to incorporate the skill of visual saccades.

  Grading for environmental factors:
- Begin in an environment with minimal distractions.
- Add peers or family members into the game for increased distractions.

Occupation-Based Visual Information Processing Activity: Dot Map

Accurate integration of fine motor coordination and visual information processing, or visual motor integration, is required for the successful completion of many occupations. The dot map activity, outlined in Chapter Seven, p. 165, can be used to support the acquisition and refinement of visual motor integration skills. Modifying the tools used can transition this task into a meaningful, occupation-based leisure activity while also addressing foundational performance patterns needed for tasks such as handwriting. Legos, within a dot map context, can be used for a child who enjoys this leisure activity.

OBJECTIVE

The objective of this activity is to enhance the child's visually guided movements for the attainment of visual motor integration. Furthermore, the child is encouraged to recognize and apply strategies for accurate completion that will support higher-level achievement.

EQUIPMENT NEEDED

- 10×10 dot map (Figure 14.9a)
- Two Legos (plate and bricks) (Figure 14.9b)
- Plastic sleeve
- Dry erase marker
- Commercial Lego mosaic kit (optional)

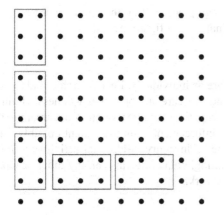

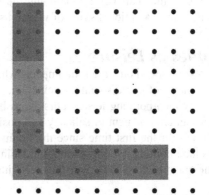

Drawn stimulus

Figure 14.9a. Lego plate drawn stimulus.

Lego construction

Figure 14.9b. Lego construction plate for the child to use to copy the pattern stimulus using Lego bricks to recreate the pattern, developing form constancy, visual motor integration, and saccades required for sustained attention during leisure pursuits.

DESCRIPTION AND SETUP

Begin with simple Lego-mosaic designs appropriate for the age and skill level of the child. The therapist should build a design on one Lego plate or draw a design using a dot map (Figure 14.9 (a)) simulating the Lego plate the child will construct on (Figure 14.9 (b)). Instruct the child to identify the beginning block by touching or circling it using a dry erase marker on the stimulus and then placing their corresponding block on their Lego plate. The child then returns to the stimulus, touching or circling the next block in the sequence and placing their corresponding block in the correct place. Continue moving back and forth between the stimulus and child's blocks until the pattern is complete. Increase the challenge of the design based on the child's performance by varying placement of lines, differing sizes of Legos, and layering the Legos.

ENDPOINT

The child should be able to copy multiple designs from a paper stimulus using a variety of Lego shapes.

ADDITIONAL GRADING STRATEGIES TO CONSIDER

Grading for client factors and performance skills:

- Choose Lego blocks most appropriate for the child's age and fine motor skill level.
- Encourage the child to build a design for the therapist to copy. The therapist should intentionally build the structure incorrectly for the student to compare, further developing visual discrimination skills.
- Use a commercial Lego mosaic kit to increase the child's interest and motivation for this activity.
- Address the foundational components of visual spatial and perceptual skills if this activity is challenging and/or frustrating for the child.

Grading for environmental factors:

- Structure the child's workspace to include only the Lego blocks needed for construction when first starting this activity.

- Increase the challenge by including multiple Lego pieces within the child's workspace. This will require additional skills of visual discrimination and figure ground.

Hobbies as Leisure

How we spend our free time impacts who we are as individuals. Leisure creates balance with other domains of work, social participation, rest, and self-care and promotes wellness within ourselves. By incorporating leisure pursuits as both occupations and goals within our treatment, OT provides an environment of saliency and positive reinforcement, with the patient possibly finding themselves for the first time since the trauma of the brain injury. Additional activities to modify can include knitting, woodworking, gardening, painting, coin collecting, or any other occupation that the client performs to create balance with life's work.

CASE SIX

Ann is a 71-year-old musician who enjoyed playing the violin. Ann fell outside of symphony hall, unable to catch herself as her hands were full with her instrument and music. She fell onto the sidewalk face-first, fracturing her right eye orbit and giving herself a left black eye. She never was officially diagnosed with a concussion, but reports symptoms that were consistent with an acquired brain injury for a short period of time thereafter. Upon diagnostic testing, it was found that she had a tear in her macula. Ann stated that prior to that, she had folds in both of her retinas. Ann had surgery to repair the macular hole, where the protocol after surgery is to lie prone for several days. Unfortunately, Ann had bronchitis at that time, which caused long bouts of coughing that led to the creation of additional scar tissue at the surgery site, impacting her full recovery.

Ann was referred to occupational therapy by her optometrist for compensatory strategies to help her to continue to read music, but she was also diagnosed with a convergence insufficiency. Functionally, Ann reported that things were twisted from what she thought was the "crater in her left retina" and telephone poles had a v-shape cut out of the middle of them. While reading music, she reported that she was "asking too much of my right eye as I am left eye dominant," resulting in strain and fatigue. When playing music with others, she wore an opaque lens; however, this made it more difficult to cue off of the violas seated to her left for timing purposes; without it, though, she reported notes were blob-like and she was unable to identify the true note from the double image. She also identified that at her performances she has had two instances of "whiteouts" when reading the music, always occurring on the top left side of her music. She did enlarge her music as much as possible, but the paper needed to pass under the stand lamp, as well as fit on the music stand and be able to be turned quickly. Ann would still skip notes and had difficulty deciphering naturals from sharps. This made playing music no longer fun for her. Additionally, Ann reported other functional deficits with depth on steps, falling twice while walking her dogs, and knocking over items with a functional reach. Objectively, Ann's BVA phoria scores showed an exophoria of 9.78pD with saccades significantly slowed and error-filled. She was also noted to have a head rotation and tilt.

Occupation-Based Visual Efficiency Activity: Symbol Tracking

The Symbol Tracking activity, described in Chapter Seven, pp. 143–146, can be adjusted to involve the reading of music notes, which are symbols in their own right. The activity can be used with music that the hobbyist already has or with new music that they have never seen. Reading music involves a multitude of performance skills with visual, motor, and cognitive demands that are integral in the successful playing of an instrument. By using accurate saccades and fixations, the music will be played correctly as long as the motor response is intact.

OBJECTIVE

The objective of Symbol Tracking is to increase the speed and accuracy of saccadic fixation while reading music along the staff.

EQUIPMENT NEEDED

- Copies of instrumental music
- Music stand or wall to place music on
- Musical instrument to play
- Copier to enlarge music as needed

DESCRIPTION AND SETUP

Enlarge the sheet music to 250% and place the sheet music at 5 feet to allow for a wider saccade and less vergence demand. Have the patient start out by stating the musical notes seen on the sheet music. Time the speed it takes to read 20 measures. Once this time is under 30 seconds, increase the demand by bringing the music closer and decreasing the size of the music. Continue this adaptation until they are able to read the music at typical stand distance without missing any notes. Add the playing of the instrument as saccades and fixations are near flawless with aloud reading.

ENDPOINT

Terminate this activity when they can read and play the given sheet music without error.

ADDITIONAL GRADING STRATEGIES TO CONSIDER

Grading for client factors and performance skills:

- Start with simpler music and upgrade to more difficult pieces with more notes.
- Start with music that only involves treble or bass clef, upgrading to music that incorporates two staffs.
- Begin with music that contains only notes that fall within the staff, upgrading the demand to music that has notes on ledger lines.
- Increase demand to music that has a faster time signature.
- Increase demand to music that has multiple repeats where the player has to go back to find where the measure starts.
- Incorporate music that has sharp and natural changes frequently for attention to detail with symbol switching.
- If a breath instrument, chunk playing time appropriately based on symptoms reported, increasing playing time as activity tolerance improves for symptom-free playing.

Grading for environmental factors:

- As noted in the task itself, change the placement of the stand to closer or farther based on the player's ability to see the notes.
- Adjust the lighting from ambient, to fluorescent, to stand lamp to allow for various lighting conditions.
- Play additional instruments with the musician for auditory integration and noise habituation.
- Have the musician stand or sit, based on if they are in a concert or rock band.

Occupation-Based Visual Information Processing Activity: Flip Flops/Reversal Sheets

When reading music, accurately interpreting note symbols is integral to knowing what note to play. Musical notes can be written with the stem up or the stem down, while connected notes can be written with the beam above or below the note. The note head can be located on the right of the stem when the connecting beam is located below the note head when playing higher octaves. This could possibly look like a flat symbol notation by someone with a saccadic dysfunction or diplopia. It is imperative that a musical hobbyist be aware of the similarities in these two symbols when reading and playing music. By using the Flip Flop activity described in Chapter Seven, p. 157, and adapting it to a sheet music creation task, intervention can prepare the music hobbyist to identify these form constancy changes that occur with reading music.

OBJECTIVE
The objective is for the music hobbyist to understand the idea of mental rotations, form constancy, and identify the meaning of shapes/notes based on their position in space and location on the staff.

EQUIPMENT NEEDED
- Eighth, quarter, half, and whole music notes in various formations, including single notes, those attached with beams, high and low octave notes made out of construction paper and laminated for strength (see Figure 14.10 for types of notes), about 3 inches in height
- Sharp, natural, and flat symbols made out of construction paper and laminated for strength, about 2 inches in height
- Wall with musical staff created out of painter's tape
- Sheet music
- Mounting putty
- Musical instrument

DESCRIPTION AND SETUP
Scatter the musical notes and symbols on the table in front of the musician. Place them face up and face down, right side up, upside down, and sideways. Have a piece of sheet music placed on the table next to the scattered notes.

Level One
Copy the sheet music. Have the musician look at the sheet music one note at a time, find the same music note scattered on the table, and place it on the created staff located on the wall. Musical notes must be flipped or rotated to match the sheet music. Repeat this activity until ten measures, or the song, completes. The staff created on the wall should match the sheet music on the table.

Level Two
Create your own score. Reset the notes so that they are scattered on the table as described above. This time, they must create a musical score using the notes scattered along the tabletop. An

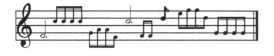
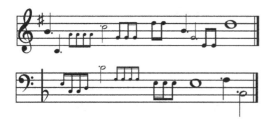

Figure 14.10. Sample sheet music with varying notes, beams, and stems depicted to allow for the development of form constancy and mental rotations.

added challenge would be to create a score from memory of a song they have previously played. They must then play the song on their instrument. This allows the musician to flip-flop notes based on the note they may need in the song, using mental rotations and form constancy skills to create a new musical piece.

Level Three
Listen to a song and create the score. Reset the notes so that they are scattered on the table as described above. This time, play a song, stopping after each measure or two. They must then find those notes played in the measure within the visual clutter of notes on the table and recreate the measure on the wall staff. Continue to play each measure, alternating with score creation on the wall, until the song is complete. This adds a level of auditory integration into the activity for extra difficulty.

ENDPOINT
The task should be done when the notes are properly arranged for each level performed, with the musician demonstrating a good understanding of form constancy and mental rotations.

ADDITIONAL GRADING STRATEGIES TO CONSIDER
Grading for client factors and performance skills:
- Have various sized notes for larger and smaller manipulations.
- Place the notes on the floor and have the musician move from the table to the floor to the wall to place the notes on the staff. This adds a cognitive demand of recalling the note and a dynamic balance component of floor-level reaching to pick up the note and bring to the wall.
- Have them recall 1 to 3 notes at a time for an additional visual memory component.
- Use various sized staffs on the wall and match the note size to the staff size.
- Have them pick up each note with different sequential opposition for fine motor control required for finger formation based on the instrument played.
- Change the complexity of the sheet music from simple to more difficult.

Grading for environmental factors:
- Add a metronome to integrate auditory timing with each fixation and movement.
- Perform the task in a distractible environment with conversation and additional noise or music.
- Play competing music to the beat of the metronome to add additional auditory distraction for integration of more complex musical pieces.
- Adjust the lighting from ambient, to fluorescent, to stand lamp to allow for various lighting conditions.
- Have the musician stand or sit based on the way they play their instrument.

The Occupational Domains of Activities of Daily Living and Instrumental Activities of Daily Living

Self-Care
Dressing is an important self-care occupation carried out by children and adults alike each day. The task of dressing begins at a young age and develops over the course of a few years as the child learns to first undress, then dress, manage clothing fasteners, don clothing with correct orientation, and tie their shoes. These complex tasks require multiple performance skills including postural strength and stability, motor planning, bilateral coordination, eye-hand coordination, etc. In addition to these skills, visual efficiency skills and visual information processing are components that also need to be evaluated and addressed for successful, independent performance in this occupation.

CASE SEVEN

John is a 10-year-old boy referred to an outpatient occupational therapy practice due to ongoing concerns with the achievement of developmental skills such as reading, writing, and completion of daily living self-care tasks. John has been evaluated by multiple professionals and has a diagnosis of developmental dyslexia, specific learning disorder, and receptive language disorder. At his recent eye exam, the optometrist identified binocular vision disorder, oculomotor dysfunction, and visuospatial deficits. In addition to his parents' concerns of reading and writing, John reportedly has difficulty with donning his clothes in the correct orientation, independently completing hygiene tasks, and managing fasteners such as shoe tying. His occupational therapy evaluation revealed age-appropriate and functional fine motor dexterity with deficits in pursuits and saccade eye movements, poor awareness of both laterality and directionality skills, and below-average visual information processing skills. Occupational therapy sessions began with targeting his accuracy in eye movements and visual spatial skill development while engaging him in the occupation of dressing.

Occupation-Based Visual Efficiency Activity: Visual Tracing

Visual tracing activities, outlined in Chapter Seven, p. 146, support the performance skills of visual fixation and pursuits necessary for the visual guidance of motor movements. Using various lines that are intertwined, the patient is encouraged to follow the line from beginning to end to connect two points. This activity can be modified using shoelaces to support the visual efficiency (fixation and pursuits) and visual information processing skills (spatial awareness) needed for independent shoe tying. Additionally, shoelaces will provide a tactile stimulus to facilitate integration of touch and vision, enhancing the child's eye-hand coordination.

OBJECTIVE

The objective of this activity is to improve visual fixation, accuracy of pursuit eye movements, and spatial relationships between shoelaces to support the visually based performance skills needed for shoe tying.

EQUIPMENT NEEDED

* 4 to 5 shoelaces, same or varying colors
* Magnetic board
* 8 to 10 magnets to tie shoelaces to

DESCRIPTION AND SETUP

Level One

Begin setup of this activity by tying each end of the shoelace to different magnets to provide stable beginning and ending points. The therapist places one magnet for each shoelace on the left side of the magnetic board. Next, intertwine the laces in an orientation similar to the visual tracing examples provided on p. 147 with the ending points of the laces on the right side of the magnetic board (Figure 14.11). Instruct the client to follow the shoelace from the beginning point to the ending point with their eyes. Next, direct the patient to move the magnets to "unwind" the shoelaces.

Level Two

Follow the directions above in Level One. As the client follows each shoelace, instruct them to verbalize whether the lace is under, over, looping around, etc. as it crosses the other laces to the ending point.

ENDPOINT

Consider terminating this activity when the client can efficiently and accurately visually follow, unwind laces, and label spatial relationships with little effort or thought.

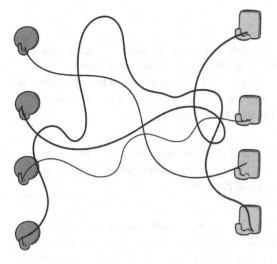

Figure 14.11. Sample shoelace magnetic board designed to develop visual fixations, saccades, and pursuits while performing a functional self-care task of shoe tying.

ADDITIONAL GRADING STRATEGIES TO CONSIDER
Grading for client factors and performance skills:
- Use larger diameter ropes to accommodate fine motor deficits.
- Utilize different colored shoelaces if the above presentation is too difficult and/or frustrating for the child.
- Encourage the child to isolate eye movements by holding their head still as they develop skills to complete this activity. Add kinesthetic feedback by placing an object on their head, such as a stuffed animal, to complete the visual tracings.
- Address foundational skills needed for this task, including postural stability, crossing midline, binocular vision stability, and spatial awareness skills.
  Grading for environmental factors:
- Begin in an environment with minimal distractions.
- Perform this activity within the context and body position the child typically uses when tying their shoes.

Occupation-Based Visual Information Processing Activity: Flip Flops
Flip Flops, outlined in Chapter Seven, p. 157, is an activity using designs and letters on a transparency sheet to further a client's understanding of spatial concepts, or directionality. Interpreting spatial concepts is not only a skill needed for identifying correct orientation of letters and words for reading and writing, but also a necessary performance skill to orient clothing for independent dressing. Using articles of clothing following the guidelines of the Flip Flops activity, one can make this task occupation-based to support the acquisition of skills necessary for independent dressing.

OBJECTIVE
The objective of this activity is to improve the child's ability to visualize spatial concepts to support independence in dressing skills with proper orientation of clothing.

EQUIPMENT NEEDED
- Articles of clothing including pants, shirts, and/or jackets

DESCRIPTION AND SETUP

Level One

Begin by laying the clothing article(s), for example jeans, on the work surface in front of the child. Direct the child to rotate the jeans to the right 90 degrees using the original jeans or to place a second pair of jeans in the new orientation (Figure 14.12). Continue with multiple possible one-step options to include rotation, flipping sideways, and flipping upside-down while assisting the child to develop a verbal strategy to identify the ending orientation.

Level Two

Instruct the child to visualize the clothing rotated and/or flipped using two or more movements and adjust the clothing or place a second article of clothing in the ending orientation. Encourage the child to verbalize the strategy they used to complete each trial.

Level Three

In this level, the therapist places the clothing (i.e., jeans) in any varying orientation, for example upside-down and rotated to the left. Direct the patient to visualize and verbalize the steps needed to orient the clothing to a position in which they can don the jeans with the correct orientation on their body.

Endpoint

Consider terminating this activity when the child is able to orient their clothing correctly and without a great deal of thought.

ADDITIONAL GRADING STRATEGIES TO CONSIDER

Grading for client factors and performance skills:

- Start with rotational patterns towards the right and left before adding in flipping patterns.
- Address the foundational skills of internal awareness of right and left sides of the body, laterality, if the child is experiencing difficulty and/or frustration with this activity.

Grading for environmental factors:

- Begin with articles of clothing with a clear front and back side before moving to a solid shirt or pants with only a tag to identify front and back sides.

Meal Preparation

Meal preparation and cooking are vital for good nutrition and health management after sustaining an acquired brain injury. Yet this task is often fatiguing and visually demanding for the concussion survivor to perform due to the alternating attention from recipe to pot or pan, the scanning for ingredients, and fixations required for eye-hand tasks such as cutting, stirring, and the flipping of food. The

 Rotate the jeans to the right 90°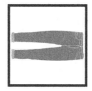

 Flip the coat over and rotate it to the left 180°

Figure 14.12. Sample articles of clothing in varying orientations to develop spatial concepts and form constancy with dressing.

amount of visual efficiency that is required for cooking cannot be underestimated, and when skills are lacking, the task can be followed by headaches, eye strain, and overall fatigue. Many times this results in ordering out and eating meals that are not helpful in healing the brain and body. Through the remediation of oculomotor skills, the occupation of cooking can become tolerated again.

Case Eight
Sally is a 39-year-old female who sustained a concussion after being rear-ended in her vehicle while at a red light, hitting the car in front of her on the driver side. Her car spun out with rotational movement, resulting in whiplash of her neck. She also possibly hit her head on the back of the head rest, resulting in a concussion. Symptoms were delayed up to a week, but she then started with a headache, poor sleeping, and blurred and double vision. Work in a factory environment was difficult with noise, frustration, and feeling off-balance. After 7 months she was referred to an optometrist who diagnosed her with a convergence insufficiency, saccadic dysfunction, exophoria, and accommodative insufficiency. Her biggest complaint, however, was that she loved to bake for her family and could no longer perform this task. When baking, she would experience severe headaches, forget ingredients, and get dizzy with frosting cakes on the lazy Susan.

Occupation-Based Visual Efficiency Activity: Rotator
The rotator activity, explained in Chapter Seven, p. 146, can be adapted to include any rotating surface, in this case a lazy Susan. The skills required to follow a lazy Susan while cake decorating include pursuits, fixations of where you want to place the decorating tip, and visual motor integration of pushing, pulling, or dotting the bag along the cake's surface.

Objective
The objective of this task is to lead the eye and hand while performing a sustained near task, developing the accuracy and speed of oculomotor movements.

Equipment Needed
- Two copies of the cake decorating sheet (Figure 14.13)
- Oaktag paper
- Tape and glue
- Lazy Susan
- Frosting
- Piping bag and tips

Description and Setup
Print off two copies of the cake decorating sheet (Figure 14.13) and tape them together on the short end. Glue these papers to the oaktag of the same size and let them dry. Once the paper is set and dry, create a tube roll with the oaktag, so again the short sides are touching, and tape together. This will provide a stable surface on which to pipe frosting. Place this tube on the lazy Susan. Place your tip and frosting in the piping bag to prepare to frost your "cake." First dot off with frosting the letters in alphabetical order, making sure to find two of each letter, rotating the lazy Susan encouraging fixations and pursuits. Encourage the baker to be in the position they would be to frost a cake, be it in standing, half bent over, or seated at a table. Next, follow with the pastry bag and tip the S pattern located on the bottom of the paper. Then pull the frosting tip along the horizontal dashes. Lastly, use a push-pull technique to cover the shapes found on the top of the cake pattern.

Endpoint
Discontinue this procedure when the baker can report single vision with accurate fixations on all targets and no complaints of dizziness.

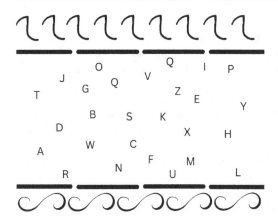

Figure 14.13. Cake decorating sheet used as a pattern for sustained near visual motor integration required for the occupation of frosting a cake.

ADDITIONAL GRADING STRATEGIES TO CONSIDER

Grading for client factors and performance skills:

- Use rice paper and place the cake pattern on a real cake.
- Have the baker come up with their own design to create on the cake.
- Change the item to be frosted including cookies or cupcakes, incorporating smaller detail and smaller visual fixations.
- Continually spin the lazy Susan for nonstop pursuits.
- Provide more complex patterns to follow with zig-zag patterns or swirls.

  Grading for environmental factors:
- Complete the task in a warmer environment due to the temperature set off by the oven.
- Perform the task in a distractible environment with conversation and additional noise or music.
- Adjust the lighting from ambient, to fluorescent, to overhead pot lights to allow for various lighting conditions.

Occupation-Based Visual Information Processing Activity: Floor Map

The Floor Map activity, as outlined in Chapter Seven, p. 153, can be used as a remedial activity allowing the practice of the performance skills of laterality, directionality, visual memory, and topographical orientation required for baking. This activity can be graded in multiple ways to ensure a client-centered, occupation-based, and just-right fit for each person needing to navigate their way around the kitchen.

OBJECTIVE

The objective of this integrative task is to improve visual fixations, allowing for starts and stops along a path, delayed recall of remembering where they left off in alternating attention tasks of reading a recipe, and finding ingredients in visual clutter using the skill of figure ground.

EQUIPMENT NEEDED

- Painter's tape
- Occupation-based activity cards
- Open wall space
- Peg design tasks
- Mounting putty

- Saccade strips
- Kitchen equipment
- Light meal prep activities (pudding, icing/frosting, grilled cheese)

DESCRIPTION AND SETUP

Create a wall maze on an open wall with painter's tape (Figure 14.14). Lines can be simple or more complex, they can overlap and be both vertical and horizontal in nature. Create occupation-based activity cards and place them at various junctions along the maze with mounting putty. These activities can include single functional tasks, like taking out the milk, or a multistep task of a quick meal prep task like making pudding. Other tasks can include performing a visual tracking/Ann Arbor task to simulate reading a recipe or performing a rotating board activity like the Fishing Game to simulate frosting a cake. One card may have the client read a simple recipe for saccades, while a card farther down the maze may have them recall the four ingredients on that card for visual memory. The options are limitless. Have the baker start at one end of the maze and follow the line with their eyes until they get to an activity card. Have them stop and read the card and perform the activity. Once the task is done, return to the maze where they left off and resume the maze. Complete all the activities located on the maze in order as they come to them.

ADDITIONAL GRADING STRATEGIES TO CONSIDER

Grading for client factors and performance skills:

- Place the activity on the floor to increase head posture of looking down or place the maze on a wall to allow for head in midline for those struggling with head and neck pain.
- Use motor input (such pointing or a laser pointer) to support guiding the eyes through visual motor integration to develop accuracy and then completing with eye movements only.
- First work accuracy of laterality and directionality, and then speed of sequencing.
- Decrease the challenge by using a large map/maze for easier saccadic movement or increase the challenge by creating a tighter maze.
- Advance the task with the use of a metronome, adding reading a saccade strip backwards compared to the direction of the maze, and then return to forward movement along the path, having the baker calling out if the map or maze turns right or left, or calling out the opposite direction the map/maze turns for cognitive flexibility and response inhibition.
- Modify map task/wall maze to incorporate visual distractions that are pertinent to what the baker needs to find in the kitchen, like pictures of measuring cups, bowls, etc.

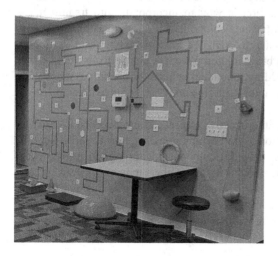

Figure 14.14. Sample wall maze with visual clutter and activity cards placed throughout to develop saccadic starts and stops, laterality and directionality, alternating attention and recall, all required for higher level independent activities of daily living.

- Use various paths to get to the same destination, adding cognitive demands of needing to pass certain target locations to be successful in the overall activity.

    Grading for environmental factors:
- Decrease distractions within the baker's immediate environment.
- Decrease ambient lighting using a flashlight or lamp to follow the map/maze for simulated low-level light tasks.
- Advance to performing skills in a busy environment adding additional distractions including music, conversations, and additional verbal requests.
- At the beginning of the task, have the baker read instructions that state when the timer goes off, they need to perform a certain task. Have the timer go off 15 minutes into the task to see if they recall the request.

The Occupational Domains of Health Management and Rest and Sleep

The final two occupational domains of the OTPF-4 that have a relationship with vision include health management, and rest and sleep. Health management incorporates activities related to maintaining health and wellness routines to be healthy enough to engage in meaningful occupations. Just by participating in vision remediation itself, the client is attempting to achieve health, well-being and participation in life, the true goal of occupational therapy's domain and process.[1] Likewise, the rest and sleep domain relates to obtaining restorative rest and sleep to aid in the active participation in activities. Without adequate rest, the body does not perform to its full potential.[9] Sleep hygiene should therefore be addressed if the client is struggling in this area in order to successfully participate in these integrated interventions, as well as life itself. While there are no activities designed within this chapter to address these domains specifically, they are inherently addressed when we acknowledge and treat the client as a whole.

As occupational therapists look at the occupational analysis of each client's needs, any comorbid and/or premorbid health condition must be considered. In the pediatric population, comorbidities such as ADHD, dyslexia, cerebral palsy, and more can affect how care is approached, as well as the outcomes of therapy. So many times, ABI patients are seen who have a comorbidity of ADHD, dyslexia, or learning disabilities on top of their new concussion or ABI that are now compounded by a visual inefficiency. Because there is no baseline of skill performance, this sometimes makes treatment more challenging in terms of knowing how they may have compensated prior to the injury. This aspect of care must be considered in order to add compensatory strategies if remediation does not resolve function.

As discussed in Chapter Ten, system integration is vital to incorporate into treatment, as vision is both a sensory component as well as a balance component when the vestibular system and proprioceptive systems are also challenged due to ABI. We must remember that vestibular ocular reflex exercises are not as effective if the brain-injured patient is unable to fixate on a target required for dynamic acuity. Therefore, by adding functional challenges, including those with positional changes, cognitive demands, and oculomotor skills, the body can begin to integrate using these skills together instead of in isolation.

Occupational therapists can also incorporate interoceptive awareness into sessions in order to enhance kinesthetic skills of eye movement and for overall symptom management. Some patients may be hyperaware of their body signals, and may have difficulty pushing through treatment when it leads to anxiety or activation of the sympathetic nervous system. Others may be hyperaware and not even feel their eyes or a headache coming on during treatment, resulting in pushing through the session only to have an increase in residual symptoms later in the day. Chemidlin[10] showed that by addressing interoceptive awareness for those with concussion, visual efficiency skills also improved with limited optometric vision remediation being performed at that time.

Throughout the engagement of occupation-based remedial vision activities, there are additional strategies that should be considered. The therapist's acknowledgment and use of these strategies or concepts can optimally support the client's performance and advanced skill development. These strategies include:

- Prescription lenses should be worn throughout all activities.
  - Client education regarding the importance of use and care of prescription lenses falls within the personal care and device management section under the occupation of health management.[1]
- Consider the client's visual efficiency skills of accommodation and vergence during setup and participation in the occupation-based activity. The therapist should relay any concerns and collaborate with the optometrist to support the client at their current level as they develop higher level performance skills.
- The peripheral visual system tells our brain *where* something is so we can efficiently and accurately move our central gaze to the target for fixation and processing. Utilizing motor input or a flashlight, by pointing to or lighting up the target and/or motion near the target can activate the peripheral system to aid in accurate eye movements.
- Interoceptive and kinesthetic awareness throughout all activities is an integral component needed to facilitate higher-level achievement. Multiple strategies can be used to support this awareness such as:
  - Video-recording the patient during the activity and replaying the video for the client can help bring awareness to challenges experienced or successes achieved. For example, specifically video-recording the client's eyes during pursuit activities can help them to see how their eyes are moving and if they moved off target during the pursuit.
  - Headlamps or flashlights can provide immediate visual feedback to the client. For instance, using a headlamp during a saccade activity to observe any head movement when isolated eye movements are expected can aid the patient in developing greater kinesthetic awareness.
  - Discuss interoceptive awareness of visual complaints such as eye strain, fatigue, blurred vision, or double vision before, during, and after the task. This is an integral piece to facilitate the client's independence in symptom and condition management for overall health management.[1] The individual must be able to report when they are experiencing fatigue or headache based on body signals in order to take appropriate breaks instead of pushing through work, exacerbating symptoms beyond recovery.
  - Ask the client to reflect on their performance and verbalize any challenges, errors, or successes. For example, after the individual completes a visual pursuit, ask them how they did and if they were able to sustain fixation throughout the pursuit or if their eyes left the target. Ask how much effort they had to put forth in order to be successful.

Summary

Functional vision deficits are highly prevalent within the populations served by occupational therapists, placing the profession in a natural role to support the identification of and provide collaborative care for these patients. Using information presented in this book, occupational therapists can begin to identify these problems and tailor occupation-based activities and tasks to incorporate remediation strategies. The activities presented in this chapter specifically not only highlight the visual skills needed for successful participation, but also offer suggestions and guidelines for adapting activities to support the development of these performance skills within the context of occupational engagement. Therefore, the activities and additional considerations described can be used merely as starting points for the occupational therapist in treating not just the oculomotor deficit, but the whole person, taking into account each occupational domain.

References

1. American Occupational Therapy Association. *Occupational Therapy Practice Framework: Domain and Process.* 4th ed. In: *Am J Occup Ther.* 2020 August; 74(Supplement 2):7412410010p1–7412410010p87. https://doi.org/10.5014/ajot.2020.74S2001.

2. Psillas, SM, Stav WB. Development of the dynamic model of occupation-based practice. *Open J Occup Ther.* 2021;9(4):1–4.

3. Reiser A, Bunin G, Scheiman M. Concussion-related vision disorder practice patterns in occupational therapy: a survey. *Open J Occup Ther.* 2020;8(4):1–20.

4. Scheiman M. *Understanding and Managing Vision Deficits: A Guide for Occupational Therapists.* 3rd ed. Thorofare, NJ: SLACK Incorporated; 2011.

5. Sharma TL. Returning to work after mild traumatic brain injury—considering the impact of employer support. *JAMA Netw Open.* 2022;5(6):e2219454.

6. Erhardt RP, Duckman RH. Visual-perceptual-motor dysfunction and its effects on eye-hand coordination and skill development. In: Gentile M, ed. *Functional Visual Behavior in Children: An Occupational Therapy Guide to Evaluation and Treatment.* 2nd ed. Bethesda, MD: American Occupational Therapy Association; 2005:180–181.

7. University of Michigan. Concussion in athletes. https://www.uofmhealth.org/conditions-treatments/brain-neurological-conditions/concussion-athletes-neurosport#:~:text=Concussions%20in%20athletes%20are%20extremely,U.S.%20from%20sports%2Drelated%20injuries.

8. Every Moment Counts. Making leisure matter. 2022. https://everymomentcounts.org/making-leisure-matter/.

9. Xue R, Wan G. Association between vision-related functional burden and sleep disorders in adults aged 20 and over in the United States. *Transl Vis Sci Technol.* 2023;12(11):3.

10. Chemidlin M. Impact of an interoception-based intervention on self-regulation in adults with mild traumatic brain injuries: A pilot study. 2022. Doctoral dissertation, Elizabethtown College.

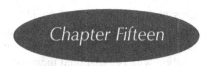

Chapter Fifteen

The Inter-Relationship Model

Mitchell Scheiman

Overview

The objective of this chapter is to describe an inter-relationship model for occupational therapists, optometrists, and other professions involved with vision rehabilitation. Pediatric occupational therapists care for children with a wide variety of problems including cerebral palsy, Down syndrome, other types of mental retardation, spina bifida, low birth weight syndrome, pervasive developmental delay, sensory integrative dysfunction, and child abuse and neglect. The most common conditions found in these children include optical problems such as hyperopia, myopia, astigmatism, strabismus, amblyopia, nystagmus, optic atrophy, and visual information processing problems.

For occupational therapists working with adults, the most common patients seen are those who have experienced cerebrovascular accident, traumatic brain injury, and spinal cord injury. Studies demonstrate that nearly half of the patients admitted to a long-term rehabilitation facility after brain injury have visual system deficits, primarily in the areas of binocular vision, accommodation, eye movement disorders, visual field deficits and neglect, strabismus, reduced visual acuity, and decreased contrast sensitivity. In recent years, occupational therapists have also become more involved in low vision rehabilitation and, in many settings, are now part of the low vision rehabilitation team.[1-3]

Whether working with children or adults, occupational therapists often manage patients who have vision disorders. Hopefully, we have demonstrated that optometry, as a result of its expansive model of vision and concern about function and performance, is the profession of choice to help occupational therapists manage patients with vision disorders.

The model we propose is one in which occupational therapists and optometrists recognize that certain patients require close interaction between the two professions to achieve maximum benefit.

Of course, the need for co-management works both ways. There are certainly patients who optometrists evaluate who should be co-managed with occupational therapists. A good example is the learning disabled child with visual information processing problems. Many of these children have difficulty with visual motor integration that interferes with handwriting and copying skills. Some optometrists may design vision therapy programs to treat these children without consultation with occupational therapists. In our experience, some of these children also have fine motor and

DOI: 10.4324/9781003526841-15

gross motor problems that could be interfering with handwriting skills, and they would benefit from an occupational therapy evaluation to evaluate these areas. Occupational therapists certainly have much broader clinical training in these areas. We believe that optometrists should seek consultation with occupational therapists in these cases. If gross and fine motor problems are present, optometrists should co-manage these patients with occupational therapists.

Inter-Relationship Model

We suggest a four-step model that can be applied to most patients seen by occupational therapists. We expect that this model will lead to the most successful management possible for learning disabled children, developmentally delayed children, and children with brain injury, cerebrovascular accident, and visual impairment.

Step One: Rule Out Vision Problems

Our first recommendation is that occupational therapists rule out vision problems in all patients before developing a treatment approach. This can be accomplished in one of two ways. Some therapists may choose to screen all patients using the screening battery presented in Chapter Six. If a patient fails any portion of this screening battery, a referral should be made to an optometrist with the education, experience, and philosophy suggested in this book. As discussed in Chapter Six, the screening battery cannot be used with all patients. Infants, preverbal children, and adults with severe perceptual, cognitive, and attention problems will be very difficult to evaluate. In such cases, a referral for a comprehensive vision examination should be made. Alternatively, some occupational therapists may make the decision to simply refer all patients for a comprehensive vision examination before initiating a therapy program.

There will certainly be many patients who return to the occupational therapist with a report that all three areas of visual function—acuity and eye health, visual efficiency, and visual information processing—are normal. This is critical information and allows the occupational therapist to confidently plan a treatment approach having eliminated vision as an issue. In this text, we have shown, however, that a large percentage of patients will have vision deficits that need to be addressed.

Step Two: Occupational Therapy Evaluation

After consultation with an optometrist, the occupational therapist can develop an appropriate evaluation to assess strengths and weaknesses of the patient. Knowing that the visual system has been adequately examined allows the therapist to select appropriate evaluation tools and more confidently interpret the results of their testing. This point has been emphasized by several authors.[4–6] They stress that normal visual information processing or visual perceptual function is dependent on normal visual acuity and visual efficiency. Scheiman and Rouse,[4] Warren,[5] and Bouska et al.[6] have all developed evaluation models that have emphasized this point. They discuss the importance of detecting and treating ocular motor, accommodative, and binocular vision disorders before the management of visual processing disorders.

In the area of low vision rehabilitation, it is recommended that the occupational therapist and appropriate vision-related rehabilitation professional jointly perform a thorough, systematic assessment of an individual's work, home, and/or school environments. The purpose of such an assessment is to determine the modifications that may be required in order to meet the daily living, safety, and accessibility needs of the individual who is visually impaired.

Step Three: Consultation

After both evaluations have been completed, the various professionals should discuss their respective test findings and conclusions. This consultation would most likely occur over the phone. The objectives of this phone consultation are to develop a complete list of deficits, to prioritize the significance of these disorders in terms of the urgency for treatment, and, finally, to develop a treatment program in which all professionals contribute when appropriate.

If vision therapy is appropriate, a decision will have to be made about who will provide the vision therapy. We have suggested in this book that in some cases vision therapy must be implemented in an optometric office and at other times vision therapy may be performed by an occupational therapist with direct supervision by the optometrist. The determining factors are the type of disorder (Table 16.1) and the developmental age or level of functioning of the patient (Table 16.2).

Generally, patients must be functioning at about a 6-year-old level to benefit from vision therapy in an optometric office. The sessions usually last about 45 minutes and require a certain level of attention and concentration. We have found that for preschool and for developmentally delayed children, certain vision conditions can be effectively treated by an occupational therapist with optometric supervision. Tracking and visual information processing problems and saccadic and pursuit disorders are included in this category. In our experience, occupational therapists are very effective with these populations and can incorporate vision therapy for these conditions into the overall occupational therapy treatment plan.

Step Four: Periodic Phone Consultation

When various professionals are providing treatment for the patient, periodic phone consultation is important to discuss progress and re-evaluation findings. In other cases, the decision may have been made initially about how to prioritize the various treatments that may be necessary. In such cases, periodic phone consultation is necessary.

Summary

Occupational therapists, whether working with children or adults, often manage patients who have vision disorders. If the four-step inter-relationship model presented in this chapter is followed, we believe that patients served by both professions will achieve maximum benefit.

Table 16.1

Conditions That Require Vision Therapy Treatment in an Optometric Office

- Amblyopia
- Strabismus
- Intermittent strabismus
- Nonstrabismic binocular vision disorders
- Accommodative disorders
- Ocular motility disorders associated with accommodative and binocular vision disorders

---

Table 16.2

Circumstances That Suggest Vision Therapy in an Occupational Therapy Setting Under Optometric Supervision

- Preschool children with other impairments and delays, very limited attention and concentration
- Older children with intellectual disability and multiple impairments
- Traumatic brain injury and cerebrovascular accident patients undergoing rehabilitation in a rehabilitation hospital

References

1. American Occupational Therapy Association. *Vision Services and Occupational Therapy*. Bethesda, MD: Author; 2000.
2. Warren M. *Occupational Therapy Practice Guidelines for Adults With Low Vision*. Bethesda, MD: American Occupational Therapy Association; 1998.
3. Kern T, Miller N. Occupational therapy and collaborative interventions for adults with low vision. In: Gentile M, ed. *A Therapist's Guide to the Evaluation and Treatment of Low Vision*. Bethesda, MD: American Occupational Therapy Association:493–536.
4. Scheiman M, Rouse MW. *Optometric Management of Learning Related Vision Problems*. 2nd ed. St. Louis, MO: CV Mosby; 2006.
5. Warren M. Identification of visual scanning deficits in adults after cerebrovascular accident. *Am J Occup Ther*. 1990;44:391–399.
6. Bouska MJ, Kauffman NA, Marcus SE. Disorders of the visual perceptual system. In: Umphred DA, Jewell MJ, eds. *Neurological Rehabilitation*. St. Louis, MO: CV Mosby; 1985:552–585.

Glossary of Key Terms

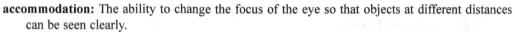

accommodation: The ability to change the focus of the eye so that objects at different distances can be seen clearly.

accommodative excess: A condition in which the amplitude of accommodation is normal, but the ciliary muscle has a tendency to spasm. Typically the problem is intermittent and variable. The individual reports that after reading for a period of time, they experience blurred vision when looking at a distant object.

accommodative infacility: A condition in which the amplitude of accommodation is normal, but the speed of the response is reduced. The most common complaint associated with accommodative facility is blurred vision when looking from near to far or far to near.

accommodative insufficiency: A condition in which the amount of accommodation available (amplitude of accommodation) is less than expected for the individual's age.

ambient processing mode: Concerned with the "where" or the location of objects. Information about movement and position of objects is transmitted to the posterior parietal cortex, which provides a reference of where objects are located in space. The ambient mode is important in posture, motion, and spatial orientation.

amblyopia: A condition in which the visual acuity is less than 20/20 and this loss of visual acuity cannot be attributed to refractive error or observable eye disease. Most people are familiar with amblyopia, which is commonly called "lazy eye" by the public. The term *lazy eye* is a misnomer and does not really describe the condition well. The eye is not lazy; it simply has not received proper stimulation.

anisometropia: A condition in which there is a significant difference in the magnitude of the refractive error between the two eyes.

anisometropic amblyopia: A condition in which the prescription in one eye is considerably stronger than the prescription in the fellow eye.

anomalous correspondence: A condition associated with strabismus in which the visual system adapts to the misalignment of the eye by altering the neurophysiology of the visual system. This adaptation eliminates double vision.

aqueous humor: A clear, watery fluid produced in the posterior chamber that fills the anterior chamber of the eye.

astigmatism: A condition in which vision is blurred and distorted at both distance and near. An astigmatic eye is not spherical. Rather, it has an oval shape and this causes the light rays entering the eye to focus at two different points.

Best's vitelliform macular degeneration: Juvenile form of macular degeneration typically inherited as an autosomal dominant trait. Onset is typically during the first decade of life. Vision loss may be mild or progress to more significant central vision loss.

congenital ocular motor apraxia: Abnormality in voluntary horizontal eye movements with reflex horizontal movements remaining intact. May be due to brain malformation or lesions.

contrast sensitivity: Contrast sensitivity tells us about the quality of the available vision. Problems associated with mobility and reduced ability to recognize faces and objects that are common after brain injury have been found to be associated with contrast sensitivity problems.

convergence excess: A condition in which the eyes have a tendency to turn inward rather than outward. Convergence excess has been found to be slightly more prevalent than convergence insufficiency in a clinical population.

convergence insufficiency: A condition in which the eyes have a tendency to drift outward when being used for near work such as reading, while at a far distance the eyes work well together. This is one of the leading causes of eyestrain and discomfort.

cornea: The anterior one-sixth of the outer coat of the eye is the transparent structure called the cornea. The cornea is an extremely important structure of the eye because it is the key optical component responsible for refraction of light that enters the eye. It is an unusual tissue because it is clear and has no blood vessels.

Crouzon syndrome: A syndrome associated with a forward-pointed skull, beak-shaped nose, underdeveloped upper jaw, widely spaced eyes (hypertelorism), protruding eyes (exophthalmos), and exotropia. Inheritance is typically autosomal dominant.

directionality: The ability of the individual to interpret right and left directions in three separate components of external space.

divergence excess: A condition in which the eyes drift outward when looking at a distance and function normally when looking at near objects.

Down syndrome: A syndrome arising from a chromosomal abnormality involving an extra chromosome 21 (trisomy 21). Associated systemic findings include developmental disability, congenital heart disease, and large protruding tongue. Ocular findings typically include a mongoloid slant of the eyes, yellowish flecks on the iris (Brushfield's spots), myopia, keratoconus, and cataracts.

eccentric fixation: Fixation with a nonfoveal point under monocular conditions. This condition is common in strabismus.

emmetropia: The term used to describe the condition in which there is an absence of refractive error.

esophoria: A condition in which the eyes have a tendency to turn in but the person is able to control this tendency.

esotropia: A condition in which the eyes turn in and the person is unable to control this tendency.

exophoria: A condition in which the eyes have a tendency to turn out but the person is able to control this tendency.

exotropia: A condition in which the eyes turn out and the person is unable to control this tendency.

focal processing mode: Made up of the foveal, parafoveal, and primary visual cortex inputs. The focal mode contributes to the "what" of vision (object recognition and identification). The focal mode is attention oriented and centers on detail in small areas of space.

fovea: The fovea is the part of the eye that contains the area of most acute vision. Whenever we look at an object we must aim the eye so that the image of the object is focused on the fovea. Smooth eye movements called pursuits and jump eye movements called saccades are both designed to allow the individual to always use the fovea.

Hallermann-Streiff syndrome: A developmental disability associated with a parrot-like facial appearance (craniofacial dysplasia), skin atrophy, and hair loss with sparse or absent eyebrows. Ocular findings may include microphthalmos and congenital glaucoma.

hemianopsia: Blindness in one-half of the visual field of one or both eyes.

holoprosencephaly: An underdeveloped prosencephalon associated with developmental disabilities and facial abnormalities including cleft lip and palate. Ocular findings may include microphthalmos, coloboma, and optic atrophy.

hyperopia: A condition in which light rays entering the eye focus behind the retina and the individual must accommodate to see clearly. This need to accommodate requires the use of muscular effort. The amount of effort necessary is greater when the individual looks at near.

isometropic amblyopia: A condition in which there is a very high refractive error in both eyes.

keratoconus: A bulging of the central cornea associated with a thinning of that region. Typically associated with significant astigmatism.

keratoglobus: An enlarged protruding cornea with thinning of the periphery of the cornea.

laterality: The ability to be internally aware of and identify right and left on one's self.

Laurence-Moon syndrome: A syndrome associated with an autosomal recessive inheritance pattern, obesity, extra digits, developmental disability, underdeveloped sexual organs, and retinitis pigmentosa.

lens: A transparent, flexible structure that is held in position by zonular fibers. It is located posterior to the iris and anterior to the vitreous humor. Like the cornea, the lens is both transparent and avascular and is another key part of the refractive system of the eye.

macrencephaly: Enlarged brain with a thickened highly convoluted cortex, associated with optic atrophy, developmental disabilities, and seizures.

Marfan syndrome: A congenital connective tissue disorder associated with a tall stature, postural abnormalities, increased length of fingers and toes, joint hyperextension, cardiovascular disease, and aneurysm of the ascending aorta. Ocular findings may include displacement (subluxation) of the lenses, cataracts, strabismus, nystagmus, myopia, and megalocornea.

microcornea: A cornea that is smaller than 10 mm in diameter. Microcornea is typically associated with myopia.

microphthalmos: A developmental abnormality resulting in a smaller than normal eye. Microphthalmos may be associated with colobomas, glaucoma, and cataracts. Refractive error is typically hyperopia.

myopia: A condition in which the light rays entering the eye focus in front of the retina. In myopia the vision is blurred at distance but clear at near.

near point of convergence: The point at which the eyes are in the position of maximum convergence. This should occur about 2 to 4 inches from the eyes.

nystagmus: A condition in which there are involuntary, rhythmic oscillations of one or both eyes.

Pierre Robin syndrome: Syndrome associated with neonatal respiratory distress, swallowing difficulties, jaw abnormalities, and low set ears. Ocular findings may include microphthalmos, glaucoma, cataracts, myopia, and strabismus.

presbyopia: A condition in which near visual acuity is decreased because of an age-related decline in accommodative ability.

pursuit dysfunction: A condition in which the individual is unable to accurately follow a moving object.

refraction: The term used to describe the evaluation of the optical system of the eye. When the optometrist performs the "refraction," they determine whether the individual is emmetropic, myopic, hyperopic, or astigmatic.

retina: The most internal coat of the eye. It is a thin, delicate membrane composed of two layers: An outer pigment cell layer and an internal neural layer.

retinoscope: An instrument used for determining the refractive power of the eye.

saccadic dysfunction: A condition in which the accuracy and speed of saccadic eye movements are reduced relative to expected findings for the individual's age.

sclera: The white, external coat of the eye that covers the posterior five-sixths of the eye.

scotoma: An isolated area of absent vision or depressed sensitivity in the visual field, surrounded by an area of normal vision.

septo-optic dysplasia (de Morsier's syndrome): Brain malformation (septum pellucidum) associated with midline facial deformities such as cleft lip and palate and growth retardation. Ocular findings may include optic atrophy, optic nerve hypoplasia (underdevelopment), coloboma, and microphthalmos.

Stargardt's maculopathy: Juvenile form of macular degeneration typically inherited as an autosomal recessive trait. Onset is typically between the ages of 8 and 16. Vision loss progresses to between 20/200 and 20/400. Peripheral vision is preserved.

stereopsis: Binocular visual perception of three-dimensional space.

Stickler syndrome: Syndrome associated with joint and hip abnormalities, progressive myopia, retinal detachment, and glaucoma.

strabismic amblyopia: Amblyopia secondary to the presence of a strabismus. The strabismus must occur early in life, involve only one eye, and be present all of the time to cause amblyopia.

strabismus: A condition in which the eyes are misaligned all or part of the time. Many types of strabismus are possible, including esotropia (eyes turn in), exotropia (eyes turn out), and hypertropia (one eye turns up).

strabismus, comitant: A strabismus that is the same magnitude in the nine diagnostic positions of gaze.

suppression: A condition usually associated with strabismus and amblyopia in which the visual system ignores the input from one eye.

Treacher Collins syndrome (Franceschetti syndrome): Syndrome associated with facial deformity, malformation of the ears associated with deafness, downward slanting eyes, segmental absence of lashes, and lid deformities.

Turner syndrome: Syndrome associated with the presence of only one X chromosome or a severe deformity of the second X chromosome in a female. Associated systemic findings include immature sexual development, pulmonary stenosis, vascular disease, and autoimmune disease. Ocular findings may include ptosis (incomplete opening of the lids), strabismus, and cataracts.

vision therapy: Also known as orthoptics, vision training, visual training, and eye training. Vision therapy is an organized therapeutic regimen utilized to treat a number of neuromuscular, neurophysiological, and neurosensory conditions that interfere with visual function. Vision therapy encompasses a wide variety of procedures to improve a diagnosed neuromuscular or neurophysiological visual dysfunction.

visual acuity: A measure of the resolving power of the eye. An individual with 20/20 acuity is considered to have normal ability to see small detail at the distance tested.

visual analysis skills: These skills contribute to the individual's ability to analyze and discriminate visually presented information, to determine the whole without seeing all of the parts, to identify more important features and ignore extraneous detail, and to use visual imagery to recall past visual information. It includes the ability of the child to be aware of the distinctive features of visual forms including shape, size, color, and orientation.

visual efficiency: Refers to the effectiveness of the visual system to clearly, efficiently, and comfortably allow an individual to gather visual information at school, work, or play. The various component skills that are important in this process are called visual efficiency skills and include the subcategories of accommodation, binocular vision, and ocular motility.

visual field: The extent of physical space visible to an eye in a given position. Its average extent is approximately 65 degrees upward, 75 degrees downward, 60 degrees inward, and 95 degrees outward.

visual motor skills: These skills are related to the individual's ability to integrate visual information processing skills with fine motor movement. Another term for visual motor integration is *eye-hand coordination.*

visual spatial skills: These skills allow the individual to develop normal internal and external spatial concepts and are used to interact with and organize the environment. They allow the individual to make judgments about location of objects in visual space in reference to other objects and to the individual's own body.

vitreous body: A colorless, transparent gel that consists of 99% water and forms four-fifths of the eyeball. In addition to transmitting light, it holds the retina in place and provides support for the lens.

yoked prisms: Yoked prisms are used to alter a patient's spatial awareness, to modify a patient's midline perception, or to change weight shifting.

Resources

Directories of Optometrists With Expertise in Vision Therapy

American Academy of Optometry (Diplomate Directory)
622 E. Washington St.
Ste. 300
Orlando, FL 32801
Phone: 877-913-4860
www.aaopt.org

OVDRA (Optometric Vision Development & Rehabilitation Association) (Locate a Doctor)
215 W. Garfield Road, Suite 260
Aurora, OH 44202
Phone: 888-268-3770 or 330-995-0718
www.covd.org

Optometric Extension Program Foundation (Find an Optometrist)
2300 York Road, Suite 113
Timonium, MD 21093
Phone: 410-561-3791
www.oepf.org

Equipment

Avanti Educational Programs
www.avantiseducation.com

Fresnel Prism & Lens Co
10810 Nesbitt Ave. S.
Bloomington, MN 55437
Phone: 800-544-4760
www.fresnel-prism.com

Finger Fitness
451 Emerson Ave.
Hamilton, OH 45013
Phone: 888-868-HAND (4263)
www.handhealth.com

Hoyle Products Inc
12563 Old Plank Dr.
New Lenox, IL 60451
Phone: 661-322-8063
https://hoyleproducts.net/

Visual Information Processing Evaluation Tests

Source	*Name of Test*
Bernell Corp	Developmental Eye Movement Test,
4016 N. Home St.	Test of Visual Perceptual Skills (TVPS)
Mishawaka, IN 46545	
Phone: 800-348-2225	
www.bernell.com	
Lafayette Instrument Co	Grooved Pegboard
3700 Sagamore Pkwy	
N. Lafayette, IN 47904	
Phone: 800-428-7545 or 765-423-1505	
https://lafayetteevaluation.com/products/	
grooved-pegboard	
Optometric Extension Program Foundation	Developmental Test of Visual Motor
1921 E. Carnegie Ave., Suite 3-L	Integration,
Santa Ana, CA 92705	Gardner Reversal Frequency Test,
Phone: 949-250-8070	Wold Sentence Copy Test
www.oepf.org	

Testing Equipment

Company
Bernell Corp
4016 N. Home St.
Mishawaka, IN 46545
Phone: 800-348-2225
www.bernell.com

Equipment
Eye patch (Black Elastic Eye Patch SF3ES)
Snellen Eye Chart (BC11931)
Red Maddox Rod (BC1200R)
Near Visual Acuity Chart (ODNVC)
Disposable penlight (WC70206, Pkg of 6)
Developmental Eye Movement Test (DEM)
Viewer-Free Random Dot Tests (SY98)
Pen-Pal Fixators (PENPALS)

Gulden Ophthalmics
225 Cadwalader Ave.
Elkins Park, PA 19027
Phone: 215-884-8105
www.guldenindustries.com

CPAC Visual Acuity Test
Fixation Sticks

Optometric Extension Program Foundation
1921 E. Carnegie Ave., Suite 3-L
Santa Ana, CA 92705
Phone: 949-250-8070

Developmental Test of
Visual Motor Integration

Vision Associates
295 NW Commons Loop, Suite 115–312
Lake City, FL 32055
Phone: 407-352-1200
www.visionkits.com

3-D Lea Symbols Set (#2516)
Lea Symbols Chart
Lea Symbols Near Vision Card

Vision Therapy Equipment

Company
Bernell Corp
4016 N. Home St.
Mishawaka, IN 46545
Phone: 800-348-2225
www.bernell.com

Item
DEM Symbol Tracking (AADSB) Letter
Tracking (AALTB)
Hart Chart
Tracing Patterns

Learning Potentials Publishers Inc
230 W. Main St.
Lewisville, TX 75057
Phone: 972-221-2564

Developing Your Child for Success by
Kenneth Lane, OD

Optometric Extension Program Foundation
1921 E. Carnegie Ave., Suite 3-L
Santa Ana, CA 92705
Phone: 949-250-8070
www.oepf.org

Visual Tracing Workbook (2)
Visual Fine Motor Workbook (2)
Rotating Pegboard
Helping Children Overcome Learning
Difficulties—Jerome Rosner

Vision Screening Report Form

Name _____ DOB __ / __ / __ Age _____

Wears glasses/contact lenses: No _____ Yes _____ Full-time _____

Distance only _____ Near only _____

Test	*Performance*	*Referral Indicated If:*
Symptom Questionnaire	_____ Significant symptoms _____ No significant symptoms	Significant symptoms are present
Visual Acuity Testing (distance) Distance _____ feet _____ with glasses _____ without glasses	Right eye 20/_____ Left eye 20/_____	20/40 visual acuity or worse in either eye A two line difference in acuity between the two eyes
Visual Acuity Testing (near) _____ with glasses _____ without glasses	Right eye 20/_____ Left eye 20/_____	20/30 visual acuity or worse in either eye A two line difference in acuity between the two eyes
Eye Alignment (distance)	_____ exophoria _____ esophoria _____ vertical phoria _____ suppression	6 exophoria or greater 4 esophoria or greater Any vertical phoria Suppression
Eye Alignment (near)	_____ exophoria _____ esophoria _____ vertical phoria _____ suppression	8 exophoria or greater 4 esophoria or greater Any vertical phoria Suppression

Test	Performance	Referral Indicated If:
Convergence	Break: _____ inches	A break greater than 4 inches
	Recovery: _____ inches	A recovery greater than 6 inches
Stereopsis	_____ Identified all three symbols	Inability to identify all three symbols
	_____ Cannot identify all three symbols	
Accommodative Amplitude	Right eye _____ diopters	2 diopters below age expected (18 minus one-third the patient's age)
	Left eye _____ diopters	
Saccades: Direct Observation		See chart below
Pursuits: Direct Observation		See chart below
Saccades: Visual-Verbal Format (DEM)	Errors _____ percentile	A score below the 15th percentile for either errors or ratio
	Ratio _____ percentile	
Visual Fields: Right Eye		Any field loss
Visual Fields: Left Eye		Any field loss
Gardner Reversal Frequency Test: Recognition Subtest	Raw score _____	A score below the 15th percentile
	Percentile _____	
TVPS: Form Constancy	Raw score _____	A score below the 15th percentile
	Percentile _____	
Developmental Test of Visual Motor Integration	Raw score _____	A score below the 15th percentile
	Percentile _____	

Northeastern State University College of Optometry Saccade Test Referral Criteria by Age and Sex

Sex	Ability	Accuracy	Head Movement
Boys	Less than 5	Less than 3	5 to 6 years: less than 2
			All other ages: less than 3
Girls	Less than 5	Less than 3	5 years: less than 2
			6 to 9 years: less than 3
			All other ages: less than 4

Northeastern State University College of Optometry Pursuit Test Referral Criteria by Age and Sex

Sex	Ability	Accuracy	Head Movement
Boys	Less than 5	5 to 6 years: less than 2	5 to 6 years: less than 2
		7 to 9 years: less than 3	7 to 9 years: less than 3
		10 years and older: less than 4	10 years and older: less than 4
Girls	Less than 5	5 to 8 years: less than 3	5 to 9 years: less than 3
		9 years and older: less than 4	All other ages: less than 4

Index

Note: **Bold** page numbers refer to tables and *italic* page numbers refer to figures.

Printed in the United States
by Baker & Taylor Publisher Services